PAEDIATRICS

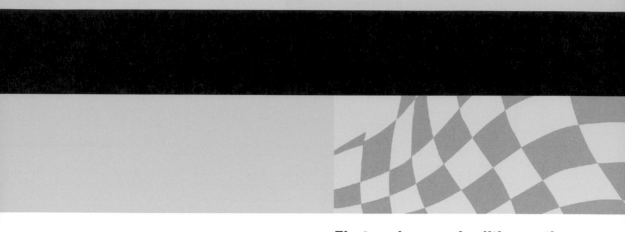

First and second edition authors:

Christine Budd

Mark Gardiner

David Pang

Tim Newson

Third edition author:

Shyam Bhakthavalsala

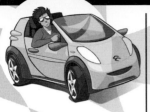

4th Edition
CRASH COURSE

SERIES EDITOR:
Dan Horton-Szar
BSc(Hons) MBBS(Hons) MRCGP
Northgate Medical Practice,
Canterbury,
Kent, UK

FACULTY ADVISOR:
Victoria Jones
BSc(Hons), MBBS, MRCPCH
Consultant Paediatrician,
North Middlesex University Hospital,
London UK

Paediatrics

Rajat Kapoor
BMedSci (Hons), BMBS, DCH, MRCPCH
Specialty Registrar,
Imperial College Healthcare NHS Trust,
London, UK

Katy Barnes
MA, MBBS Specialty Registrar,
Barts Health NHS Trust,
London UK

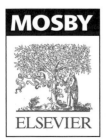

MOSBY
ELSEVIER

Edinburgh London New York Oxford Philadelphia St Louis Sydney Toronto 2013

MOSBY
ELSEVIER

Content Strategist: Jeremy Bowes
Content Development Specialist: Fiona Conn
Project Manager: Andrew Riley
Designer: Christian Bilbow
Icon Illustrations: Geo Parkin
Illustration Manager: Jennifer Rose

First edition 1999
Second edition 2004
Third edition 2008
Fourth edition 2013
   Reprinted 2013, 2014

ISBN: 978-0-7234-3635-5

British Library Cataloguing in Publication Data
A catalogue record for this book is available from the British Library

Library of Congress Cataloging in Publication Data
A catalog record for this book is available from the Library of Congress

Notices

Knowledge and best practice in this field are constantly changing. As new research and experience broaden our understanding, changes in research methods, professional practices, or medical treatment may become necessary.

Practitioners and researchers must always rely on their own experience and knowledge in evaluating and using any information, methods, compounds, or experiments described herein. In using such information or methods they should be mindful of their own safety and the safety of others, including parties for whom they have a professional responsibility.

With respect to any drug or pharmaceutical products identified, readers are advised to check the most current information provided (i) on procedures featured or (ii) by the manufacturer of each product to be administered, to verify the recommended dose or formula, the method and duration of administration, and contraindications. It is the responsibility of practitioners, relying on their own experience and knowledge of their patients, to make diagnoses, to determine dosages and the best treatment for each individual patient, and to take all appropriate safety precautions.

To the fullest extent of the law, neither the Publisher nor the authors, contributors, or editors, assume any liability for any injury and/or damage to persons or property as a matter of products liability, negligence or otherwise, or from any use or operation of any methods, products, instructions, or ideas contained in the material herein.

Series editor foreword

The *Crash Course* series first published in 1997 and now, 16 years on, we are still going strong. Medicine never stands still, and the work of keeping this series relevant for today's students is an ongoing process. These fourth editions build on the success of the previous titles and incorporate new and revised material, to keep the series up to date with current guidelines for best practice, and recent developments in medical research and pharmacology.

We always listen to feedback from our readers, through focus groups and student reviews of the *Crash Course* titles. For the fourth editions we have completely re-written our self-assessment material to keep up with today's 'single-best answer' and 'extended matching question' formats. The artwork and layout of the titles has also been largely re-worked to make it easier on the eye during long sessions of revision.

Despite fully revising the books with each edition, we hold fast to the principles on which we first developed the series. *Crash Course* will always bring you all the information you need to revise in compact, manageable volumes that integrate basic medical science and clinical practice. The books still maintain the balance between clarity and conciseness, and provide sufficient depth for those aiming at distinction. The authors are medical students and junior doctors who have recent experience of the exams you are now facing, and the accuracy of the material is checked by a team of faculty advisors from across the UK.

I wish you all the best for your future careers!

Dr Dan Horton-Szar
Series Editor

Preface

The new edition of *Crash Course: Paediatrics* has been reformatted compared to previous editions to provide a structure for history and examination at the beginning of the book. The self assessment section has been updated to include 'single best answer' and 'extended matching' questions to reflect the current form of assessment.

This edition continues to provide a practical approach to paediatrics and the hints and tips boxes have been revised to reflect this. The booked is aimed at the undergraduate but would be a great resource for foundation trainees or specialty doctors embarking on a career in paediatrics.

Rajat Kapoor
Katy Barnes
Victoria Jones

Acknowledgements

We would like to thank our families for their continuous support.

Rajat Kapoor
Katy Barnes
Victoria Jones

Contents

Contents

Contents

History and examination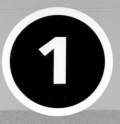

● Objectives

At the end of this chapter you should be able to:
- Take a detailed and appropriate paediatric history
- Perform a structured clinical examination
- Perform a routine neonatal examination
- Document your history, findings and conclusions appropriately

The art of taking a history from, and examining, a child shares some principles with the corresponding process in adult medicine. The young infant and neonate present special challenges, whereas the older child can often be clerked in a similar manner to an adult. Most clinicians are concerned that children might not cooperate and communicate during the clinical assessment.

In many cases, the history will come predominantly from the parents but it is important not to overlook a communicating child, as he or she might offer essential information. This is especially important in cases of child protection.

A problem-based approach

It is important to include a summary of clinical problems and proposed management at the end of your clerking in the notes. This is important, even when you are still a student – you may not always be right but it is never too early to train yourself to think like a doctor. Failure to include a problem list and management plan is a common criticism of new foundation doctors.

PAEDIATRIC HISTORY TAKING

The overall format is similar to that in adult medicine but it is important to establish a rapport with parent(s) and child at an early stage. Ignoring the child when taking a history wastes a valuable opportunity to alleviate the anxiety that the child will have in this unfamiliar situation.

COMMUNICATION

Ask the parents to help if the child is upset or shy.

The beginning

- Introduce yourself to the parents and the child. It is important to find out the name and sex of the child at this point. Do not be afraid to clarify the gender of the child if not obvious from the name as it is better to check than to get it wrong.
- Make sure you know who is accompanying the child; many parents are not married or the child might have been taken to hospital by a relative.
- A young person may prefer to be seen alone if appropriate. The consultation can therefore be shared with the parent/carer(s) for part of it and the other period with the child alone.
- The parental responsibility of the child is especially important when dealing with cases concerning child protection or consent.
- It may be necessary to enrol the help of linkworkers to translate to obtain a thorough and accurate history from the parent/carer(s). This is of paramount importance when dealing with suspected child abuse.

Presenting complaint

Open-ended questions to start will put the parents at ease and at this point they might volunteer both the presenting symptoms and the symptoms that caused them most anxiety. Often the symptoms that they are worried about are not the symptoms that most concern the doctor.

Once the main symptoms are established and the relevant body system has been identified, details such as the nature of onset, duration and precipitating factors should be obtained by specific questioning. Associated symptoms and previous illnesses should be asked for at this stage.

Past history

Most children are healthy and have only minor illnesses in the past history but an increasing number with significant illnesses such as extreme prematurity, leu-kaemia and cardiac disease are surviving to older ages. Ask about:

- Immunizations.
- Hospital admissions.

Birth

(Please refer to later section on Neonatal history.)

Developmental history

- Age at reaching milestones.
- Concerns about vision and hearing.

Family and social history

- Ask about any illnesses that run in the family and about recent infectious contacts.
- Make a family tree and ask about parental consanguinity (this increases the incidence of autosomal recessive conditions, which often present with neurological or metabolic problems).
- Social circumstances: smoking, housing, pets, parental occupations and any difficulties at home. The family might be under the care of a social worker.
- Travel history: include foreign travel and contacts.
- For adolescents, it is important to enquire about sexual history, alcohol and drug use.

Systems review

A systems review is not performed routinely because, with experience, the history of the presenting complaint should cover all relevant systems. However, a formal review of systems can be useful if the doctor feels that something might be missing in the history.

The history does not stop at one sitting – repeat questioning might produce information that was not volunteered the first time. There is no shame in reviewing the history and many parents do not give a complete picture at the beginning.

HINTS AND TIPS

It is essential to review the personal child health record (or 'Red Book') for all infants and young children with respect to immunizations and development.

NEONATAL HISTORY

When taking a neonatal history, more emphasis should be on the details of the birth. Many maternal conditions affect the newborn infant and the details of delivery and resuscitation are essential.

Pregnancy

- Maternal medical history, e.g. diabetes, HIV.
- Medication taken during pregnancy including illicit drugs.
- Alcohol and smoking.
- Complications of pregnancy, e.g. pre-eclampsia.
- Results of any amniocentesis, chorionic villus biopsy and ultrasound reports.

Maternal infections

Most mothers in the UK are tested in the antenatal period for HIV, hepatitis B, syphilis and rubella. Ask if a high vaginal swab was taken for group B streptococci and maternal fever.

Birth

Important facts:

- Duration or rupture of membranes.
- Gestational age at delivery.
- Mode of delivery.
- Resuscitation of the baby (if needed).
- Birthweight.
- Any problems encountered after birth, e.g. feeding, jaundice or admission to the neonatal unit.

EXAMINATION

Older children are usually cooperative and an approach similar to that used in adults can be employed; young children and infants might be frightened and rather less cooperative. Examination in these age groups is therefore much more opportunistic. It is important to let the parents help you. They are the people the child is most comfortable with and it should be no surprise if a child is unwilling to let a total stranger approach if the parents are absent.

In children, most of the examination findings are obtained by observing the child interact with their environment. Watching a child play will give you almost all the information you need about his or her neurology.

HINTS AND TIPS

Examination of the child begins as they enter the room or when they play. Observing their spontaneous movements will provide more information than asking them to perform.

General examination

- Weight and height – plot on a growth chart with head circumference in infants.
- Temperature.
- Colour.
- Posture, movements and conscious level.
- Rashes.

Respiratory system

Count the respiratory rate. Note the different normal values with age (Fig. 1.1). Note any cyanosis or finger clubbing.

Listen for
- Stridor (inspiratory) or wheeze (expiratory) sounds.
- Cough and its nature: barking cough is suggestive of croup.

Look for
- Nasal flaring and use of accessory muscles.
- Intercostal and subcostal recession.
- Chest shape abnormalities and Harrison's sulci.

Percuss
This is more useful in children >5 years and can give additional information to auscultation alone.

Auscultate
This can be done at any time that is suitable because the crying child will make auscultation impossible. Often, upper airway sounds will predominate and mask lung sounds. Listen for:

- Intensity of breath sounds on both sides.
- Presence of bronchial breath sounds.
- Wheeze and crackles.
- Ratio of inspiration to expiration.

Cardiovascular system

Similar to adults except that it is done as soon as the child is settled and not crying (Fig. 1.2). Innocent murmurs are common in children and should be distinguished from pathological murmurs (Fig. 1.3). Palpation of the

Fig. 1.1 Respiratory rates at different ages	
Age	Upper limits (breaths per minute)
Neonate	60
Infant	40
Young child	30
Older child	20

Fig. 1.2 Normal heart rates in children	
Age	Beats per minute
<1 year	120–160
2–5 years	90–140
5–12 years	80–120
>12 years	60–100

Fig. 1.3 Features of innocent heart murmurs
Changes with posture
Localized
Asymptomatic
Normal cardiac examination
Systolic only
No thrill

femoral pulse in neonates is mandatory to detect coarctation of the aorta. Hepatomegaly is one of the signs of cardiac failure. In contrast to adults, children with cardiac failure do not show signs of lung crepitations or sacral oedema.

Do not forget to measure blood pressure.

Abdomen

Observe for jaundice and abdominal distension. The liver is usually palpable during infancy. It is common for most infants to have a distended abdomen before they are walking. This alone is not pathological.

Palpate
The child must be as relaxed and as comfortable as possible. An unsettled anxious child will unconsciously tense their abdominal muscles.

- Abdominal masses: the liver is usually palpable until puberty.
- Peristalsis: this might represent obstruction or pyloric stenosis.
- Inguinal herniae.
- Umbilical herniae are common and not pathological.
- Watch the child's face for any sign of tenderness.

Nervous system

Most children will give you a lot of information in their play and the examiner must observe how the child interacts with his or her surroundings. The assessment of the cranial nerves, tone, reflexes, power, coordination and sensation must be tailored to the individual child. Observe:

- The gait as the child walks in.
- Posture at rest.
- Level of alertness or conscious level.

Important points:

- In infants, palpation of the fontanelle, sutures and measurement of the head circumference are essential (Fig. 1.4).
- Presence of primitive reflexes in neonates and infants.
- The plantar reflexes are predominantly extensor (down-going) in infants under 6 months and the transition to flexor might be asymmetrical.

Ear, nose and throat

This is often done at the end because it causes the most distress to the child (Fig. 1.5). It is vital that the examiner is helped by a parent who can hold the child still.

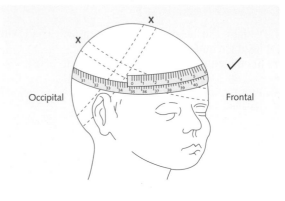

Occipital   Frontal

Fig. 1.4   Measuring head circumference

The neck should be palpated for lymphadenopathy and then the ears should be examined. Looking at the throat should be done at the end because a wooden tongue depressor might be needed to visualize the throat.

Never examine the throat if upper airway obstruction is suspected, e.g. epiglottitis or severe croup.

Fig. 1.5   Throat examination. Holding a young child to examine the throat. The mother has one hand on the head and the other across the child's arms. Remember to have a throat swab with you if pus or exudate are seen to avoid examining the throat again and upsetting the child or infant

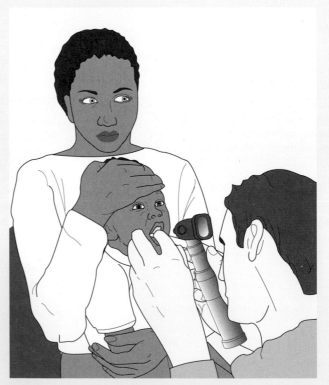

Holding a young child to examine the throat. The mother has one hand on the head and the other across the child's arms

THE NEONATAL EXAMINATION

All neonates should undergo a full examination within 24 hours. This allows any abnormalities to be detected early and also reassures parents of the numerous common normal variants that are found (Fig. 1.6).

Vital signs

Look at the baby's:

- Colour.
- Heart rate.
- Respiratory rate.
- Weight and head circumference.

Skin

Observe:

- Many neonates show some jaundice but this is pathological if seen in the first day or if severe.
- Erythema toxicum is a benign condition affecting approximately 50% of all infants. It presents as macular lesions with a central yellow papule.
- Cyanosis can be difficult to detect and should be observed on the tongue and lips. Peripheral cyanosis without central cyanosis is not pathological (acrocyanosis).

Fig. 1.6 Routine neonatal examination

- Birthweight and centile
- Colour
- Skin lesions
- Palpate fontanelle and sutures
- Measure occipitofrontal head circumference
- Check eyes for cataract, red reflex
- Examine facies for dysmorphic features
  - Down syndrome
- Check palate
- Observe breathing rate and chest wall movement
- Palpate praecordium
- Auscultate the heart
  - Count heart rate
  - Heart murmurs (see Hints and Tips box)
- Palpate abdomen
  - Liver 1–2 cm. Spleen tip may be palpable
- Inspect the umbilical cord
- Palpate the femoral pulses
- Inspect genitalia for
  - Inguinal herniae
  - Hypospadias
  - Undescended testes and anus for patency
- Check hips for congenital dislocation (see Hints and Tips box)
- Assess muscle tone
- Pick up the baby and hold in ventral suspension
- Inspect back and spine for midline defects
- Moro reflex

- Pallor might represent anaemia or illness; plethora might be due to polycythaemia.
- Mongolian blue spots must be documented because they appear identical to bruising. They are commoner in Afro-Caribbean babies and usually resolve by 1 year.
- Mottling is often seen in healthy infants and alone is not suggestive of pathology.
- Vascular lesions such as strawberry haemangiomas and port wine stains.

> **HINTS AND TIPS**
>
> Note all Mongolian blue spots for future reference. Ideally, these should also be documented in the personal child health record book.

Head

Note the shape and size of the head and fontanelle. The sutures should be palpable and head trauma from delivery may manifest as:

- Caput succedaneum: diffuse swelling that crosses the suture lines. It resolves in several days.
- Cephalohaematoma: this never crosses the suture lines and is caused by subperiosteal haemorrhage; 5% are associated with fractures.

Neck

Sternocleidomastoid tumours or thyroglossal cysts might be palpable as neck lumps in the midline. The clavicles might be fractured but no treatment is necessary. Palpable lymph nodes are found in 33% of all neonates.

Face

Observe for symmetry when the infant cries or yawns. Facial nerve palsy is common after forceps delivery and is self-limiting:

- Eyes: look for the red reflex (if absent think of retinoblastoma) and evidence of conjunctivitis. Occasionally, the red reflex may be difficult to see in which case it may be useful to check the mother's red reflexes for comparison. A blue sclera is normal in <3 months.
- Ears: look at the position and for any skin tags.
- Mouth: loose natal teeth need removal. Palpate *and* look at the palate for cleft palate.

Chest

These often cause concern amongst parents but have no clinical significance:

- Pectus excavatum.
- Breasts and milk production: caused by maternal oestrogens.

Note that the normal respiratory rate in newborns is 40–60 breaths/minute and heart rate is 120–160 beats/minute. Commonly, periodic breathing can be seen, during which there are pauses lasting less than 10 seconds. This is normal and more common in pre-term infants.

Auscultation for breath sounds and heart sounds should be done when the infant is quiet.

- Breath sounds: listen for presence and symmetry.
- Heart sounds: listen for the quality and intensity of the heart sounds.
- Murmurs might be heard but their presence does not always indicate heart disease.

HINTS AND TIPS

Murmurs are not always heard in the first 24–48 hours of life and cardiac problems do not usually present at this early stage.

The femoral pulses should be palpated and, if weak or absent, might indicate coarctation of the aorta.

Abdomen

Many infants have a small degree of abdominal distension and this is a normal finding. Observe for:

- Abdominal wall defects.
- Scaphoid abdomen suggests diaphragmatic hernia.
- Examine the umbilicus for three vessels. Single umbilical artery is associated with renal abnormalities. Also look for discharge and inflammation.
- Check for hypospadias and good urinary stream in case of underlying renal pathology.

Genitalia

The clitoris and labia are normally enlarged and vaginal bleeding might be observed. This is due to maternal oestrogen withdrawal and requires no treatment.

In boys, the testes should be palpable and phimosis is normal. The foreskin should never be retracted. A good urinary stream should be observed.

Anus

Check for patency of anus and that meconium is seen to be exiting from the anus to exclude any suspicion of a fistula; meconium should be passed in the first 24–48 hours. A delayed passage of meconium may indicate underlying pathology, e.g. cystic fibrosis or Hirschsprung's disease.

HINTS AND TIPS

Urine should be passed within 24 h and meconium within 48 h.

Extremities

Examine all digits and for palmar creases. Supernumary digits (polydactyly) and abnormal fusion of the digits (syndactyly) are often familial.

Trunk and spine

Hips

Palpate the vertebrae, looking for scoliosis. Any abnormal pigmentation, dimples or hairs over the lumbar region should raise the suspicion of spina bifida. A sacral dimple is common and usually normal if the base is seen.

The Barlow and Ortolani tests should be performed. In the Barlow test, backward pressure is applied to the head of each femur in turn, and a subluxable hip is suspected on the basis of palpable partial or complete displacement. The Ortolani test consists of forward pressure applied to each femoral head in turn, in an attempt to move a posteriorly dislocated femoral head back into the acetabulum. Palpable movement suggests that the hip is dislocated or subluxed, but reducible. Observe for leg length discrepancy and range of abduction; only gentle force is needed.

Nervous system

The spontaneous movements of the infant should be observed and then examination of:

- Tone: look for both hypo- and hypertonia.
- Reflexes: both primitive and deep tendon reflexes.
- Cranial nerves.

A fine tremor and ankle clonus for 5–10 beats is normal.

MEDICAL SAMPLE CLERKING

A sample medical clerking is shown in Fig. 1.7. It illustrates some of the points discussed earlier in this chapter.

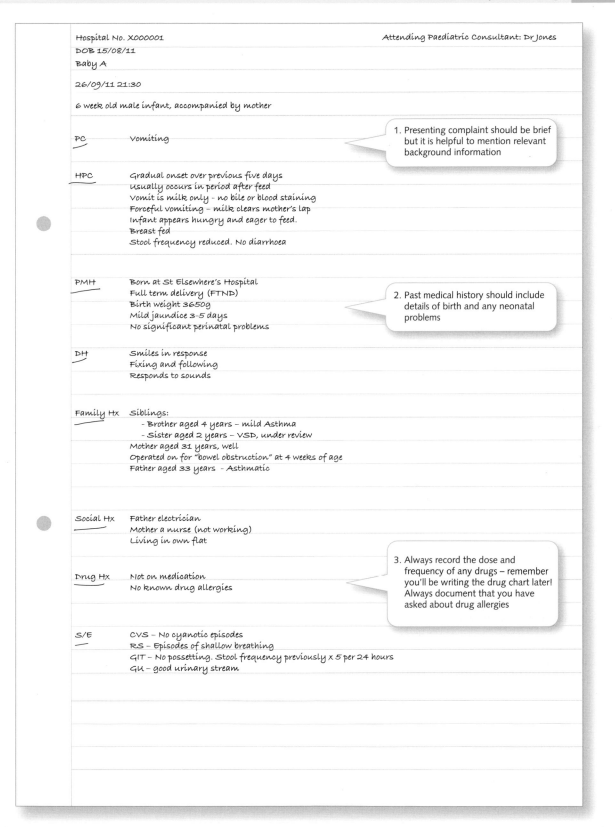

Hospital No. X000001   Attending Paediatric Consultant: Dr Jones
DOB 15/08/11
Baby A

26/09/11 21:30

6 week old male infant, accompanied by mother

PC   Vomiting

> 1. Presenting complaint should be brief but it is helpful to mention relevant background information

HPC   Gradual onset over previous five days
            Usually occurs in period after feed
            Vomit is milk only - no bile or blood staining
            Forceful vomiting - milk clears mother's lap
            Infant appears hungry and eager to feed.
            Breast fed
            Stool frequency reduced. No diarrhoea

PMH   Born at St Elsewhere's Hospital
            Full term delivery (FTND)
            Birth weight 3650g
            Mild jaundice 3-5 days
            No significant perinatal problems

> 2. Past medical history should include details of birth and any neonatal problems

DH   Smiles in response
            Fixing and following
            Responds to sounds

Family Hx   Siblings:
                - Brother aged 4 years – mild Asthma
                - Sister aged 2 years – VSD, under review
            Mother aged 31 years, well
            Operated on for "bowel obstruction" at 4 weeks of age
            Father aged 33 years - Asthmatic

Social Hx   Father electrician
            Mother a nurse (not working)
            Living in own flat

Drug Hx   Not on medication
            No known drug allergies

> 3. Always record the dose and frequency of any drugs – remember you'll be writing the drug chart later! Always document that you have asked about drug allergies

S/E   CVS – No cyanotic episodes
            RS – Episodes of shallow breathing
            GIT – No possetting. Stool frequency previously x 5 per 24 hours
            GU – good urinary stream

Fig. 1.7   Clerking

Continued

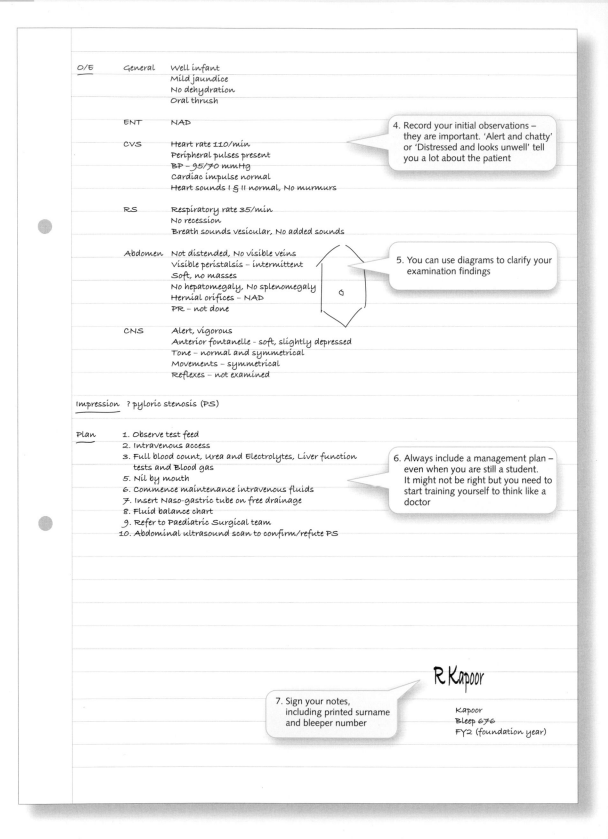

O/E   General   Well infant
Mild jaundice
No dehydration
Oral thrush

ENT   NAD

> 4. Record your initial observations – they are important. 'Alert and chatty' or 'Distressed and looks unwell' tell you a lot about the patient

CVS   Heart rate 110/min
Peripheral pulses present
BP – 95/70 mmHg
Cardiac impulse normal
Heart sounds I & II normal, No murmurs

RS   Respiratory rate 35/min
No recession
Breath sounds vesicular, No added sounds

Abdomen   Not distended, No visible veins
Visible peristalsis – intermittent
Soft, no masses
No hepatomegaly, No splenomegaly
Hernial orifices – NAD
PR – not done

> 5. You can use diagrams to clarify your examination findings

CNS   Alert, vigorous
Anterior fontanelle - soft, slightly depressed
Tone – normal and symmetrical
Movements – symmetrical
Reflexes – not examined

Impression   ? pyloric stenosis (PS)

Plan
1. Observe test feed
2. Intravenous access
3. Full blood count, Urea and Electrolytes, Liver function tests and Blood gas
5. Nil by mouth
6. Commence maintenance intravenous fluids
7. Insert Naso-gastric tube on free drainage
8. Fluid balance chart
9. Refer to Paediatric Surgical team
10. Abdominal ultrasound scan to confirm/refute PS

> 6. Always include a management plan – even when you are still a student. It might not be right but you need to start training yourself to think like a doctor

R Kapoor

> 7. Sign your notes, including printed surname and bleeper number

Kapoor
Bleep 676
FY2 (foundation year)

Fig. 1.7 Clerking—cont'd

Developmental assessment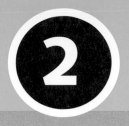

At the end of this chapter you should be able to:
- Take a basic history in a child presenting with delayed development
- Perform a simple developmental assessment
- Identify a child with developmental delay

Growing up involves the acquisition of new abilities and skills, as well as physical growth. The process by which an immobile, incontinent and speechless baby develops into a mobile, communicating, socially interactive and (hopefully!) well-behaved child involves a complex interaction between genes (nature) and environment (nurture).

Much study over many years has established the average rate and pattern of development and identified a very wide range of normal variation. A child might be far from average but still normal. A major challenge is to distinguish such normal variation from a significant problem requiring active intervention.

Developmental screening is offered routinely to all children in the UK. It is one component of child health surveillance, which also encompasses physical health and growth. In October 2009, the Department of Health published the Healthy Child Programme: pregnancy and the first 5 years of life. It differs from the previous child surveillance schedule in several aspects: greater focus on antenatal care, major emphasis on support for both parents, early identification of at-risk families, new vaccination programmes and new focus on changed public health priorities.

The aim is to identify developmental problems at an early stage to allow appropriate intervention. Any delay might be global or specific (see Chapter 11) but it is important to bear in mind the close interrelationships involved, e.g. hearing impairment can cause a delay in speech and language, with consequent disruption of social interaction and behaviour.

Clinical assessment of a child's developmental status is based on a thorough history, physical examination, and observation of the child's performance and play.

HISTORY

Certain aspects of the history clearly assume special importance in assessing development. In particular, it is important to enquire about and document 'risk factors'

that contribute to vulnerability and poor outcome (Fig. 2.1). The history should therefore include inquiry into:

- Pregnancy and birth.
- Developmental milestones: depending on age.
- Family and social history.
- Specific parental concerns.
- Parent-held personal child health record.

Milestones reflect the average age that a child acquires a particular ability:
- Motor problems often manifest in the first year.
- Talking and coordination problems often manifest in the second year.
- Behavioural and social problems often manifest in the third year.

EXAMINATION

Four aspects of development are routinely assessed:

- Gross motor.
- Fine motor and vision.
- Hearing and speech.
- Social behaviour and play.

Routine surveillance is carried out during well-recognized stages of development and covered in Chapter 26.

Newborn

Gross motor

- Symmetrical movements in all four limbs.
- Normal muscle tone.

Fig. 2.1 Risk factors for development
Prematurity
Perinatal asphyxia
Dysmorphology
Psychosocial deprivation

Fine motor and vision

- Fixes on mother's face and follows through 90°.

Hearing and speech

- Cries.
- All newborn babies are tested as part of the Newborn Hearing Screening Programme (NHSP). The automated otoacoustic emission (AOAE) screening test is used which is a simple, painless test that produces immediate results and can be carried out while the baby is asleep. If two AOAE test results are unsatisfactory, an automated auditory brainstem response (AABR) test is then performed.

Social

- Responds to being picked up.

Six to eight weeks: the supine infant

Gross motor

- Good head control when pulled up to sitting (Fig. 2.2).
- When held in ventral suspension holds head transiently in horizontal plane (Fig. 2.3).
- Presence of the Moro response.

HINTS AND TIPS

The Moro response consists of extension of the arms, then brisk adduction towards the chest when the infant is startled or the baby's head allowed to drop back slightly. It should be symmetrical and should have disappeared by 6 months. Persistence of this or any of the primitive reflexes beyond 6 months might indicate a cerebral disorder.

Fine motor and vision

- Stares at and follows mother's face.

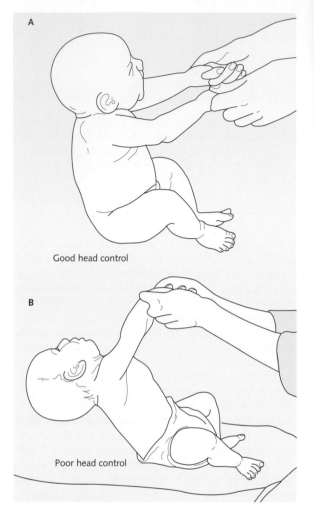

Fig. 2.2 (A) Good head control compared with (B) poor head control at 6 weeks

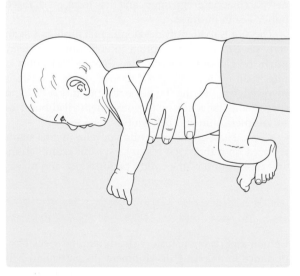

Fig. 2.3 Ventral suspension at 6 weeks

Hearing and speech

- Coos.
- Startles to loud noises.

Social

- Smiles in response.

At 4–6 months the ability to roll, sit and use of both hands is dependent on the disappearance of primitive reflexes and the appearance of head and trunk righting.

Twelve months

Gross motor

- Crawling and pulling to stand.
- Some children will be walking (approx. 50%).

Fine motor and vision

- Pincer grip (Fig. 2.4).
- Turns pages (many at a time).
- Points to objects.

Hearing and speech

- Uses single words, e.g. mama, dada.
- Understands simple commands.

Social

- Finger feeds.
- Waves goodbye.
- Demonstrates separation anxiety.
- Responds to name.

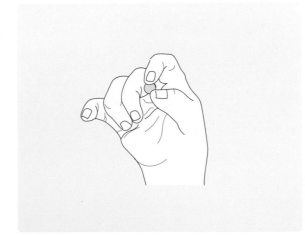

Fig. 2.4　Pincer grip

Thirty months: the communicating child

Gross motor

- Uses stairs holding banister.
- Jumps with both feet.
- Kicks a ball.

Fine motor and vision

- Threads beads on a string.
- Builds a six–eight-brick tower.
- Copies a line.

Speech and language

- Short sentences.
- Can name some colours.
- Can name parts of the body.

Social

- Toilet trained: dry by day.
- Dresses with help.
- Plays with other children.

Five years: the school-aged child

Gross motor

- Skips.
- Catches a ball.
- Heel–toe walking.

Fine motor and vision

- Draws a man with all features.
- Copies alphabet letters.
- Snellen's chart test (by name or matching).

> **HINTS AND TIPS**
>
> Hand preference develops at 18–24 months and is fixed at 5 years. Handedness in <1 year indicates a problem with the non-dominant side.

Hearing and speech

- Comprehensive speech.

Social

- Plays games.
- Learning to read.
- Can tell the time.

SIGNS OF ABNORMAL DEVELOPMENT: 'LIMIT AGES'

Fig. 2.5 lists the worrying signs at the ages given. Any parental or carer concerns about their infant or child's development (developmental progress or regression) should be taken seriously and warrants prompt assessment and referral to the local community paediatric team. Recognition by a parent or carer that their infant or child's development is abnormal when compared to their sibling(s) or a friend's child is also significant and further assessment is also indicated.

HINTS AND TIPS

Management options for concern over development:
- Review history and examination and assess if no delay, specific delay or global delay. This will depend upon what setting you are in and what tools are available to you, e.g. clinic or emergency department.
- Refer to local community paediatrician if you have concerns.
- Community team may then arrange appropriate investigations, e.g. audiology testing, blood tests, imaging, etc. with appropriate follow-up.

HINTS AND TIPS

Babies who were preterm need their development corrected for their gestational age but this becomes less important after 2 years of age.

Fig. 2.5 Worrying signs at various ages

Age	Developmental sign
Worrying signs	
6–8 weeks	Asymmetrical Moro Excess head lag No visual fixation/following No startle or quietening to sound No responsive smiling
8 months	Persisting primitive reflexes Not weight-bearing on legs Not reaching out for toys Not fixing on small objects Not vocalizing
10 months	Unable to sit unsupported
1 year	Showing a hand preference Not responding to own name
18 months	Not walking No pincer grip Persistence of casting
3 years	Inaccurate use of a spoon Not speaking in sentences Unable to understand simple commands Unable to use the toilet alone Not interacting with other children

Further reading

Department of Health, Healthy Child Programme: pregnancy and the first five years of life. http://www.dh.gov.uk/en/ Publicationsandstatistics/Publications/ PublicationsPolicyAndGuidance/DH_107563.

Investigations  **3**

Objectives

At the end of this chapter you should be able to:
- Interpret the results of common blood tests
- Understand the indications, advantages and disadvantages of common imaging studies
- Understand the indications for certain special investigations and their interpretation

Investigations are often used to confirm, or refute, a clinical diagnosis that is uncertain or to monitor the progress of a disease or its treatment. They should be performed only when there are specific indications, not as a 'routine'. In all cases, the potential benefits must be weighed against any associated pain or discomfort.

HINTS AND TIPS

There is no such thing as a 'routine investigation' – always consider how the result will affect your practice. Tests should be done for the benefit of the patient, not the doctor.

In this chapter, the indications for and interpretation of the following common and important special investigations are considered.

BLOOD TESTS

Venous or capillary blood is usually satisfactory and can be obtained by venepuncture or capillary sampling. Arterial blood sampling is only occasionally necessary for determination of oxygenation but pulse oximetry will often suffice. With experience, skill and local anaesthetic cream, blood can be obtained quickly and with minimal discomfort from most infants and children.

HINTS AND TIPS

Once a suitable vein for venepuncture has been identified, local anaesthetic cream can be applied and fixed to the skin with an occlusive dressing. Anaesthetic cream is appropriate for any child over 1 month of age and can take 30–40 minutes to take effect. Alternative analgesic options include ethyl chloride spray (or 'cold spray') coupled with distraction techniques.

Blood tests fall into the following general categories (see Fig. 3.1 for clinical chemistry reference values):

Haematology

Full blood count

This provides information on:
- Haemoglobin, Hb (g/dL).
- Total white cell count, WBC ($\times 10^9$/L).
- Platelet count ($\times 10^9$/L).

HINTS AND TIPS

Haemoglobin concentration and white cell counts must be interpreted in relation to age:
- Hb concentration is high at birth (15–19 g/dL) and falls to a nadir at 3 months (9–13 g/dL).
- The total white cell count is high at birth and rapidly falls to normal adult levels. There is a relative lymphocytosis during the first 4 years of life after the neonatal period.

It can also provide:
- Red cell indices: mean cell volume (MCV) (fl), mean cell haemoglobin (MCH) (pg), mean cell haemoglobin concentration (MCHC) (%).
- Reticulocytes (%).
- Differential white cell count: neutrophils, lymphocytes, eosinophils, monocytes (% or 10^9/L).

The examination of the film allows evaluation of:
- Red cell morphology (Fig. 3.2).
- Differential white cell count.
- Platelet numbers and morphology.
- Presence or absence of abnormal cells (e.g. blast cells).

See also Fig. 3.3, which shows important abnormalities that can be identified from a full blood count (FBC).

13

Fig. 3.1 Normal ranges for blood tests (normal range for some tests varies between laboratories and must be checked with the local laboratory)

Clinical chemistry			
Test	**Normal range (plasma or serum)**		
Sodium		133–145 mmol/L	
Potassium	Infant	3.5–6.0 mmol/L	
	Child	3.3–5.0 mmol/L	
Urea	Neonate	1.0–5.0 mmol/L	
	Infant	2.5–8.0 mmol/L	
	Child	2.5–6.5 mmol/L	
Creatinine	Infant	20–65 µmol/L	
	1–10 years	20–80 µmol/L	
Osmolality		275–295 mosm/kg	
Calcium (total)	24–48 h	1.8–3.0 mmol/L	
	Child	2.15–2.60 mmol/L	
Calcium (ionized)	24–48 h	1.00–1.17 mmol/L	
	Child	1.18–1.32 mmol/L	
Phosphate	Neonate	1.4–2.6 mmol/L	
	Infant	1.3–2.1 mmol/L	
	Child	1.0–1.8 mmol/L	
Alkaline phosphatase	Neonate	150–700 U/L	
	1–12 months	250–1000 U/L	
	2–9 years	250–850 U/L	
	Years	Females	Males
	10–11	250–950 U/L	250–730 U/L
	14–15	170–460 U/L	170–970 U/L
	>18	60–250 U/L	50–200 U/L
Albumin	Neonate	25–35 g/L	
	Child	35–55 g/L	
Creatine kinase	Infant/child	60–300 U/L	
Glucose	1 day	2.2–3.3 mmol/L	
	>1 day	2.6–5.5 mmol/L	
	Child	3.0–6.0 mmol/L	
Iron	Infant	5–25 µmol/L	
	Child	10–30 µmol/L	
Ferritin	Child	<150 µg/L	
C-reactive protein		<10 mg/L	
Blood gas (arterial, not preterm)	pH	7.35–7.45	
	pO_2	11–14 kPa (82–105 mmHg)	
	pCO_2	4.5–6.0 kPa (32–45 mmHg)	
	Bicarbonate	18–25 mmol/L	
	Base excess	−4 to +4 mmol/L	

Sickle test

This is a screening test for the sickle cell trait or disease. Sickle cells are seen when the blood is deoxygenated with Na_2HPO_4. The percentage of haemoglobin S in the blood is useful in monitoring sickle cell disease and in the management of associated complications and blood transfusions.

HINTS AND TIPS

Structure of haemoglobin:
- Fetal haemoglobin (HbF): $\alpha_2 \gamma_2$
- Adult haemoglobin: HbA, $\alpha_2 \beta_2$; HbA2 $\alpha_2 \delta_2$
- Sickle haemoglobin (HbS): $\alpha_2 \beta_2{}^s$

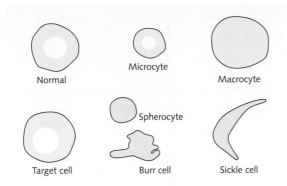

Fig. 3.2   Red cell morphology

Fig. 3.3   Important problems identifiable on full blood count

Anaemia, e.g. iron deficiency
Thrombocytopenia, e.g. idiopathic thrombocytopenic purpura
Neutropenia, e.g. immunosuppression
Pancytopenia, e.g. bone marrow failure
Neutrophil leucocytosis, e.g. bacterial infection
Lymphocytosis, e.g. *Bordetella pertussis*

Haemoglobin electrophoresis

The pattern of haemoglobin electrophoresis at different ages (birth and adult) and in different haemoglobino-pathies is shown in Fig. 3.4.

Coagulation studies

To evaluate a bleeding disorder it is necessary to measure platelets as well as prothrombin time (PT), activated partial thromboplastin time (APTT) and thrombin time (TT). The interpretation of these tests is covered in Chapter 22.

von Willebrand's disease (VWD) and disseminated intravascular coagulation (DIC)

These topics are discussed in Chapter 22.

Biochemical analysis

Urea and electrolytes

Urea and electrolytes (U&E) (urea, Na^+, K^+, Cl^-) are the most commonly requested biochemical analysis and can be useful in a host of circumstances including:

- Dehydration-diarrhoea, vomiting.
- Ill patients on IV fluids – monitoring electrolyte status.
- Diabetic ketoacidosis.
- Renal disease.
- Diuretic therapy.

Urea

Urea is a major metabolite of protein catabolism. It is synthesized in the liver and excreted by the kidneys. The plasma concentration is influenced by:

- State of hydration.
- Protein intake.
- Catabolism.
- Glomerular filtration rate (GFR).

The creatinine concentration is a more reliable indicator of renal function. The most commonly encountered cause of a raised plasma urea is dehydration.

Sodium (Na^+)

Changes in the plasma sodium concentration can reflect changes in either the sodium or water balance. Causes are shown in Figs 3.5 and 3.6.

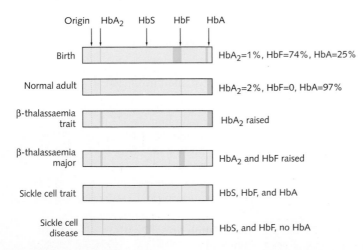

Fig. 3.4   Haemoglobin (Hb) electrophoresis

Fig. 3.5 Causes of hyponatraemia (Na$^+$ <130 mmol/L)

Mechanism	Cause
Water excess	Iatrogenic: excess hypotonic IV fluids Water retention due to inappropriate ADH secretion, e.g. postoperative, meningitis, head injury
Sodium depletion	Diarrhoea Diuretics Adrenal insufficiency (rare) Cystic fibrosis/sweating (rare)

Fig. 3.6 Causes of hypernatraemia (Na$^+$ >150 mmol/L)

Mechanism	Cause
Water deficit	Diarrhoea Diabetes insipidus Excessive insensible water loss, e.g. overhead heater
Sodium excess	High solute intake Iatrogenic: excess hypertonic IV fluids Child abuse: salt poisoning (rare)

Fig. 3.7 Causes of hypokalaemia (K$^+$ <3.4 mmol/L)

Mechanism	Cause
Potassium depletion	Diarrhoea Diuretics
Inadequate intake	Daily need 2–3 mmol/kg
Redistribution	Metabolic alkalosis Glucose and insulin

Fig. 3.8 Causes of hyperkalaemia (K$^+$ >5.5 mmol/L)

Mechanism	Cause
Failure of renal excretion	Renal failure Adrenocortical insufficiency
Redistribution	Metabolic acidosis, e.g. diabetic Ketoacidosis
Excess intake	Iatrogenic
Tissue injury	Hypoxia, catabolism
Artefact	Haemolysed specimen

Concerning plasma sodium:
- Artefactually low plasma Na$^+$ concentration can occur with hyperlipidaemia, e.g. in diabetic ketoacidosis, parenteral feeding.
- A normal plasma Na$^+$ concentration might be found in salt depletion or overload if associated parallel changes in body water have occurred.
- Rapid falls in plasma Na$^+$ can cause cerebral oedema.

Potassium (K$^+$)

This is a predominantly intracellular cation. Plasma concentration is therefore influenced by exchange with the intracellular compartment as well as the whole-body potassium status. The causes of changes in plasma potassium are shown in Figs 3.7 and 3.8.

Concerning plasma potassium:
- The intracellular K$^+$ concentration is very high: >100 mmol/L.
- Acidosis brings K$^+$ out of cells in exchange for H$^+$.
- Haemolysis releases K$^+$ from red cells and causes artefactual hyperkalaemia.
- ECG changes may occur with changes in plasma K$^+$ concentration.

Chloride (Cl$^-$)

Hypochloraemia is seen particularly in vomiting associated with pyloric stenosis and leads to a metabolic alkalosis.

Creatinine

Creatinine is a naturally occurring substance that is formed in muscles. The normal plasma concentration increases with age as muscle mass increases with growth. The plasma concentration of creatinine is a useful indirect measure of the GFR. In renal failure, the creatinine concentration increases steadily by more than 3 mmol/L/day.

Liver function tests

The basic biochemical tests of liver function include bilirubin, enzymes and albumin and are outlined below.

Bilirubin
- Conjugated and unconjugated.

Enzymes
- Aspartate transaminase (AST).
- Alanine transaminase (ALT).
- Alkaline phosphatase (ALP).
- γ-Glutamyltranspeptidase (γGT).

Additional investigations, which are useful for evaluating hepatic function (and are deranged in liver failure), include:

- Coagulation tests: PT, APTT.
- Ammonia.
- Glucose.

Bilirubin

Clinical evaluation of the severity of jaundice is unreliable, so it is important to document plasma levels of unconjugated and conjugated bilirubin. The normal proportion of conjugated bilirubin should not exceed 10% in infants. The causes of hyperbilirubinaemia are considered elsewhere (see Chapter 12).

> **HINTS AND TIPS**
>
> Excess conjugated hyperbilirubinaemia is a worrying sign in young infants as it might indicate biliary atresia.

Liver enzymes

Transaminases (aminotransferases)

These intracellular enzymes occur in many tissues including the liver, heart and skeletal muscle. Normal plasma activity reflects release of enzymes during cell turnover and increases occur with tissue injury. Elevated serum aminotransferase activity is therefore primarily seen in hepatocyte damage, e.g. hepatitis (infection, drugs).

> **HINTS AND TIPS**
>
> Raised transaminases indicate hepatocellular damage.

However, elevation is not a specific marker of primary hepatocellular disease as it occurs in other forms of hepatobiliary disease (e.g. biliary atresia, cholecystitis) and also in non-hepatic conditions such as myocarditis and pancreatitis.

AST is the more sensitive indicator of liver injury but ALT is more specific.

Alkaline phosphatase

Isoenzymes of alkaline phosphatase are widely distributed in many organs including liver and bone. Normal activity levels change markedly throughout childhood and reference ranges are both age- and method-dependent. Activity is increased in:

- Biliary obstruction: intrahepatic or extrahepatic.
- Hepatocellular damage.
- Increased osteoblastic activity, e.g. rickets, normal growth and pubertal growth spurt.

γ-Glutamyltranspeptidase

Serum activity is commonly raised in liver disease especially when there is cholestasis. It might also be raised in the absence of liver disease in patients taking certain drugs, e.g. phenytoin, phenobarbital and rifampicin (as a result of enzyme induction).

Fig. 3.9 Causes of hypoalbuminaemia (albumin <30 g/L)

Causes of hypoalbuminaemia (<30 g/L)	
Type	Cause
Decreased synthesis	Chronic liver disease Malnutrition (protein–energy malnutrition) Malabsorption
Increased losses	Nephrotic syndrome Burns Protein-losing enteropathy

Albumin

Albumin is synthesized in the liver and is the main contributor to plasma oncotic pressure. It also has an important role as the protein to which many circulating substances are bound such as:

- Bilirubin.
- Calcium.
- Drugs.
- Hormones.

Albumin has a long half-life of about 20 days.

Plasma albumin levels are a useful indicator of hepatic function. Low levels occur in several important clinical contexts (Fig. 3.9).

Prolonged hypoalbuminaemia (e.g. in nephrotic syndrome) is associated with oedema because fluid leaks into the extravascular space and hypovolaemia triggers renal salt and water retention.

Glucose

Blood glucose concentrations are normally maintained within fairly narrow limits, which are lower in the newborn. Blood glucose can be estimated very rapidly at the bedside using test sticks but values should be verified by laboratory investigation.

> **HINTS AND TIPS**
>
> Always measure the blood glucose urgently in a fitting or unconscious child.

Common causes of hyperglycaemia in children are insulin-dependent type 1 diabetes mellitus, sepsis and glucocorticoid use. There are, however, many causes of hypoglycaemia (Fig. 3.10).

Calcium and phosphate

Disorders of calcium and phosphate metabolism in childhood are uncommon and usually reflect abnormalities in the major controlling hormones, vitamin D and parathormone. Laboratory estimations provide a measure of both total and ionized calcium. Changes in

Fig. 3.10 Causes of hyperglycaemia and hypoglycaemia

Hyperglycaemia	Hypoglycaemia
Diabetes mellitus • IDDM (most common) • Secondary – pancreatic disease, Cushing syndrome Stress-related, e.g. postconvulsive Iatrogenic • Drugs, e.g. corticosteroids • Total parenteral nutrition	Neonatal • Infant of diabetic mother • Small for gestational age Postneonatal • Ketotic hypoglycaemia • Hyperinsulinaemia – known diabetic, pancreatic tumour (rare) • ↓GH, ACTH, cortisol – hypopituitarism (rare), adrenal failure (rare)

Fig. 3.11 Causes of hypocalcaemia and hypercalcaemia

Hypocalcaemia	Hypercalcaemia
Rickets (low phosphate, high alkaline phosphatase) Hypoparathyroidism, e.g. DiGeorge syndrome Hypoalbuminaemia	Hyperparathyroidism Syndromic (Williams syndrome) Vitamin D excess

plasma albumin concentration affect total calcium levels independently of ionized calcium, leading to misinterpretation if serum albumin is outside the normal range. Therefore, the total calcium concentration needs to be corrected to give the expected value if albumin were in the normal range. Major causes of hypercalcaemia and hypocalcaemia are shown in Fig. 3.11.

Blood gases and acid–base metabolism

Metabolism generates acid, which is eliminated via the lungs as carbon dioxide and via the kidneys as hydrogen ions. Acidosis, from whatever cause, is a much more common problem than alkalosis. Ideally, estimations of blood gas and acid–base status are made on an arterial sample but capillary or venous blood can be used.

Where the main concern is oxygenation, non-invasive pulse oximetry is a valuable alternative to arterial blood gas analysis.

The pattern of changes seen in different forms of acidosis and alkalosis are shown in Fig. 3.12.

Common clinical contexts in which these disturbances occur include:

- Respiratory acidosis: hypoventilation (e.g. respiratory distress syndrome, severe asthma, neuromuscular diseases).

Fig. 3.12 Acid–base disturbances

	pH	$PaCO_2$	HCO_3^-
Acidosis			
Respiratory	Low	High	Normal or high (compensation)
Metabolic	Low	Normal or low (compensation)	Low
Alkalosis			
Respiratory	High	Low	Normal or low (compensation)
Metabolic	High	Normal or high (compensation)	High

- Metabolic acidosis: diabetic ketoacidosis, hypoxia, circulatory failure.
- Respiratory alkalosis: hyperventilation, e.g. hysterical (rare in children), iatrogenic (ventilated patients).
- Metabolic alkalosis: pyloric stenosis.

Immunology

Tests of the immune system carried out on the blood might be required in the following clinical contexts:

- Immunodeficiency.
- Autoimmune disease.
- Infection: diagnostic serology, acute-phase reactants.

Tests for immunodeficiency

Immunodeficiencies can be primary or secondary. The inherited primary deficiencies are rare; secondary causes are far more common (Fig. 3.13).

Immunodeficiency should be suspected in the following clinical circumstances:

- Recurrent severe infections.
- Infections with atypical organisms.

Fig. 3.13 Causes of immunodeficiency

Primary
Primary antibody deficiencies:
• Common variable immune deficiency
• X-linked antibody deficiency
• IgG subclass deficiency
• Specific antibody deficiency
• Selective IgA deficiency
Severe combined immunodeficiency
Chronic granulomatous disease
Secondary
Malnutrition
Infections, e.g. HIV, measles
Immunosuppressive therapy, e.g. steroids, cytotoxic drugs
Hyposplenism, e.g. sickle cell disease, splenectomy

- Common infections with a severe or atypical clinical course.
- Failure to thrive.

Basic screening tests of immune function should include:

- Immunoglobulins.
- FBC including differential WCC and T lymphocyte subsets.
- HIV test

Immunoglobulins

Serum immunoglobulin levels vary with age. Maternally transferred IgG is present at high levels at birth but has mostly disappeared by 6 months of age. This decline occurs before endogenous synthesis has fully developed, creating a physiological trough between 3 and 6 months of age. This is shown in Fig. 3.14.

IgG is the major immunoglobulin in normal human serum, accounting for about 70% of the total pool. There are four distinct subclasses (IgG-1 to IgG-4), which have different functions. Specific IgM changes are very useful in the diagnosis of viral infections, e.g. rubella.

> **HINTS AND TIPS**
>
> - IgG2 is the most common subclass deficiency and might be associated with IgA deficiency. The total IgG level might be normal. It causes recurrent respiratory infections, e.g. sinusitis, pneumonia.
> - Selective IgA deficiency is common (1:700 population) and might cause no symptoms.

Differential white cell count

Immunodeficiency caused by marrow-suppressive cytotoxic or immunosuppressive therapy is related to the absolute neutrophil count. Patients with absolute neutrophil counts below $1.0 \times 10^9/L$ are at increased risk of Gram-negative septicaemia.

Lymphocyte subsets

Lymphocytes are further subdivided into T cells and B cells. T cells are categorized into:

- Cytotoxic T cells (TC), which are mostly $CD8^+$.
- Helper T cells (TH), which are mostly $CD4^+$.

Cytotoxic T cells recognize infected target cells and lyse them. Helper T cells secrete regulatory molecules (lymphokines) that affect other T cells and cells of various lineages.

Monitoring absolute numbers of $CD4^+$ helper cells is useful in monitoring the progression of HIV-related diseases.

Autoantibodies

Autoimmune disease is uncommon in childhood but includes such entities as juvenile chronic arthritis (JIA), systemic lupus erythematosus (SLE) and autoimmune thyroiditis causing juvenile hypothyroidism.

The following tests might be of value:

Antinuclear antibodies

Antinuclear antibodies (ANA) are a broad group of antibodies present in 5% of normal children and induced by a wide spectrum of inflammatory conditions.

- High titres of ANA occur in 95% of SLE patients.
- The presence of ANA in subgroups of JIA is a risk factor for chronic anterior uveitis.

SLE is associated with antibodies against specific nuclear antigens such as double-stranded DNA.

Rheumatoid factors

Rheumatoid factors (RFs) are IgM autoantibodies against IgG. They should not be used to screen for JIA because they are neither sensitive nor specific. The majority of children with JIA are rheumatoid factor negative. Rheumatoid factors can be useful as a prognostic indicator in polyarticular JIA (their persistent presence is a poor prognostic factor).

Thyroid antibodies

Thyroid microsomal (peroxisomal) and thyroglobulin titres should be measured in suspected autoimmune thyroiditis.

Diagnostic serology

This is most widely used in the diagnosis of viral infections but is also of value in certain specific non-viral infections such as *Mycoplasma pneumoniae*, group A β-haemolytic streptococci and *Salmonella* spp.

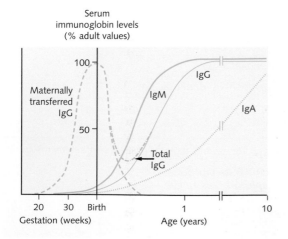

Fig. 3.14 Serum immunoglobulin (Ig) levels in fetus and infant

Viral antibody tests

Serological diagnosis depends on the detection of virus antibody. Diagnosis of recent infection requires the demonstration of a rising titre of specific IgM between the acute phase and convalescence. Methods used include:

- Immunofluorescence.
- Enzyme-linked immunoabsorbent assay (ELISA).
- Radioimmune assay (RIA).

Epstein–Barr virus

Specific Epstein–Barr virus (EBV) serology is the most reliable diagnostic test. Antibodies to viral capsid antigen (VCA) are detected. IgG anti-VCA merely indicates a past infection. A positive IgM to VCA is diagnostic and is found early in the disease.

Tests for heterophile antibody, which agglutinates sheep red blood cells, are the basis of slide agglutination tests (monospot and Paul–Bunnell). However, this antibody does not appear until the second week or even later, and may not be produced at all in young children.

Mycoplasma pneumoniae

Diagnosis of infection with *Mycoplasma pneumoniae* is most quickly established by acute and convalescent serology: a four-fold rise in complement-fixing antibodies is diagnostic.

Antistreptolysin O titre

Estimation of antibody to streptolysin O is a useful means of retrospectively diagnosing infection by group A β-haemolytic streptococci. The antistreptolysin O test (ASOT) is a valuable investigation in the evaluation of:

- Suspected acute nephritis.
- Rheumatic fever.
- Scarlet fever.

Acute-phase reactants

An inflammatory stimulus provokes the production of proteins in the liver known as the acute-phase reactants. This response is documented by the measurement of:

- C-reactive protein (CRP).
- Erythrocyte sedimentation rate (ESR).

The response is non-specific and does not help in identifying aetiology. However, if acute phase reactants are elevated at the onset of disease, serial measurements are useful for monitoring progress.

The response times vary:

- CRP: elevated within 6 hours.
- ESR: peaks at 3–4 days.

Microbiology

Blood is normally sterile. Transient asymptomatic bacteraemia can occur after dental treatment, or invasive procedures such as catheterization. However, bacteraemia leading to septicaemia and shock can accompany a number of important childhood diseases such as pneumonia, meningitis and typhoid fever.

Blood culture should be taken under the following circumstances:

- Pyrexia of unknown origin.
- Clinical signs of septicaemia.
- Febrile illness: in an immunodeficient child (e.g. sickle-cell disease, nephrotic syndrome, neutropenia) or in patients with a central catheter.
- Investigation of specific infections: meningitis, pneumonia, pyelonephritis, enteric fever.

The most common pathogens recovered from the blood are shown in Figs 3.15 and 3.16. Most significant isolates will be obtained within 48 hours of inoculation, especially in septic neonates.

Upper respiratory culture

- Nasopharyngeal aspirates are best for diagnosing viral respiratory tract infections. They are sent for immunofluorescence and results are usually back on the same day. Rapid antigen tests for influenza are available and can offer a bedside diagnosis.
- Throat swabs are useful to diagnose pharyngeal infections.
- A pernasal swab is used to diagnose pertussis infection.

Fig. 3.15 Common causes of septicaemia in children after the newborn period

Streptococcus pneumoniae
Neisseria meningitidis
Staphylococcus aureus
Salmonella spp.
Haemophilus influenzae type B

Fig. 3.16 Common causes of septicaemia in the newborn

Group B streptococcus
Staphylococcus aureus
Coagulase-negative staphylococci
Coliforms
- Enterococcus
- *E. coli*
- *Klebsiella*

URINE TESTS

Urine samples are examined in the following ways:

- Dipsticks (sticks are available that test for: protein, glucose, ketones, blood, pH, urobilinogen, leucocytes and nitrites).
- Microscopy and culture (bacteria are easily identified on microscopy of an uncentrifuged sample; a centrifuged sample is necessary to examine the urinary sediment).

Dipstick testing

In certain clinical contexts, urine testing by dipstick is mandatory. These include:

- History of polyuria, polydipsia: diabetes mellitus?
- Generalized oedema: nephrotic syndrome?

Microscopy and culture

Microscopy is required to look for casts and red cells in suspected glomerular disease, and is combined with culture in the investigation of suspected urinary tract infection (UTI). (Methods of urine collection are discussed in Chapter 19).

In UTI, pus cells and bacteria might be seen on microscopy. However, pyuria can occur with fever in the absence of UTI, and cell lysis might obscure pyuria if the sample is not examined immediately. The urine white cell count is not therefore a reliable feature in the diagnosis of UTI.

A mixed growth in the absence of pyuria usually represents contamination. Confident diagnosis of a UTI requires a bacterial culture of more than 10^8/L colony-forming units of a single species in a properly collected specimen.

CEREBROSPINAL FLUID

Cerebrospinal fluid (CSF) is usually obtained by lumbar puncture. This is the critical investigation for the diagnosis of meningitis. The CSF can be evaluated in several ways including (Fig. 3.17):

- Appearance.
- Pressure.
- Microbiology: microscopy (white cell count/mm^3, organisms – Gram stain or acid-fast?), culture and sensitivity.
- Biochemistry: protein (g/L), glucose (mmol/L).
- Rapid diagnostic techniques: countercurrent immunoelectrophoresis, latex agglutination, polymerase chain reaction.

HINTS AND TIPS

Concerning meningitis:
- Consent must be gained from the child's parent or carer prior to performing a lumbar puncture, explaining the risks and benefits of the procedure.
- Infants might have non-specific clinical signs; a high index of suspicion is therefore required, and a low threshold for performing a lumbar puncture.
- A missed diagnosis can be catastrophic.

HINTS AND TIPS

Lumbar puncture is contraindicated in the following circumstances:
- Signs of raised intracranial pressure.
- Focal neurological signs.
- Rapidly deteriorating conscious level.
- Bradycardia.
- A coagulation defect.
- Skin infection at the lumbar puncture site.
- Petechiae.

Appearance

Normal CSF is clear. If the cell count increases to more than 500 cells/mm^3, it becomes turbid. Typically, this occurs in bacterial meningitis.

Fig. 3.17 A summary of the content and appearance of cerebrospinal fluid in different types of meningitis

A summary of the content and appearance of CSF in different types of meningitis				
Type	Appearance	WBC (mm^3)	Protein (g/L)	Glucose
Normal CSF (not neonatal)	Clear	0–5	0.15–0.4	>50% blood glucose
Bacterial meningitis	Turbid	500–10 000 polymorphs	0.4–3	Low
Viral meningitis	Clear	<1000	<10	Normal
TB meningitis	Clear/viscous	Up to 500 Usually <100	>10	Low

Microbiology

Microscopy

Normally, a few (<5 cells/mm^3) white cells can be found in CSF. The presence of polymorphs is always abnormal except in the neonatal period when up to 30 white cells/mm^3 can be physiological. In the early stages of meningitis, white cells might not be detectable but classically very high counts are found.

Spun CSF is routinely Gram stained:

- Gram-negative cocci: *Neisseria meningitidis*.
- Gram-positive cocci: *Streptococcus pneumoniae*.
- Gram-negative coccobacilli: *Haemophilus influenzae*.

Culture and sensitivity

This is always carried out even if the sample is clear and no white cells were detected on microscopy. Viral studies should be sent in encephalitis.

Biochemistry

Protein

Protein content of the CSF rises in bacterial meningitis. Note that in neonates the normal levels are high compared with older children and adults.

Glucose

Normal CSF glucose is approximately two-thirds of the blood glucose level. In bacterial meningitis, it drops to less than 40% of the blood glucose level. It is essential to take a capillary glucose sample at the time of the lumbar puncture (LP).

Rapid diagnostic techniques

Bacterial antigens can now be detected by sensitive and rapid tests including:

- Countercurrent immunoelectrophoresis.
- Latex agglutination.

Sufficient antigen remains present even after treatment with antibiotics has been initiated and when direct culture is no longer possible. Unfortunately, neither test is reliable at detecting group B meningococcus, which is the most common type in the UK.

Polymerase chain reaction and DNA hybridization

New techniques that detect bacterial DNA, and viral DNA or RNA are being used more frequently. They rely on the use of polymerase chain reaction (PCR) techniques to amplify tiny amounts of DNA or RNA of pathogens. They can therefore detect pathogens without the need for culture and are reliable even after administration of antibiotics (e.g. 16S rDNA).

IMAGING

All the major imaging methods are used in paediatric practice:

- Ionizing radiation: X-rays: simple or computed X-ray tomography and nuclear medicine.
- Ultrasound.
- MRI.

The main circumstances in which each of these tests can be used are described in the following sections.

X-rays

Most commonly requested are:

- Chest X-ray (CXR).
- Plain abdominal X-ray (AXR).
- Skull X-ray (SXR).
- Computed tomography (CT).

Chest X-ray

When inspecting a CXR, adopt a systematic approach for viewing and presentation:

- Check patient name, date, L/R orientation, posterior–anterior (PA), or anterior–posterior (AP).
- Note any striking abnormalities.
- Heart and mediastinum.
- Lung fields and pulmonary vessels.
- Diaphragm and subdiaphragmatic areas.
- Bony thorax.
- Soft tissues.

HINTS AND TIPS

The cardiac shadow is not always reliable in diagnosing heart disease. Look at the lung fields and hilar shadows.

Indications for doing a CXR

Acute:

- Complicated pneumonia.
- Severe bronchiolitis.
- Asthma: severe or first presentation.
- Cardiac failure.
- Foreign body inhalation.
- Non-accidental injury (old fractures).

Non-urgent investigation of:

- Cervical lymphadenopathy.
- Tuberculosis (TB).
- Cystic fibrosis.
- Cardiac disease.
- Malignant disease.

Abdominal X-ray

Supine AP is the standard plain film. An erect AP (or decubitus) often adds little to diagnosis. There is wide variation in the normal appearance of these X-rays.

The checklist for an AXR includes:

- Check patient name, date, erect, or supine.
- Note striking abnormalities.
- Hollow organs: stomach, bowel and bladder.
- Solid organs: liver, spleen and kidneys.
- Diaphragm.
- Bones.

Indications for doing an AXR

- Suspected bowel obstruction.
- Suspected bowel perforation (erect AP film).
- Refractory constipation or if diagnostic uncertainty.

Skull X-ray

The most common indication for skull radiography used to be head injury but CT scanning provides much more useful information. These days, its primary use is in the diagnosis of non-accidental injury and craniosynostosis.

> **HINTS AND TIPS**
>
> The presence of a skull fracture and/or neurological signs increases the likelihood of intracranial damage.

Computed tomography

CT scanning uses multidirectional X-rays that, instead of falling onto film, are quantified by a detector and fed into a computer. Different readings are produced as the X-ray beam rotates round the body and the information is then presented as a two-dimensional image.

CT is a useful and widely available imaging modality for evaluating brain, chest and abdominal disorders. These include:

- Brain: intracranial haemorrhage (e.g. head injury), tumours, intracranial calcification (e.g. tuberous sclerosis).
- Chest: mediastinal masses (e.g. lymphoma), lungs (e.g. bronchiectasis).
- Abdomen: masses (e.g. neuroblastoma or Wilms'), injury (e.g. splenic rupture).

CT accurately assesses the nature of a mass, e.g. fluid, fat, necrosis or calcification. Disadvantages include a lack of contrast between different organs. Intravenous contrast enhances the resolution between tissue planes. CT scans are a quick and readily available

investigation but less good for defining structures when compared to MRI scans.

> **HINTS AND TIPS**
>
> Stabilization of any ill child must be done prior to a CT scan.

Ultrasound

Ultrasound scanning (USS) uses ultra-high frequency sound waves to provide cross-sectional images of the body. In addition, Doppler ultrasound can be used for estimating the direction and velocity of blood flow.

The advantages of USS include:

- Non-invasive – no ionizing radiation involved.
- Portable equipment.

Body tissues reflect sound waves to different degrees and are therefore said to be of different echogenicity:

- Hyperechoic tissues appear white (e.g. fat).
- Hypoechoic tissues appear dark (e.g. fluid).

Ultrasound does not penetrate gas or bone and is therefore less useful for assessment of bony lesions. Intracranial contents are only accessible to ultrasound examination in young infants in whom the anterior fontanelle is still open.

The main applications include:

- Antenatal ultrasound.
- Cranial ultrasound in the neonate.
- Abdominal and renal ultrasound.
- Hip ultrasound.

Antenatal ultrasound

Initial ultrasound screening is carried out at 12 weeks (in some units) with a detailed scan at 18–20 weeks' gestation. Antenatal USS allows:

- Estimation of gestational age (less than 20 weeks).
- Identification of multiple pregnancies.
- Monitoring of fetal growth.
- Detection of structural malformations.
- Amniotic fluid volume estimation.

Neonatal cranial ultrasound

This is useful for the detection and evaluation of intracranial pathology (Fig. 3.18), including:

- Intracranial haemorrhage, e.g. intraventricular haemorrhage (IVH).
- Periventricular leucomalacia.
- Hydrocephalus.
- Cerebral malformations.

Fig. 3.18   (A) A parasagittal neonatal cranial ultrasound scan showing extensive intraventricular haemorrhage. (B) Coronal ultrasound scan of a neonatal brain with hydrocephalus

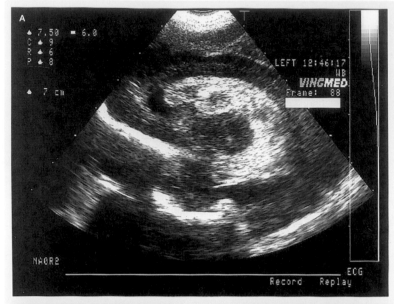

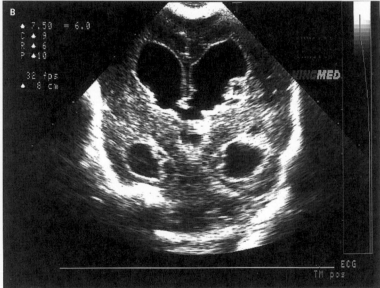

A cranial ultrasound is performed in all preterm babies under 32 weeks and should be repeated to look for haemorrhages and leucomalacia.

Abdominal and renal ultrasound

Abdominal ultrasound is useful in the evaluation of:

- Abdominal pain: acute (e.g. identification of appendix abscess, intussusception).

- Vomiting infant: ultrasound is the imaging of choice in pyloric stenosis.
- Liver disease: provides information on size and consistency of both the liver and spleen. The gall bladder and extrahepatic bile ducts can be visualized.

Renal ultrasound is very useful in the investigation of disorders of the genitourinary tract (Fig. 3.19). It provides information on:

- Kidney size.
- Structural abnormalities of the urinary tract, e.g. hydronephrosis, hydroureter, or increased bladder size.
- Gross renal scarring.

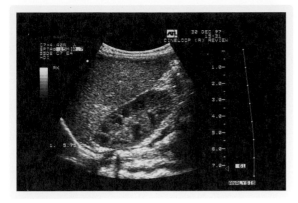

Fig. 3.19 Normal renal ultrasound. Normal prominent pyramids are demonstrated

- Renal calculi.
- Tumours (e.g. Wilms').

Hip ultrasound

Ultrasound is a useful modality for the investigation of hip disease. It is the imaging method of choice for assessing neonatal hip instability and is more reliable than plain radiography up to the age of 6 months. It allows evaluation of:

- Acetabular morphology.
- The degree to which the acetabulum covers the femoral head.

Ultrasound is also useful in the investigation of suspected hip pathology in young children. Even small effusions can be detected, and needle aspiration can be carried out under ultrasound guidance.

Magnetic resonance imaging

Magnetic resonance imaging (MRI) has several distinctive features that confer a number of useful advantages:

- No ionizing radiation.
- Images can be obtained in any plane.
- Excellent soft tissue contrast.

It is the imaging modality of choice for many disorders of the brain and spine (in which sagittal views are particularly useful). MRI is also helpful in the evaluation of musculoskeletal disorders. It has not replaced other approaches, such as CT or ultrasound, in the imaging of many thoracic and abdominal disorders. Its main disadvantage in children is the need for sedation or general anaesthesia to enable the child to remain still for a sufficient period.

At the end of this chapter, you should be able to:
- Assess a child with fever
- Understand the common types of rash in children
- Identify the warning signs in a child with fever and rash
- Learn a systematic approach to a child with petechial rash

THE FEVERISH CHILD

Fever is a common presenting symptom in children and can be a major challenge to paediatricians. Most fevers are due to benign, self-limiting viral infections but skill is needed to distinguish these from serious infection (Fig. 4.1). The latter has the potential to deteriorate rapidly so it is essential that it is identified as early as possible.

Fever is defined as a central temperature of greater than 38°C. Electronic tympanic membrane thermometers correlate moderately well with rectal temperature and are adequate for most practical purposes.

History

How long has the child been febrile?

A duration of more than a week requires further evaluation and diseases such as tuberculosis (TB), Kawasaki's disease, malaria, typhoid, autoimmune non-infectious disorders and malignancy should be excluded.

Are there any localizing symptoms?

An infection in certain systems will advertise itself:
- Cough or coryza: suggest respiratory tract infection.
- Vomiting and diarrhoea: suggest gastrointestinal tract infection, although vomiting alone is non-specific.
- A painful limb: suggests infection of the bones or joints.
- Lower abdominal pain: suggests urine infection but lobar pneumonia can also present this way.
- Headache, photophobia and neck pain: suggest meningism.

Younger children (<2 years of age) might not localize symptoms and fever might be the only symptom.

Has there been recent foreign travel?

Malaria or typhoid can be overlooked if recent travel abroad is not disclosed in the history.

Examination

Is the child systemically unwell?

The active, playing and communicative child is unlikely to have sepsis. However, any ill child must have an assessment of the airway, breathing and circulation, and of the vital signs. Clues to serious sepsis include (see also Fig. 4.6, later in this chapter):
- Poor peripheral perfusion.
- Persistent tachycardia.
- Lethargy or irritability.

Are there local signs of infection?

Tonsillitis, otitis media, pneumonia, meningitis and septic arthritis can all be revealed on examination (Fig. 4.2); a rash might be diagnostic. Look for a bulging fontanelle in meningitis.

Investigations

In a well child in whom a confident clinical diagnosis has been possible, no investigation is required. However, certain investigations are appropriate in any ill febrile child. These include:
- Markers of inflammation: white cell count (raised or low in overwhelming sepsis), differential (neutrophil predominance in bacterial infection) and C-reactive

Fig. 4.1 Common causes of a fever	
Minor illnesses	**Major illnesses**
Upper respiratory infection	Meningitis
Non-specific viral infections and rashes	Pneumonia
Gastroenteritis without dehydration	Urinary tract infection Septicaemia

- A 'septic screen'; infants suspected of severe infection without localizing signs on examination are investigated with a standard battery of investigations before starting antibiotic therapy. These include: blood culture, full blood count (FBC), CRP, lumbar puncture, urine sampling and CXR.

Aide-memoire to identify serious sepsis

ILLNESS – Irritability, Lethargy, Low capillary refill, Neutropenia or neutrophilia, Elevated or low temperature suggests Serious Sepsis.

Management

If a benign viral infection is suspected then only symptomatic therapy is needed. In the very young, or those who look ill, antibiotics are started before the results of diagnostic testing are available because quickly ruling out serious infection is often impossible; treatment can be tailored when the results are back. Treating the fever with antipyretics might reduce febrile convulsions.

Pyrexia of unknown origin

The designation pyrexia of unknown origin (PUO) should be reserved for a child with a documented protracted fever (more than 7 days) and no diagnosis despite initial investigation (Fig. 4.3). It is frequently misapplied to any child presenting with a fever of which the cause is not immediately obvious. Most are infectious and 40–60% will resolve without diagnosis. Particular patterns of fever and response to treatment can be helpful in making important diagnosis (e.g. Kawasaki disease, juvenile chronic arthritis).

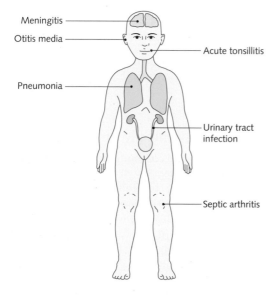

Fig. 4.2 Fever: important sites of local bacterial infection

protein. These are useful if there is uncertainty in diagnosis or for serial measurement of a septic child; however, they cannot rule out serious infection.

> **HINTS AND TIPS**
>
> A seriously ill child might initially have normal blood inflammatory markers.

- Samples for microbiological examination: blood cultures, urine for microscopy and culture, throat swab and cerebrospinal fluid. Polymerase chain reaction (PCR) is becoming increasingly useful as it provides high sensitivity and specificity.
- Imaging: a chest X-ray (CXR) is useful if there is no clear focus but is not required if a clinical diagnosis of an uncomplicated pneumonia has been made.

Fig. 4.3 Causes of pyrexia of unknown origin	
Type	**Cause**
Infective	Pyelonephritis
	Osteomyelitis
	Abscesses
	Endocarditis
	Tuberculosis
	Typhoid
	Cytomegalovirus (CMV)
	Human immunodeficiency virus (HIV)
	Hepatitis
	Malaria
Inflammatory	Kawasaki disease
	Rheumatoid arthritis
	Crohn's disease
Malignancy	Leukaemia, lymphoma
Factitious fever	Only recorded by patient

THE CHILD WITH A RASH

Children often present with a rash that might, or might not, be associated with systemic signs. An exact diagnosis is often not possible but a few rashes are associated with serious systemic disease. Careful clinical history and examination are again essential and investigation is reserved only for certain cases.

History

The history of a rash should ascertain the following:

- Duration, site of onset, evolution and spread.
- Does it come and go (e.g. urticaria)?
- Does the rash 'itch' (e.g. eczema, scabies)?
- Has there been any recent drug ingestion or exposure to provocative agents (e.g. sunlight, food, allergens, detergents)?
- Are any other family members or contacts affected (e.g. viral exanthems, infestations; see Chapter 15)
- Are there any other associated symptoms (e.g. sore throat, upper respiratory tract infection)?
- Is there any family history (e.g. atopy, psoriasis)?

Examination

Check for non-dermatological features such as:

- Fever.
- Mucous membranes.
- Lymphadenopathy.
- Splenomegaly.
- Arthropathy.

Describe the rash in 'dermatological language', observing the morphology, arrangement and distribution of the lesions.

Morphology

Describe the shape, size and colour of the lesions. There might be:

- Macules, papules or nodules.
- Vesicles, pustules or bullae.
- Petechiae, purpura or ecchymoses.

Arrangement

Are the lesions scattered diffusely, well circumscribed or confluent?

Distribution

The distribution is important (Fig. 4.4). It can be local or generalized (flexor surfaces: eczema; extensor surfaces: Henoch–Schönlein purpura (HSP) or psoriasis) or

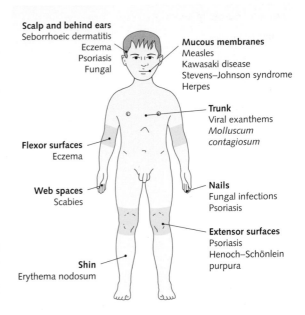

Fig. 4.4 Distribution of rashes

Scalp and behind ears
Seborrhoeic dermatitis
Eczema
Psoriasis
Fungal

Mucous membranes
Measles
Kawasaki disease
Stevens–Johnson syndrome
Herpes

Trunk
Viral exanthems
*Molluscum
contagiosum*

Flexor surfaces
Eczema

Nails
Fungal infections
Psoriasis

Web spaces
Scabies

Extensor surfaces
Psoriasis
Henoch–Schönlein
purpura

Shin
Erythema nodosum

might involve mucous membranes (measles, Kawasaki disease, Stevens–Johnson syndrome).

Palpation

Feel the rash for scale, thickness, texture and temperature; dry skin suggests eczema.

Investigations

Investigations are rarely required but might include skin scrapings for fungi or scabies.

Causes of a rash

The main causative categories are shown in Fig. 4.5.

Diagnostic features of the more common generalized rashes

The common generalized rashes are: maculopapular rash, vesicular rash, haemorrhagic rash and urticarial rash.

Maculopapular rash

This is most likely to be caused by a viral exanthem but might be a drug-induced eruption. Common diagnostic features are:

- Measles: prodrome of fever, coryza and cough. Just before the rash appears, Koplik's spots appear in the mouth. The rash tends to coalesce.

Fig. 4.5 Causes of a rash

Type	Cause
Infection	Viral
	Toxin-related
	Streptococcal
	Meningococcal
Infestations	Scabies
Dermatitis	Eczema
	Vasculitis
Allergy	Drug-related
	Urticaria
Haematological	Bleeding disorders

- Rubella: discrete, pink macular rash starting on the scalp and face. Occipital and cervical lymphadenopathy might precede the rash.
- Roseola infantum: occurs in infants under 3 years. After 3 days of sustained fever, a pink morbilliform (measles-like) eruption appears as the temperature subsides. It is caused by human herpesvirus (HHV)-6 or HHV-7.
- Enteroviral infection: causes a generalized, pleomorphic rash and produces a mild fever.
- Glandular fever: symptoms include malaise, fever and exudative tonsillitis. Lymphadenopathy and splenomegaly are commonly found.
- Kawasaki disease: causes a protracted fever, generalized rash, red lips, lymphadenopathy and conjunctival inflammation.
- Scarlet fever: causes fever and sore throat. The rash starts on the face and can include a 'strawberry' tongue.

Vesicular rash

Common causes of vesicular rash are:

- Chickenpox: successive crops of papulovesicles on an erythematous base; the vesicles become encrusted. Lesions present at different stages. The mucous membranes are involved.
- Eczema herpeticum: exacerbation of eczema with vesicular spots caused by a herpes infection.

Haemorrhagic rash

Due to extravasated blood these lesions do not blanch on pressure. Lesions are classified by size:

- Petechiae (smallest).
- Purpura.
- Ecchymoses (largest).

Common diagnostic features are:

- Meningococcal septicaemia: petechial or purpuric rash (might be preceded by maculopapular rash).
- Acute leukaemia: look for pallor and hepatosplenomegaly.
- Idiopathic thrombocytopenic purpura: the child looks well but might have petechial rash with, or without, nose bleeds.
- Henoch–Schönlein purpura: distribution is usually on the legs and buttocks. Arthralgia and abdominal pain might be present.
- Bleeding disorders: haemophilia, von Willebrand disease and Ehlers–Danlos usually present with easy bruising and prolonged bleeding following trivial trauma.

HINTS AND TIPS

Take care to consider suspected non-accidental injury in cases of traumatic or non-traumatic bruising.

HINTS AND TIPS

Non-blanching or rapidly spreading rash should be treated as meningococcal sepsis until proven otherwise.

Urticarial rash

Urticaria (hives), a transient, itchy rash characterized by raised weals, appears rapidly and fades; it can recur. Causes include:

- Food allergy, e.g. shellfish, eggs, cows' milk.
- Drug allergy, e.g. penicillin: note that <10% of penicillin allergies are unsubstantiated.
- Infections, e.g. viral: this is the most common and is often self-limiting.
- Contact allergy, e.g. plants, grasses, animal hair.

Two other distinctive rashes that occur in childhood and require special consideration are erythema multiforme and erythema nodosum.

Erythema multiforme

A distinctive, symmetrical rash characterized by annular target (iris) lesions and various other lesions including macules, papules and bullae. The severe form with mucous membrane involvement is Stevens–Johnson syndrome. Causes include infections (most commonly herpes simplex, mycoplasma or Epstein–Barr virus) and drugs. Mostly it is idiopathic and self-limiting.

Erythema nodosum

Red, tender, nodular lesions usually occur on the shins. Important causes include streptococcal infections and TB.

THE CHILD WITH FEVER AND PETECHIAL RASH

The most important differential diagnosis in this common scenario is serious sepsis especially meningococcal disease which requires immediate treatment. Other differential diagnoses are covered under haemorrhagic rash above.

The majority of children presenting with fever and petechiae do not have serious sepsis. In June 2010, the National Institute for Health and Clinical Excellence (NICE) published guidance on bacterial meningitis and meningococcal septicaemia in children and young people. Within these guidelines is a section on the management of petechial rash (see Further reading).

Indicators of serious sepsis

(See also Figs 4.6 and 4.7.)

- Unwell child: tachycardia, tachypnoea, cold extremities, poor capillary refill, irritability, lethargy.
- Spreading petechiae or purpura.
- Abnormal blood results WCC <5 or >20; neutrophilia or neutropenia; high CRP.

Fig. 4.6 Worrying signs of serious bacterial sepsis

All children less than 3 months old
Bulging fontanelle
White cell count greater than 20×10^9/L or less than 4×10^9/L
Presence of shock
Decreased conscious level or lethargy
Persistent tachycardia
Apnoea
Non-blanching rash

Fig 4.7 'Traffic light' system for identifying likelihood of serious illness.

	Green – low risk	Amber – intermediate risk	Red – high risk
Colour	Normal colour of skin, lips, and tongue	Pallor reported by parent or carer	Pale, mottled, ashen or blue
Activity	Responding normally to social cues Content, smiling Stays awake or awakens quickly Strong normal cry or not crying	Not responding normally to social cues Waking only with prolonged stimulation Decreased activity Not smiling	No response to social cues Appears ill to a healthcare professional Unable to rouse or if roused does not stay awake Weak, high-pitched or continuous crying
Respiratory	–	Nasal flaring Tachypnoea: 6–12 months of age: RR* >50 breaths per minute >12 months of age: RR* >40 breaths per minute Oxygen saturation ≤95% in air Crackles	Grunting Tachypnoea (RR* >60 breaths per minute) Moderate or severe chest indrawing
Hydration	Normal skin and eyes Moist mucous membranes	Dry mucous membrane Poor feeding in infants CRT† ≥ 3 seconds Reduced urine output‡	Reduced skin turgor

Continued

	Green – low risk	Amber – intermediate risk	Red – high risk
Other	None of the amber or red symptoms or signs	Fever for $\geq$ 5 days	0–3 months of age, temperature $\geq$ 38 °C 3–6 months of age, temperature $\geq$ 39 °C
		Swelling of limb or joint Non-weight-bearing/not using an extremity	Non-blanching rash Bulging fontanelle Neck stiffness Status epilepticus Focal neurological signs Focal seizures
		A new lump >2 cm	Bile-stained vomit

Fig 4.7 'Traffic light' system for identifying likelihood of serious illness—cont'd

*RR = respiratory rate.
†CRT = capillary refill time.
‡In infants, ask about wet nappies.

Data from NICE, 2007b at: http://www.cks.nhs.uk/feverish_children_risk_assessment/evidence/references#
Adapted from National Institute for Health and Clinical Excellence (NICE) guidance on feverish illness in children, May 2007: http://www.nice.org.uk/guidance/CG47)

Management of early meningococcal disease/ septicaemia

Principles of management are:

- Oxygen, obtaining good venous access, immediate administration of fluid resuscitation, administration of a third generation cephalosporin (cefotaxime 50 mg/kg or ceftriaxone 80 mg/kg), early senior intensive care input.
- Investigations: full blood count, blood culture, coagulation screen, meningococcal PCR, C-reactive protein, renal function, liver function and throat swab.

Further reading

National Institute for Health and Clinical Excellence (NICE), May 2007. Guidance on feverish illness in children. http://www.nice.org.uk/guidance/CG47.

National Institute for Health and Clinical Excellence (NICE), June 2010. Guidance on the management of bacterial meningitis and meningococcal septicaemia. http://www.nice.org.uk/guidance/CG102.

Heart, lung or ENT problems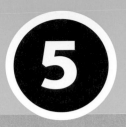

● **Objectives**

At the end of this chapter, you should be able to:
- Understand common cardiac and respiratory symptoms and signs
- Evaluate a child with a murmur
- Identify respiratory distress in a child
- Differentiate stridor from wheeze
- Understand common upper airway symptoms

HEART

Congenital heart malformations account for most of the cardiovascular disease seen in paediatric practice. Rare causes include rheumatic fever, viral myocarditis or pericarditis and arrhythmias. Kawasaki disease is now the leading cause of acquired heart disease in children in the developed world. Heart disease presents in a limited number of ways:

- An abnormality detected on prenatal ultrasound.
- A murmur noted on routine examination in an asymptomatic infant or child.
- Arrhythmia and/or syncope.
- Sudden collapse.
- Cardiac failure with or without low cardiac output.

History

Cardiac symptoms include:
- Poor feeding, cough, sweating and difficulty breathing – cardiac failure in babies.
- Syncope: caused by arrhythmias and on rare occasions by severe aortic stenosis (AS).
- Older children might describe palpitations.
- Older children may complain of chest pain (although rarely signifies cardiac disease).
- Recurrent chest infections.
- Failure to thrive.
- Rapid weight gain from oedema.

HINTS AND TIPS

Inappropriate weight gain may be a sign of cardiac failure in infants.

Examination

The major physical signs are:
- Cyanosis.
- Murmurs.
- Signs of cardiac failure.

Cyanosis

Several varieties of congenital heart disease might present with central cyanosis (a 'blue' baby) at, or soon after, birth. Central cyanosis is visible if the concentration of deoxygenated haemoglobin (Hb) in the blood exceeds 5 g/dL. Peripheral cyanosis – blueness of the hands and feet (due to a sluggish peripheral circulation) – can be a normal finding in newborn babies within the first 24 hours of birth and in babies who are cold, crying or unwell from some non-cardiac cause.

Central cyanosis due to congenital heart disease is distinguished from that due to respiratory disease by the failure of right radial artery pO_2 to rise above 15 kPa after breathing 100% O_2 for 10 min. This is known as the nitrogen washout test. Differential cyanosis in the limbs indicates the presence of right to left shunting across the ductus arteriosus.

Causes

In most patients, there is an abnormality that allows a portion of the systemic venous return to bypass the lungs and enter the systemic circulation directly (i.e. a right to left shunt). These can be classified as:

1. Lesions with abnormal mixing: desaturated systemic venous blood is mixed with oxygenated pulmonary venous blood so that the blood discharged into the systemic circulation is not fully saturated. Pulmonary vascularity is increased and pulmonary plethora is apparent on chest X-ray (CXR), e.g. transposition of the great arteries (TGA) (Fig. 5.1).

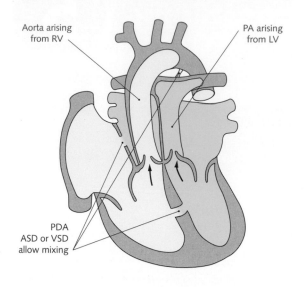

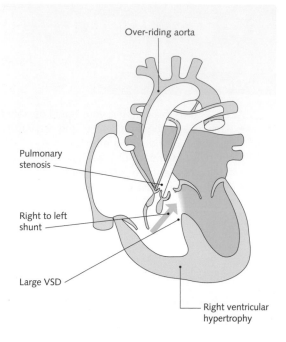

Fig. 5.1 Transposition of the great arteries. There has to be mixing between the two circulations to be compatible with life. As the foramen ovale and the ductus arteriosus begin to close, progressive cyanosis develops

Fig. 5.2 Tetralogy of Fallot: the stenosis of the pulmonary valve causes resistance to flow and shunting of blood through the large ventricular septal defect

2. Lesions with inadequate pulmonary blood flow: these infants often have right outflow tract obstruction and depend on blood flowing to the lungs from left to right across a patent ductus arteriosus (PDA). Severe cyanosis develops when the duct closes, pulmonary vascularity is diminished and oligaemic lung fields are apparent on CXR, e.g. Fallot's tetralogy (Fig. 5.2).

Murmurs

Cardiac murmurs are common in children of all ages. The majority of these are not associated with pathology (innocent murmurs) and clinical examination will allow most to be distinguished from structural cardiac disease.

Evaluation of a murmur

A murmur is merely one component of the information obtained by examination of the cardiovascular system and cannot be interpreted in isolation. Important features of a murmur include:

- Timing: is it systolic or diastolic? (most murmurs in children are systolic; diastolic murmurs are rare and always pathological).
- Character: is it pansystolic or ejection systolic?
- Loudness: this is graded out of 6; grade 4 and above can be palpated (thrill).
- Radiation: a murmur that radiates from its site of maximal loudness is more likely to be significant.

Innocent murmurs

> **HINTS AND TIPS**
>
> The hallmarks of an innocent murmur are:
> - An asymptomatic child.
> - A normal cardiovascular examination including normal heart sounds.
> - Systolic or continuous (a diastolic murmur by itself is never innocent).
> - No radiation.
> - Variation with posture.

In most children with a murmur, the heart is normal and the murmur is innocent. Innocent murmurs are generated by turbulent flow in a structurally normal cardiovascular system (CVS). There are two main varieties of innocent murmur, the ejection murmurs and the venous hums.

The ejection murmurs are:

- Generated in the outflow tract of either side of the heart.
- Soft, blowing, systolic.
- Heard in the second or fourth left intercostal space.

The venous hums:

- Are generated in the head and neck veins.
- Are continuous low-pitched rumble.
- Are heard beneath the clavicle.
- Disappear on lying flat.

An innocent murmur is more likely to be noted during tachycardia, e.g. with fever, anaemia or exercise, and it is therefore important to reassess for persistence of the murmur at a later stage following recovery of an acute illness.

Significant murmurs

A murmur with any of the following features is significant:

- Symptoms: syncope, episodic cyanosis.
- CVS signs: abnormal pulses, heart sounds, blood pressure (BP) or cardiac impulse.
- Murmur: diastolic, pansystolic, radiating to the back or associated with a thrill.

Significant murmurs, which can be difficult to distinguish from an innocent murmur, include those caused by pulmonary stenosis (PS) and PDA. Refer for echocardiography if in doubt.

Cardiac failure

Cardiac failure is less commonly seen in paediatric practice and is usually encountered during infancy. The clinical features are different from those in adults, i.e. areas of dependent oedema do not occur. Feeding is the only exertion they undertake and, not being ambulant bipeds at this time of life, their ankles do not swell up.

Clinical features of cardiac failure

- Symptoms: the parents might notice poor feeding and breathlessness, excessive sweating and recurrent chest infections. There might be failure to thrive.
- Signs: tachycardia, cool periphery, tachypnoea and hepatomegaly. CVS signs can include a third heart sound, murmur and abnormal pulses (Fig. 5.3).

Causes of cardiac failure

This may be due to pressure overload (obstructive lesions) or volume overload (left to right shunts):

- Obstructive lesions usually present in neonates (e.g. severe coarctation of the aorta (COA) or hypoplastic left heart syndrome).
- Volume overload usually presents in infants. The left to right shunt increases (e.g. ventricular septal defects (VSD), PDA) as the pulmonary vascular resistance falls.

Cardiac failure can be confused with the more common respiratory causes of tachypnoea, e.g. bronchiolitis or wheezing associated with a viral infection. A CXR will clarify the situation. Less common causes of cardiac failure include supraventricular tachycardia and viral myocarditis.

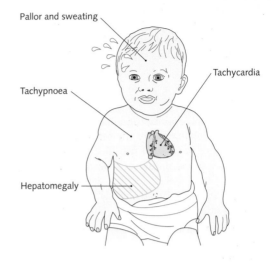

Fig. 5.3 Signs of cardiac failure in an infant

Investigations for cardiac failure

Useful investigations include the following:

- CXR will show an enlarged heart with pulmonary congestion.
- Electrocardiogram (ECG) will be suggestive of the underlying heart defect.
- Echocardiography shows the underlying heart defect, as well as poor contractility of the ventricles.

LUNG

Several noises of great diagnostic value emanate from the respiratory tract. A cough is the most obvious. Stridor and wheeze – two other noises associated with breathing and caused by airway narrowing – are also of vital importance.

Paediatric airway anatomy

The paediatric airway differs from the adult and older child:

- Tongue is larger.
- Larynx is higher, more anterior and funnel shaped.
- Trachea is shorter.

- Narrowest portion is at cricoid (vocal cords in adults).
- Epiglottis is horseshoe-shaped.

Neonates are obligate nose breathers until 5 months of age, although 40% of term babies will convert to oral breathing if nasal obstruction occurs. See Chapter 1 for physiological respiratory differences.

Respiratory distress

This term is loosely applied to indicate an increased work of breathing. This may be in the form of fast breathing; use of accessory muscles of breathing – intercostal and subcostal recessions, flaring of alae nasi; cyanosis and grunting.

Tachypnoea (fast breathing) is usually a rate (in breaths per minute) of:

- >60 in neonates.
- >50 in infants.
- >40 in under 5 s.
- >30 in older children.

Cough, stridor and wheeze

Cough

A cough is a reflex, involuntary explosive expiration that is a primary defence mechanism of the respiratory tract. In most instances, cough is due to an acute upper respiratory viral infection, but there are important causes of chronic cough. The cough itself is rarely diagnostic except in two instances:

1. The 'barking' cough of croup (acute laryngotracheobronchitis).
2. The paroxysmal prolonged bouts of coughing, sometimes ending in a sharp intake of breath (the 'whoop'), that occur in pertussis (whooping cough) and certain viral infections.

History of cough

Find out the following information:

- Duration of the cough: this is usually brief, e.g. less than 1 week. A chronic cough (>3 weeks duration) indicates chronic infection, suppurative lung disease, postviral cough, receptor sensitivity, asthma, whooping cough, inhaled foreign body or TB. Abrupt onset of symptoms, sometimes with a history of choking, suggests inhaled foreign body.
- Type of cough – whether dry, moist or productive: the majority are dry (e.g. postviral infection, asthma); a moist or productive cough raises the possibility of suppurative lung disease, e.g. cystic fibrosis (a productive cough is rare in children as sputum produced is swallowed).

Fig. 5.4 Causes of cough

Type of cough	Cause	Clues to diagnosis
Acute	Viral respiratory infection	Coryzal symptoms
	Bronchiolitis	Wheeze in <1 year
	Pneumonia	Fever and dyspnoea
	Foreign body	Sudden onset
Chronic	Asthma	Associated wheeze
	Tuberculosis	Tuberculosis contact
	Pertussis	Lymphocytosis, apnoea
	Suppurative lung disease, e.g. cystic fibrosis	Productive cough

- Association with wheeze: cough without wheeze in children is rarely due to asthma.
- Trigger factors: passive smoking, exposure to daycare, nocturnal cough or cough on exposure to animals and atopy.

Common causes of a cough are shown in Fig. 5.4. Note that many children with neurological disorders, e.g. severe cerebral palsy, cannot cough well and this is one of the reasons for their susceptibility to respiratory infections.

Apnoea

This is the cessation of breathing for at least 10 seconds or associated with a fall in heart rate. Its presence can signify significant respiratory or neurological disease and acute life-threatening events, especially in infants. It is common in preterm infants due to immaturity of the respiratory centres.

Stridor and wheeze

Differences between stridor and wheeze

Stridor is a noise associated with breathing due to narrowing of the extrathoracic airway, i.e. the upper airway; wheeze is a noise associated with breathing due to narrowing of the intrathoracic airway. Either noise can occur at any phase of the respiratory cycle. The differences are:

- Stridor is usually worse on inspiration when extrathoracic airways naturally collapse.
- Wheeze is usually worse on expiration when intrathoracic airways naturally collapse.

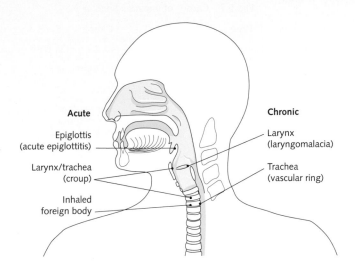

Fig. 5.5 Causes of stridor

It is very important to make a clear distinction between these signs as the likely cause and management of stridor is very different from that of wheeze. Stridor implies an upper airway obstruction, which could be life threatening.

Stridor

> **COMMUNICATION**
>
> A parent will often find it difficult to distinguish between the sounds of stridor and wheeze. Do not be afraid to ask them to try and impersonate what their infant or child sounded like or to attempt to replicate the sounds yourself.

There are two types of stridor: the acute and the persistent (Fig. 5.5).

Causes of acute stridor are:

- Acute laryngotracheobronchitis (croup).
- Acute epiglottitis.
- Inhaled foreign body.
- Angioneurotic oedema (rare), anaphylaxis.

Causes of persistent stridor in an infant are:

- Laryngomalacia ('floppy' larynx).
- Anatomical obstructions, e.g. vascular ring (rare).

The different features of epiglottitis and croup reflect the differences in pathology. In epiglottitis, there is rapid onset of supraglottic swelling (the swollen epiglottis is painful and makes swallowing difficult) and bacteraemia. In croup, involvement of the larynx generates the characteristic hoarse voice and barking cough (Fig. 5.6).

Fig. 5.6 Comparison of epiglottitis and croup

Features of epiglottitis	Features of croup
Appearance: toxic	Appearance: well
Cough: slight/absent	Cough: barking
Voice: muffled	Voice: hoarse
Hyper-reactive cough receptors	Usually after upper respiratory tract infection
Drooling: yes	Drooling: no
Able to drink: no	Able to drink: yes

> **HINTS AND TIPS**
>
> Laryngomalacia is the most common congenital laryngeal abnormality that is present at birth and tends to resolve by 12–18 months of age. It usually does not require any specific treatment but symptoms can be more pronounced during an intercurrent illness, when sleeping or when lying flat.

Wheeze

The usual causes are viral lower respiratory tract infections and asthma. In children <1 year old, the tiny airways are easily narrowed by oedema and secretions, making wheeze a common feature of infections that involve the bronchi and bronchioles. In children >5 years old, asthma is the most common cause of wheeze. Asthma might have its onset in the first year of life; however, it can be difficult to distinguish from the episodic wheezing induced by recurrent viral infections of the lower respiratory tract and so diagnosis should not be made hastily.

Less common causes of recurrent or acute wheezing in childhood include:

- Cystic fibrosis associated with failure to thrive and frequent chest infections.
- Laryngeal pathology: abnormal voice or cry.
- Gastro-oesophageal reflux: excessive vomiting.
- Inhaled foreign body: sudden onset is the clue.

HINTS AND TIPS

Respiratory distress may be due to a cardiac cause. History of an underlying heart problem, failure to thrive, presence of murmurs, abnormal position of the cardiac apex, hepatomegaly and cyanosis not improving despite 100% oxygen should alert to the possibility of a heart defect.

EAR, NOSE AND THROAT

Infections of the ears and the throat are very common in childhood and ear, nose and throat (ENT) examination is therefore essential in any febrile child.

HINTS AND TIPS

A small child might not localize pain to the ear. The ears must be examined carefully in any febrile child.

Ear

Pain or discharge

Earache is usually caused by infection of the middle ear (acute otitis media). Less common causes include otitis externa, a foreign body or referred pain from teeth. A discharge might be of wax or purulent material (from otitis externa, otitis media with perforation or a foreign body).

Hearing impairment

Hearing impairment is classified into two main types: conductive and sensorineural hearing loss (SNHL). The causes of both are illustrated in Fig. 5.7.

- Conductive hearing loss is very common and usually due to otitis media with effusion (OME, also known as 'glue ear'). Over half of all preschool children have at least one episode of OME. A much smaller percentage has persistent OME with hearing impairment, which can delay language acquisition.

Fig. 5.7 Causes of impaired hearing

Type	Cause
Conductive	Otitis media with effusion
	Foreign body
	Wax
Sensorineural	Congenital infection Prematurity (<32/40) Risk factors:hypoxia jaundice ototoxic drugs Meningitis Genetic (rare)

Impedance tests are used to assess middle ear function (Fig. 5.8); they are not a direct measure of hearing.

HINTS AND TIPS

Any child with delayed speech must have a hearing test:
- Speech uses frequencies of 400–4000 Hz.
- Hearing thresholds (in decibels = db):
>70 db = profound hearing loss.
20–70 db = mild/severe hearing loss.
<20 db = normal hearing.

- Sensorineural hearing loss is less common. Universal newborn screening is now performed in the UK (Fig. 5.9). Not all cases will be detected in the neonatal period as, for example, congenital infections and some genetic causes of SNHL are progressive and cannot be detectable at this age.
- Acquired hearing loss occurs after CNS infections, e.g. meningitis, and all affected children should have their hearing tested after the acute illness has resolved (Fig. 5.10). Treatment with cochlear implantation might be required.

HINTS AND TIPS

- Parental suspicions about possible hearing loss should be taken seriously, with early referral for audiological testing.
- Children with significantly impaired language development, behavioural problems or those with a history of repeated middle ear disease should also be referred.

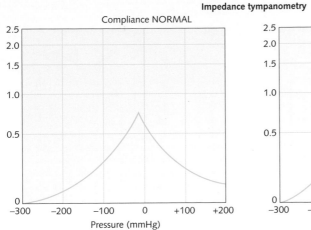
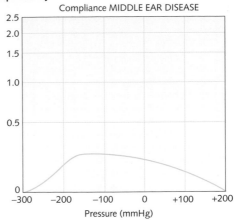

Fig. 5.8 Impedance tympanometry. This tests for middle ear disease. Sound is transmitted across the tympanic membrane if it is compliant (i.e. equal pressure either side). The test measures reflected sound at different pressures. In serous otitis media, compliance is reduced at all pressures because of the fluid present, resulting in a flattened curve

Fig. 5.9	Tests of auditory function	
Age	**Test**	**Indication**
Newborn	Otoacoustic emission Brainstem-evoked potential audiometry response cradle	Presence of high-risk factors, e.g. prematurity Newborn screening
7–9 months	Checklist in personal child health record book	
18–24 months	Speech discrimination tests Threshold audiometry (<3 years) Impedance audiometry	Children with suspected hearing loss Children with repeated middle ear disease
School entry	'Sweep test' (modified pure tone audiogram – Fig. 5.10)	Screen all children

Nose

Noses can discharge or bleed. The common cold accounts for most acute watery discharges. A chronic discharge might be due to allergic rhinitis or a unilateral foreign body.

Causes of epistaxis (nose bleeds) include:

- Trauma.
- Nose picking.
- Bleeding disorders (especially thrombocytopenia).

Throat

Sore throat (pharyngitis)

- Constitutional upset, tonsillar exudate and lymphadenopathy suggest a bacterial infection: group A β-haemolytic streptococcus is a common pathogen ('strep throat').
- Rarely, a peritonsillar abscess (quinsy) might develop and require incision and drainage.
- Epstein–Barr virus (infectious mononucleosis) is an important cause of exudative tonsillitis.

Snoring and obstructive sleep apnoea

Snoring is a common symptom in children but in some is associated with significant obstructive sleep apnoea (OSA). History of apnoea with arousals during sleep and unusual sleep positions can indicate OSA. Daytime symptoms include chronic mouth breathing, behavioural problems and occasionally daytime sleepiness. Severe OSA can result in failure to thrive, right heart failure and cor pulmonale. Those children at high risk of OSA include children with craniofacial problems and Down syndrome.

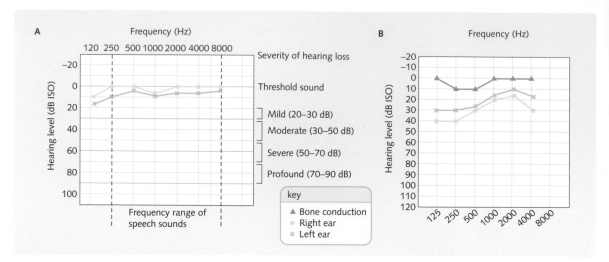

Fig. 5.10 Audiogram demonstrating: (A) normal hearing and (B) bilateral conductive hearing loss. In (B), there is a 20–40 dB hearing loss in both the right and left ears

Further reading

National Institute for Health and Clinical Excellence (NICE), February 2008. Guidance on surgical management of children with otitis media with effusion (OME). http://www.nice.org.uk/CG60.

Gut or liver problems  6

At the end of this chapter, you should be able to:
- Understand common symptoms of gastrointestinal disease
- Assess a child with a gastrointestinal complaint
- Differentiate among common gastrointestinal problems

GUT

Disorders of the gut present with a limited number of symptoms, including abdominal pain, vomiting, diarrhoea or constipation, failure to thrive and bleeding.

Abdominal pain

Acute abdominal pain

The most important issue is to identify conditions needing urgent surgical or medical intervention (Figs 6.1 and 6.2).

History

In babies, abdominal pain is inferred from episodic screaming and drawing up of the legs. In older children, important features in the history are:

- Duration: pain lasting more than 4 hours is likely to be significant.
- Location: pain further away from the umbilicus is more likely to be significant (early appendicitis is an exception to this).
- Nature: constant or intermittent/colicky.
- Associated symptoms: vomiting (bilious suggests obstruction), stools (pain and bloody stools suggest intussusception in an infant, inflammatory bowel disease in older children), dysuria (urinary tract infection (UTI)), cough (pneumonia), anorexia (a normal appetite is reassuring).

Physical examination

Careful systemic examination is vital to avoid traps for the unwary. Look for:

- Fever: may be present in appendicitis, mesenteric adenitis, UTI and pneumonia.
- Jaundice: infectious hepatitis or biliary colic causes abdominal pain.

- Rash: the abdominal pain of Henoch–Schönlein purpura (HSP) might precede the characteristic purpuric rash.
- Respiratory tract: is there a pneumonia?
- Hernial orifices: is there a strangulated hernia?
- Genitalia: is there a torsion of the testis?

> **COMMUNICATION**
>
> Asking the child to 'blow up their tummy' and 'suck in their tummy' can help you to assess severity of the pain before you touch the abdomen.

Investigations

- Urinalysis: dipstick for glucose and ketones, urine microscopy and culture.
- Full blood count (FBC): a neutrophilia might be present in pneumonia or a UTI. It may be mildy raised in acute appendicitis.
- A sickling test should be considered in children of African or Afro-Caribbean origin.
- Urea and electrolytes (U&E) and glucose: abnormalities must be identified and corrected and diabetic ketoacidosis excluded.
- Imaging: a plain abdominal film is rarely helpful unless obstruction is suspected. Abdominal ultrasound or computed tomography may be used to aid the diagnosis of appendicitis.

Recurrent abdominal pain

In most children, recurrent abdominal pain does not have an organic cause and a diagnosis of 'functional' abdominal pain can be made without investigations (Fig. 6.3).

If a diagnosis of functional abdominal pain is made, it is important to emphasize that the pain is often real and not faked, but without an identifiable physical cause.

Fig. 6.1 Surgical causes of acute abdominal pain

Acute appendicitis
Malrotation and volvulus
Intussusception
Torsion of testes
Strangulated inguinal hernia

Fig. 6.2 Medical causes of acute abdominal pain

Abdominal causes	Systemic causes
Colic (diagnosis of exclusion)	Diabetic ketoacidosis
Constipation	Sickle cell disease
Mesenteric adenitis	Henoch–Schönlein purpura
Gastroenteritis	Lower lobe pneumonia
Acute pyelonephritis/urinary tract infection	
Pancreatitis	

Fig. 6.3 Features of 'functional' recurrent abdominal pain

• Pain usually periumbilical
• No associated appetite loss or bowel disturbance
• Family history of migraine, irritable bowel syndrome or recurrent abdominal pain
• Healthy, thriving child with normal physical examination

Fig. 6.4 Rare 'organic' causes of recurrent abdominal pain

Recurrent urinary tract infection
Urinary calculus
Helicobacter pylori gastritis
Inflammatory bowel disease
Malrotation with intermittent volvulus
Recurrent pancreatitis

There is a long list of rare causes of recurrent abdominal pain (Fig. 6.4). Careful history and examination will usually provide a clue. Further investigations to exclude a possible organic cause may include:

- Urine microscopy and culture.
- Plain abdominal film.
- Abdominal ultrasound.
- Full blood count (FBC), inflammatory markers.
- *Helicobacter pylori* stool antigen.

HINTS AND TIPS

- Acute appendicitis is uncommon under 2 years.
- Consider intussusception in vomiting infants aged 6–18 months.
- Not all abdominal pain originates in the abdomen.
- Diabetic ketoacidosis may be associated with abdominal pain.
- Consider gynaecological causes in a teenage girl.

Vomiting

Vomiting is a non-specific symptom associated with a variety of conditions but can also be a normal finding in babies. A complete clinical assessment often distinguishes the normal possets from serious pathology. Vomiting may also indicate disease outside the gastrointestinal tract.

History

Important points to establish include:

- Does the vomit contain blood or bile? Biliary vomiting suggests obstruction until proved otherwise.
- Is it projectile? It is quite common for babies to posset and bring up small quantities of milk. Projectile vomiting, on the other hand, may indicate pyloric stenosis.
- Duration: is vomiting an acute or a persistent problem?
- Associated symptoms: is vomiting accompanied by fever, abdominal pain, constipation or diarrhoea?

Examination

Examine for the following:

- Signs of dehydration.
- Fever.
- Abdominal distension (visible peristalsis), tenderness or masses.
- Hernial orifices and genitalia.

Common and important causes are discussed below.

The neonate

Vomiting can be a sign of systemic infection (e.g. meningitis, UTI) or an inborn error of metabolism.

Surgical causes include bowel obstruction, which can be anywhere along the length of the bowel. This is often associated with abdominal distension and no bowel motions.

Causes of small bowel obstruction include:

- Duodenal atresia (associated with Down syndrome).
- Malrotation with volvulus.
- Strangulated inguinal hernia.
- Meconium ileus due to cystic fibrosis.

Causes of large bowel obstruction include:

- Hirschsprung's disease (absence of the myenteric plexus in the rectum and colon).
- Imperforate anus or rectal atresia.

Necrotizing enterocolitis tends to occur in preterm neonates and can affect small or large bowel.

Infants: 1 month to 1 year

The commonest cause of persistent vomiting in infants is gastro-oesophageal reflux due to functional immaturity of the lower oesophageal sphincter that resolves spontaneously. Thickening the feeds may help. Severe reflux might be complicated by failure to thrive, oesophagitis and recurrent aspiration pneumonia.

Acute medical causes of vomiting include:

- Gastroenteritis.
- Respiratory tract infections, tonsillitis and otitis media.
- UTI.
- Meningitis.

Important surgical causes include pyloric stenosis and intussusception:

- Pyloric stenosis causes non-bilious projectile vomiting, more common in boys between the age of a few weeks and 3 months.
- The peak age of intussusception is around 6–9 months. Associated with episodic severe abdominal pain, irritability and is associated with pallor eventually shock and passage of bloodstained 'redcurrant jelly' stools.

Older children

Acute vomiting can occur in infections as described or might be one of the symptoms of acute appendicitis or abdominal migraine. Rare but important causes include raised intracranial pressure, malrotation of the intestine, inborn errors of metabolism. A more chronic picture is seen in eating disorders and cyclical vomiting.

Haematemesis

The differential diagnosis for vomiting blood varies with age. In the first few days of life it may be caused by swallowed maternal blood. Later on it can be due to oesophagitis and gastritis. Haematemesis can also occur due to a tear in the oesophageal mucosa due to forceful vomiting (Mallory–Weiss syndrome) or may be following a nosebleed due to swallowed blood.

Diarrhoea

Acute diarrhoea

The most common cause is infective viral gastroenteritis. It commonly occurs in combination with vomiting. Always take a travel history.

Some infections cause pathology in the lower gastrointestinal (GI) tract. In this case, there might be no vomiting, and diarrhoea – often with blood and mucus – dominates the clinical presentation (Fig. 6.5). Bloody diarrhoea should raise suspicion of specific pathogens and of non-infective conditions such as intussusception and inflammatory bowel disease.

HINTS AND TIPS

Bloody diarrhoea – consider:
- Infective causes: *Campylobacter*, *Shigella*, amoeba.
- Intussusception: especially 6–9 months.
- Haemolytic-uraemic syndrome: check renal function and blood pressure.
- Inflammatory bowel disease.

Fig. 6.5 Causes of acute diarrhoea
Infective causes of acute diarrhoea
Viral
Rotavirus
Small round structured virus (SRSV)
Adenovirus
Bacterial
E. coli
Campylobacter spp.
Salmonella spp.
Shigella spp.
Vibrio cholerae
Protozoa
Giardia lamblia
Entamoeba histolytica
Cryptosporidium parvum

Fig. 6.6 Assessment of dehydration

Assessment of dehydration (adapted from NICE guidance)			
Signs and symptoms	Not dehydrated	Dehydrated	Shocked
Urine output	Normal	Reduced	Reduced
Extremities	Warm	Warm	Cool
Sunken eyes or depressed fontanelle	Absent	Present	Present
Skin turgor	Normal	Reduced	Reduced
Heart rate	Normal	Increased	Increased
Respiratory rate	Normal	Increased	Increased
Capillary refill time	Normal	Normal	Prolonged
Appearance	Alert	Alert/lethargic	Lethargic
NICE, National Institute of Health and Clinical Excellence			

On examination, high fever suggests a bacterial gastroenteritis. Assessment of dehydration is vital (Fig. 6.6).

Chronic diarrhoea

The most common cause of persistent loose stools in a well, thriving, preschool child is so-called 'toddler diarrhoea'. A maturational delay in intestinal motility causes intermittent explosive loose stools with undigested vegetables often present ('peas and carrots' syndrome). An acute diarrhoeal episode might become protracted (duration >2 weeks) because of transient secondary lactose intolerance. Watery diarrhoea returns when a normal diet, including milk, is reintroduced. Stools give a positive Clinitest result for reducing substances.

Chronic diarrhoea in a child who has faltering growth raises the possibility of several important diagnoses (Fig. 6.7). A description of the stools might suggest steatorrhoea (pale, bulky and offensive) and the presence of blood or mucus suggests infective causes or inflammatory bowel disease.

Fig. 6.7 Causes of chronic diarrhoea

Infective causes	Giardiasis
	Amoebiasis
Food allergy or intolerance	Cow's milk protein allergy
	Lactose intolerance
Malabsorption	Coeliac disease
	Cystic fibrosis
Inflammatory bowel disease	Crohn's disease
	Ulcerative colitis

Physical examination

This includes assessment of dehydration (including weight) and then identifying the cause of diarrhoea. Look for any evidence of malabsorption – anaemia, poor weight gain, abdominal distension and buttock wasting. A thriving child with no associated symptomatology is unlikely to have significant disease. Faecal soiling due to constipation and overflow can be mistaken for diarrhoea.

Investigations

These are directed towards the suspected cause:

- Stool microscopy and culture if bacterial cause suspected.
- Tests for reducing substances and faecal fats if considering malabsorption.
- Coeliac antibodies.
- Endoscopy and colonoscopy if inflammatory bowel disease suspected.

Constipation

The term 'constipation' refers to delay or difficulty in passing stools for more than 2 weeks. It might be accompanied by soiling caused by involuntary passage of faeces (overflow incontinence).

> **HINTS AND TIPS**
>
> Bowel habit varies enormously and so a deviation from the norm is more of a concern than the actual frequency of defaecation.

Fig. 6.8	Organic causes of constipation
Local causes	Hirschsprung's disease Neuromuscular disorders, e.g. cerebral palsy
Systemic causes	Hypothyroidism Coeliac disease Food allergies (non IgE mediated)

Fig. 6.10 Red flag signs and symptoms
Symptoms started within first few weeks of life
Passage of meconium >24 hours of life
Faltering growth
Delayed walking or lower limb abnormal neurology
Distension of abdomen and or vomiting
Child protection concerns

In infants and children constipation is often acute and transient. Constipation might follow an acute febrile illness and can be prolonged if the hard stools cause a small, superficial anal tear.

Organic causes of constipation are rare (Fig. 6.8). An organic cause is more likely in infants, with onset at birth or when constipation is accompanied by faltering growth.

In childhood, a common cause of chronic constipation is so-called 'simple' constipation (Fig. 6.9) associated with acquired megacolon. Short-segment Hirschsprung's disease might present late and should be considered in severe or intractable constipation. Red flag signs and symptoms are listed in Fig. 6.10.

History

Enquire about:
- Frequency and consistency of stools.
- Presence of pain or blood on defaecation.
- Presence or absence of soiling.
- Any history of delay in passage of meconium.

Physical examination

Check for the following:
- Systemic signs of faltering growth.
- Abdominal distension, palpable descending colon.
- Presence of anal fissure.

Digital rectal examination is not a routine part of the examination in idiopathic constipation and should only be perfomed if there is suspicion of an underlying disorder.

Faltering growth

Faltering growth is used to describe a child who is not meeting their expected growth potential. It usually relates to weight gain but may also encompass linear growth.

The rate of weight gain obtained by plotting serial weights on a centile chart over a period of time is more important, since a single observation is difficult to interpret. It is imperative to remember that birth weight is determined by the intrauterine environment, and the weight of a large infant may drop from its birth centile to a lower, genetically determined centile (catch down) in the first year.

> **HINTS AND TIPS**
>
> Poor weight gain is a common cause of parental anxiety. If the child's growth steadily follows the centile curve, it is likely to be normal. Normal small infants have small appetites, a feature that can cause inappropriate parental anxiety

> **HINTS AND TIPS**
>
> Recognition of the constitutionally small child:
> - Small parents.
> - Low birth weight for gestational age.
> - Proportionally small: low centile for height, weight and head circumference.
> - Normal height and weight velocities.
> - Healthy child.
> - Normal physical examination.

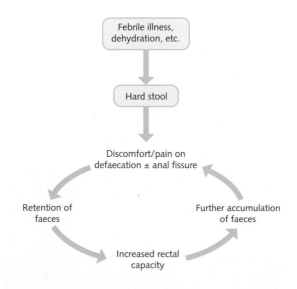

Fig. 6.9 The cycle of simple constipation

Fig. 6.11 Causes of faltering growth
Organic causes of faltering growth
Inadequate food intake: • Breast feeding – inadequate supply, poor technique • Formula feeding – milk too dilute • Anorexia: due to chronic illness • Unable to feed: cleft palate, cerebral palsy • Vomiting: gastro-oesophageal reflux
Malabsorption: • Coeliac disease • Cystic fibrosis • Short gut (postoperative) • Cow's milk protein allergy
Increased energy requirements: • Chronic illness – cystic fibrosis, congenital heart disease, chronic renal failure

Globally, the most common cause of faltering growth is inadequate intake of food (i.e. starvation). In the UK, many cases have a non-organic cause and are associated with psycho-social and environmental deprivation. Organic causes include inadequate food intake, defective absorption of food from the gastrointestinal tract (malabsorption), increased energy expenditure (Fig. 6.11).

Following a thorough assessment, investigations should be targeted towards the most likely cause. The constitutionally small normal child should be recognized (see Hints and tips box) and non-organic failure to thrive can be positively diagnosed. A brief hospital admission to document weight gain on a measured dietary intake might be helpful.

LIVER

Liver disease is uncommon in childhood and usually manifests as jaundice or hepatomegaly.

Jaundice

Jaundice is a yellowish discolouration caused by an increase in circulating bilirubin. The bilirubin can be unconjugated or conjugated, depending on the aetiology (Fig. 6.12). Mild jaundice is best detected in the sclerae rather than the skin.

Infectious hepatitis is the most common cause of acute jaundice in the older child. However, jaundice is encountered most commonly in the newborn period, at which time its usual cause is physiological liver disease but occasionally may be severe liver disease requiring early recognition and intervention (see Chapter 12).

Jaundice after infancy

Jaundice in childhood usually has an infective cause. Viral hepatitis accounts for most, but other pathogens can involve the liver. Infective hepatitis can be caused by:

- Hepatitis viruses: hepatitis A is the most common cause of jaundice after the neonatal period.
- Epstein–Barr virus (EBV).
- Malaria or bilharzia.

Liver injury can be caused by a variety of drugs (e.g. sodium valproate, halothane) and, in overdose, paracetamol and iron are toxic to the liver. Jaundice with pallor suggests a haemolytic episode (e.g. glucose-6-phosphate dehydrogenase deficiency, sickle cell disease or haemolytic-uraemic syndrome).

Hepatomegaly after infancy

Isolated hepatomegaly is uncommon. In association with jaundice, the causes include biliary atresia and infective hepatitis. In babies, hepatomegaly is an important feature of cardiac failure.

Hepatosplenomegaly can occur in malaria, in advanced liver disease and in a number of important haematological diseases (e.g. leukaemia, sickle cell disease and thalassaemia) and rare storage disorders (e.g. mucopolysaccharidosis).

Fig. 6.12 Bilirubin metabolism

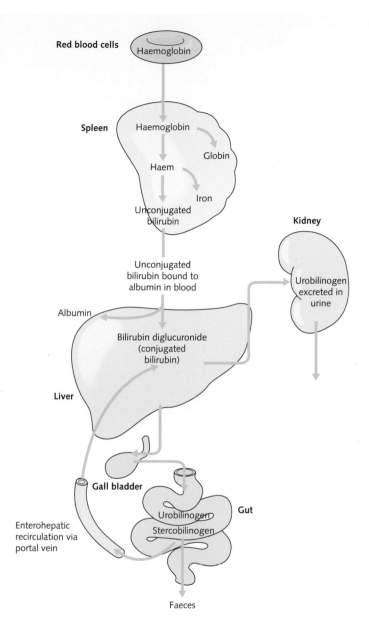

47

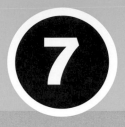

At the end of this chapter, you should be able to:
• Identify the common abnormalities in urinalysis
• Identify the common causes of haematuria and proteinuria

In the infant or younger child, urinary tract infection (UTI) is the most common disorder encountered and it often presents without specific symptoms or signs. Urine abnormalities might also indicate renal pathology. Important symptoms are:

• Polyuria (frequency) or enuresis: suggesting UTI or diabetes mellitus. Polyuria means increased urine output due to a diuresis (diabetes mellitus, diabetes insipidus) or due to increased water intake, whereas frequency does not necessarily mean an increased urine output.
• Dysuria: suggesting UTI.
• Oliguria: suggesting dehydration or acute renal failure.
• Discoloured urine (Fig. 7.1).
• Fever with or without rigors: rule out UTI or pyelonephritis.

HINTS AND TIPS

• Polyuria and polydipsia suggest diabetes mellitus – test the urine for glucose and ketones and check blood sugar.
• Excessive drinking is a more common cause of polyuria and polydipsia in a toddler than diabetes insipidus.
• Polyuria might present as secondary enuresis.

Important signs are:

• Hypertension: suggesting glomerulonephritis.
• Oedema: suggesting nephrotic syndrome.
• Palpable bladder or kidneys: suggest anatomical abnormalities.

HAEMATURIA

Test strips are very sensitive. Haematuria should be confirmed by urine microscopy and is defined as >10 red blood cells (RBCs) per high power field. The causes are listed in Fig. 7.2.

History

Find out the following:
• Duration.
• Dysuria and frequency: suggest UTI.
• Associated loin pain: suggests pyelonephritis if associated with fever or renal stones, especially if the pain is colicky.
• Recent foreign travel: suggests schistosomiasis or malaria.
• Recent sore throat or skin infection: suggests post-streptococcal glomerulonephritis.
• Family history of haematuria or deafness: suggests Alport syndrome.

Examination

Examine for:
• Fever: suggests UTI.
• Oedema: suggests nephrotic syndrome. In nephritis oedema is usually mild though haematuria is more common.
• Hypertension: suggests acute nephritis/chronic renal scarring or chronic renal insufficiency.
• Typical rash and joint swelling: suggests Henoch–Schönlein purpura.
• Bruises and purpura: suggests idiopathic thrombocytopenic purpura.
• Abdominal mass: suggests Wilms' tumour.

HINTS AND TIPS

Urinary tract infection can present with fever and no clues to its origin, especially in infants and young children. Urine microscopy and culture should be undertaken in any infant with unexplained fever.

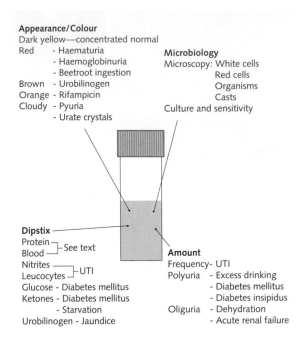

Appearance/Colour
Dark yellow—concentrated normal
Red   - Haematuria
          - Haemoglobinuria
          - Beetroot ingestion
Brown - Urobilinogen
Orange - Rifampicin
Cloudy - Pyuria
          - Urate crystals

Microbiology
Microscopy: White cells
                    Red cells
                    Organisms
                    Casts
Culture and sensitivity

Dipstix
Protein ┐
Blood   ├ See text
Nitrites ┐
Leucocytes ┘ UTI
Glucose - Diabetes mellitus
Ketones - Diabetes mellitus
            - Starvation
Urobilinogen - Jaundice

Amount
Frequency- UTI
Polyuria - Excess drinking
            - Diabetes mellitus
            - Diabetes insipidus
Oliguria - Dehydration
            - Acute renal failure

Fig. 7.1   Information available from urine

Investigations

The choice of investigations depends on the renal pathology suspected:

- Microscopy and culture of urine.
- Imaging: nuclear medicine and ultrasound scans.
- Haematology: full blood count (FBC), coagulation screen and sickle cell screen.
- Biochemistry: urea and electrolytes (U&E), creatinine (Cr), Ca^{2+}, PO_4^{3-} and urate.
- Throat swab.
- Antistreptolysin O titre (ASOT), C3 and hepatitis B antigen.

Transient, benign haematuria can occur but is a diagnosis of exclusion. A renal biopsy might be indicated in the following situations:

- Persistent haematuria for >6 months.

Fig. 7.2   Causes of haematuria

Glomerular	Non-glomerular
Presence of red cell or white cell casts and proteinuria suggests a glomerular source of the blood – glomerulonephritis: • Acute, poststreptococcal • Henoch–Schönlein nephritis • IgA nephropathy (Berger's disease) • Alport syndrome (familial deafness and nephritis)	Infection: • Bacterial urinary tract infection • Tuberculosis • Schistosomiasis Trauma Stones Wilms' tumour Bleeding disorders, esp. thrombocytopenia

Fig. 7.3   Causes of proteinuria

Transient	Persistent
Fever Exercise Orthostatic – proteinuria During the day (stops when recumbent at night)	Nephrotic syndrome (>1 g/m^2/24 h) Urinary tract infection Glomerulonephritis

- Unexplained abnormal renal function.
- Chronic glomerulonephritis.

PROTEINURIA

Transient, mild proteinuria frequently occurs in children with viral infections and is self-limiting. In contrast, nephrotic syndrome causes persistent heavy proteinuria. The causes of proteinuria are listed in Fig. 7.3. Normal children produce <60 mg/m^2/24 h of protein in the urine.

Definition

- Early morning urine protein/creatinine ratio >20 mg/mmol.
- Greater than 5 mg/kg in a 24 h urine sample.

Examination

Physical examination should include evaluation for signs of renal disease (especially the nephrotic syndrome); these include:

- Oedema: especially periorbital, scrotal and ankle.
- Ascites.
- Pleural effusions (unusual).
- Blood pressure: low or high.

Investigations

The investigations include:

- Urine dipstix (Fig. 7.4).
- Early morning protein:creatinine ratio.
- Renal function: U&E, Cr.
- Plasma albumin and lipids.
- Midstream urine for microscopy, culture and sensitivity.
- Throat swab, ASOT, anti-DNaseB.
- Complement C3, C4.

Fig. 7.4   Albustix values

Stix reading	Albumin concentration g/L
+	0.3
+ +	1.0
+ + +	3.0
+ + + +	>20

Objectives

At the end of this chapter, you should be able to:
- Understand the common types of paroxysmal events in children
- Take a history and examine a child with suspected epilepsy
- Understand the common causes of headache
- Evaluate an unconscious child

Important symptoms are:
- Paroxysmal episodes (fits, faints and funny turns).
- Headache.
- Vomiting and ataxia.

Important signs are:
- Focal neurology.
- Altered consciousness or coma.

Global or specific developmental delay can be a manifestation of neurological disease, as can abnormalities of head size or shape; these are discussed in Chapters 11 and 20.

FITS, FAINTS AND FUNNY TURNS

Transient episodes of altered consciousness, abnormal movements or abnormal behaviour are a common presenting problem. The first task is to distinguish true epileptic seizures (fits) from faints and funny turns. An accurate witness account is essential.

History

Provoking events

Exactly when and where the episode occurred and what the child was doing just before.

Description of the episodes

Get an exact description of:
- Any altered consciousness or awareness?
- Abnormal movements involving limbs or face (unilateral or bilateral?)?
- Altered tone (rigidity or sudden fall?)?
- Altered colour (pallor or cyanosis?)?
- Eye movements (did they 'roll up'?)?

- Duration of the episode?
- Any trigger, e.g. flashing lights or breath-holding?

Other important features to establish include:
- Birth history, any developmental delay, any recent head injury?
- Family history: both epilepsy and febrile convulsions run in families.

The key differential diagnoses for epileptic seizures are listed in Fig. 8.1, and described below.

> **COMMUNICATION**
>
> While taking history, it is useful to go through the event from the beginning. Parents can often demonstrate the fit. It is extremely useful if parents can record the event on video (e.g. on mobile phone).

Seizures

> **HINTS AND TIPS**
>
> - A 'seizure' is a transient episode of abnormal and excessive neuronal activity in the brain.
> - The term 'epilepsy' refers to the tendency to recurrent seizures.

Generalized tonic-clonic seizures

These are characterized by:
- Tonic phase of rigidity with loss of posture followed by clonic movements of all four limbs.
- Loss of consciousness.
- Duration: 2–20 minutes.
- Postictal drowsiness.

Febrile seizures are usually of this sort.

Fig. 8.1 Differential diagnosis of seizures by age

Age	Differential diagnosis
Infants	Jitteriness Benign myoclonus Apnoeas Gastro-oesophageal reflux
Toddlers	Breath-holding attacks Reflex anoxic seizures Rigors Masturbation
Children	Vasovagal syncope (faints) Tics Day-dreaming Migraine Panic attacks, tantrums Night terrors

HINTS AND TIPS

Meningitis or encephalitis must be considered in all children with fever and seizure. Febrile convulsions are a diagnosis of exclusion.

Absence seizures

These are characterized by:

- Brief unawareness lasting a few seconds.
- No loss of posture.
- Immediate recovery.
- Might be very frequent.
- Associated with automatisms (e.g. blinking and lip-smacking).

Partial seizures

These are characterized by:

- Involvement of only a part of the body.
- May be associated with an aura.
- May spread to involve the entire body – secondary generalization.
- Consciousness may be retained (simple partial seizure) or impaired (complex partial seizures).

Faints (vasovagal syncope)

Features include:

- Usually occur in teenagers.
- Provoked by emotion, hot environment.
- Preceded by nausea and dizziness.
- Sudden loss of consciousness and posture.
- Rapid recovery.

Funny turns

Breath-holding attacks

These have the following characteristics:

- They are provoked by temper or frustration usually in children between 6 months and 6 years of age.
- The screaming toddler holds his or her breath in expiration, goes blue, then limp and then makes a rapid spontaneous recovery.

HINTS AND TIPS

It is important to advise parents not to reinforce these behaviours by paying too much attention to the child. Support groups such as 'STARS' can help parents with reflex anoxic seizures and breath-holding attacks.

Reflex anoxic seizures

These have the following characteristics:

- They are provoked by pain (usually a mild head injury) or fear.
- The infant or toddler becomes pale and loses consciousness (reflecting syncope, secondary to vagal-induced bradycardia).
- The subsequent hypoxia might induce a tonic-clonic seizure.

Rigors

Rigors are transient exaggerated shivering in association with high fever.

Examination

The well child

Physical examination is often normal in idiopathic epilepsy (the majority). However, particular attention should be paid to:

- Skin: neurocutaneous syndromes are associated with epilepsy, especially tuberous sclerosis and neurofibromatosis.
- Optic fundi: fundal changes may occur in congenital infections and neurodegenerative diseases.

The convulsing child

Physical examination of an infant or child presenting acutely with generalized tonic-clonic seizures (convulsions) has a different emphasis, reflecting the likely causes (Fig. 8.2). Important features on examination include:

Fig. 8.2	Causes of acute seizures	
Common	**Uncommon**
Febrile seizures	Meningitis/encephalitis
Epilepsy	Head injury
Hypoglycaemia	Hyponatraemia Cerebral tumour or malignant infiltration

- Fever: febrile convulsions or intracranial infection.
- Anterior fontanelle: tense or bulging if the intracranial pressure (ICP) is raised.
- Meningism.
- Optic fundi: papilloedema in raised ICP (signs of congenital infections and neurodegenerative diseases).
- Focal neurological signs.
- Altered level of consciousness.

HEADACHE

An acute headache commonly occurs as a non-specific feature of any febrile illness but can be a feature of meningitis. Recurrent headaches are very common in children and their causes range from the trivial to the sinister (Fig. 8.3); serious causes are rare. Red flag symptoms for headaches in children are laid out in Fig. 8.4; children displaying these symptoms may need imaging.

History

Important features include:
- Site: frontal, temporal, bilateral or unilateral?
- Intensity: severe, throbbing?
- Duration and frequency?
- Provoking factors: stress, food?
- Associated symptoms: weakness, paraesthesia, nausea or vomiting?
- Ongoing illness: e.g. fever (meningitis), diabetic ketoacidosis (cerebral oedema)?

Simple tension headaches

These are characterized by the following:
- Symmetrical and band-like in nature.
- Gradual onset, duration less than 24 hours.

Fig. 8.4	Red flag symptoms, headache in children
Sudden onset, severe headache
Headache lasting several days or progressing in severity
Weight loss
Associated with straining, e.g. coughing, or increased by lying down
Morning headache, especially associated with vomiting
Seizures or focal neurology

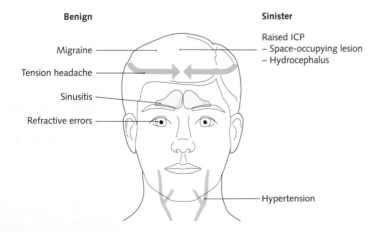

Fig. 8.3 Causes of recurrent headache

- No associated nausea or vomiting.
- Often recur frequently.
- Affect 10% of school children.

Migraine

- Can be unilateral and throbbing in nature.
- With or without visual aura, area of visual loss or fortification spectra.
- Associated nausea, vomiting, abdominal pain.
- Duration several hours.
- Trigger factors – stress or relaxation, foods (cheese, chocolate).
- Family history.

HINTS AND TIPS

Migraine can be classified as:
- Common: no aura.
- Classical: aura preceding headache.
- Complex: associated neurological deficit, e.g. hemiplegia, ophthalmoplegia.

Headache from raised intracranial pressure

- Worse in recumbent position, i.e. during the night or early morning.
- Associated with nausea and vomiting.
- Pain is usually mild and diffuse.
- Personality changes may develop.

Examination

Attention should be paid to the following signs in a child with recurrent headache:

- Blood pressure: hypertension (e.g. aortic coarctation is a rare cause of headache).
- Pulse: radial-femoral delay (coarctation).
- Visual acuity: refractive errors cause headache.
- Papilloedema: a late sign of raised ICP.
- Focal neurological deficit: especially cerebellar signs (posterior fossa tumour).

HINTS AND TIPS

Headache is rarely caused by a brain tumour but 70% of children with a brain tumour present with headache. The headache might wake the child at night, is worst in the morning and associated with vomiting. Most are in the posterior fossa and cause raised intracranial pressure.

THE UNCONSCIOUS CHILD

The acute development of a diminished level of consciousness is a medical emergency. In the majority of cases a systemic problem rather than a primary brain disorder is responsible (Fig. 8.5). The cause might be evident from the history but, if not, clinical evaluation is the key after emergency management. For investigation and management see Chapter 29. It is important not to perform lumbar puncture in an acutely comatose child as raised intracranial pressure is likely. It can always be performed later if a diagnosis is required.

Examination

Systemic examination

The priorities are:

- ABC: Airway, Breathing, and Circulation.
- Temperature.
- Blood glucose.
- Hypertension, bradycardia, irregular respiration (signs of coning).
- Signs of physical abuse or injury.

Neurological examination

For a neurological examination, check the AVPU score. There are four categories:

- A = Alert.
- V = responds to Voice.
- P = responds to Pain (the Glasgow Coma Scale (GCS) is usually less than 8 at this point).
- U = Unresponsive.

Fig. 8.5 Causes of coma

Cause	Differential diagnosis
Infection	Meningitis Encephalitis
Trauma	Head injury
Metabolic	Hypoglycaemia
Primary CNS disorder	Seizures
Drugs	Opiates Lead

When a child is comatose:
- Establish the degree of unconsciousness (use the GCS or AVPU).
- Assess and treat the ABCs and hypoglycaemia.
- Look for signs of raised intracranial pressure.
- Establish the possible causes and decide which need immediate treatment.

Check also:
- The Glasgow Coma Scale score (Fig. 8.6).
- The pupils: these might be small (suggests opiate or barbiturate poisoning), large (suggests a postictal state) or unequal (suggests severe head injury or intracranial haemorrhage).
- For meningism.
- The fontanelle.

Fig. 8.6 The Glasgow Coma Scale: top score = 15

	Glasgow Coma Scale		
Score	Eye opening	Best motor response	Best verbal response
1	No response	No response	No response
2	Open to pain	Extension	Non-verbal sounds
3	Open to verbal command	Inappropriate flexion	Inappropriate words
4	Open spontaneously	Flexion with pain	Disorientated and conversing
5		Localizes pain	Orientated and conversing
6		Obeys command	

Further reading

National Institute for Health and Clinical Excellence (NICE), January 2004. Clinical Guideline 137. The epilepsies: the diagnosis and management of the epilepsies in adults and children in primary and secondary care. http://guidance.nice.org.uk/CG137/NICEGuidance/pdf/English.

National Institute for Health and Clinical Excellence (NICE), May 2007. Clinical Guideline. Feverish illness in children: assessment and initial management in children younger than 5 years. http://www.nice.org.uk/nicemedia/pdf/CG47Guidance.pdf.

Musculoskeletal problems

Objectives

At the end of this chapter, you should be able to:
- Assess a limping child
- Understand the common causes of limb and joint pains
- Understand the normal postural variations in children

Disorders of the musculoskeletal system can present in a variety of ways. The common presenting symptoms include:

- Limb or joint pain.
- Fever.

Important signs are:

- Limp.
- Altered posture.
- Point tenderness.
- Reduced range of movement.

LIMP

A limp is an abnormality of gait (the term applied to the rhythmic movement of the whole body in walking). It can be painful or painless, and the cause varies with age (Fig. 9.1).

HINTS AND TIPS

- The most common cause of an acute limp in a well child is 'irritable hip'.
- The diagnoses not to miss are septic arthritis, osteomyelitis and slipped upper femoral epiphysis.

History

The history should establish:

- Duration: chronic pain is unlikely to be caused by infection.
- Any prodromal illness (e.g. sore throat) or trauma.
- Presence and location of any pain.
- Any history of trauma.

Examination

Physical examination can begin by observing the child walking, if this can be done without distress. Important physical signs include:

- Fever: suggests bone or joint infection.
- Skin rashes.
- Range of movement.
- Point tenderness or signs of inflammation.
- Unequal leg length.
- Spinal abnormality, e.g. hairy patch.
- Neurological signs: check tone, power and tendon reflexes.

Investigations

Useful investigations may include:

- Imaging: X-rays above and below the focal point, ultrasound of the joint, MRI scan.
- Nuclear medicine: isotope bone scans.
- Full blood count, acute phase reactants.
- Blood cultures (if febrile).
- Aspiration of the joint.

THE PAINFUL LIMB

Pain in a limb can arise from the bone, joint or soft tissues. In the lower limbs, pain might be associated with a limp (see above). Pain in a joint (arthralgia) is considered separately.

Recurrent limb pain

So-called 'growing pains' are common in the lower limbs. Their features are listed in Fig. 9.2.

An important rare cause of limb pain, especially at night, is malignant deposits in the bone (e.g. leukaemia). Vitamin D deficiency may also be a cause of non-specific limb pain in children, especially in 'at-risk' ethnic groups.

Limb pain of acute onset

In a young infant this might present as pseudoparalysis. Important causes include:

Fig. 9.1 Causes of a limp

Age group	Cause
All ages	Trauma Septic arthritis/osteomyelitis
1–2 years	Congenital dislocation of the hip (developmental dysplasia of the hip) Cerebral palsy
3–10 years	Transient synovitis (irritable hip) Perthes' disease Rarities: • Juvenile idiopathic arthritis (JIA) • Leukaemia
11–15 years	Slipped upper femoral epiphysis Osgood–Schlatter's disease Rarities: • Bone tumours • JIA • Hysteria

Fig. 9.2 Features of growing pains

Common between 3–5 years of age and 8–12 years of age
Occurs in evening and night
Predominantly lower limbs
Normal examination
Never:
Functional disability
Limp
Morning symptoms
Always in one leg only

Fig. 9.3 Causes of acute monoarthralgia

Cause	Clinical clues
Septic arthritis	Fever and inability to move
Irritable hip	Recent cold
Haemophilia	Easy bruising
Juvenile idiopathic arthritis (JIA)	Chronic pain and swelling
Trauma	Immediate symptoms – no chronicity

Fig. 9.4 Causes of polyarthritis

Type	Cause
Inflammatory	Juvenile idiopathic arthritis (JIA) Systemic lupus erythematosus (SLE) Henoch–Schönlein purpura
Infectious/reactive	Viral Mycoplasma Rheumatic fever

HINTS AND TIPS

Septic arthritis is a medical emergency – joint destruction can occur within 24 hours if untreated. X-rays are not helpful in early diagnosis and aspiration of the joint space followed by prompt intravenous antibiotics is indicated if septic arthritis is suspected.

- Trauma.
- Osteomyelitis or septic arthritis.
- Sickle cell disease ('painful crisis').
- Meningococcal sepsis.

Trauma is usually accidental (e.g. sports injury) but non-accidental injury should also be a consideration. Osteomyelitis usually presents with a painful, immobile limb in a febrile child. The long bones around the knee are the most common site of infection.

THE PAINFUL JOINT

Arthralgia usually reflects inflammation, i.e. arthritis. Diagnostic possibilities depend on whether the presentation is acute or insidious, and whether one or several joints are involved. Causes of an acutely painful joint are shown in Fig. 9.3.

Polyarthritis might have an acute onset but is more likely to run a chronic and relapsing course. Causes to consider are shown in Fig. 9.4.

Inequalities of limb length

This is caused by shortening or overgrowth in one or more bones in the leg. Causes include trauma, neuromuscular disorders and congenital malformations. Treatment is surgical.

NORMAL POSTURAL VARIANTS

These are common and most resolve without treatment (Fig. 9.5). They include:

- Bow legs (genu varum): common in infants and toddlers up to 2 years.

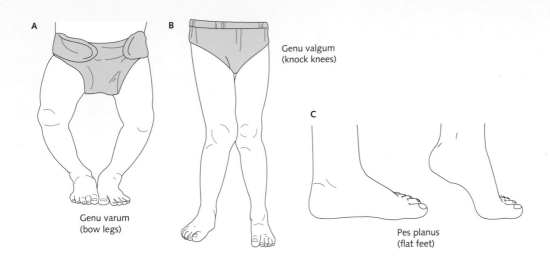

Fig. 9.5 Normal postural variants: (A) genu varum (bow legs), (B) genu valgum (knock knees), (C) pes planus (flat feet). Note the medial longitudinal arch appears when standing on tiptoe

- Knock knees (genu valgum): the physiological knock-knee pattern is seen during the third and fourth years.
- Flat feet (pes planus): often present in toddlers.
- Intoeing: metatarsus varus in infants, medial tibial torsion in toddlers, femoral anteversion in children (Fig. 9.6).

Pathology should be suspected if there is:
- Rapid or severe progression.
- A positive family history.
- Asymmetry.
- Association with any abnormal signs.
- A posture variant outside the age range for normal limits.

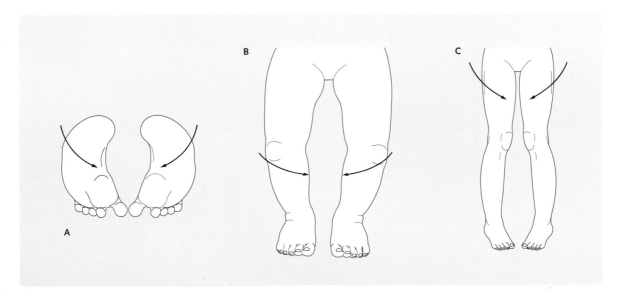

Fig. 9.6 Causes of intoeing: (A) metatarsus varus, (B) medial tibial torsion, (C) femoral anteversion

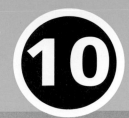
Objectives

At the end of this chapter, you should be able to:
- Assess a child with anaemia
- Understand the coagulation cascade
- Evaluate a child with excessive bleeding
- Evaluate a child with splenomegaly or hepatosplenomegaly
- Understand the common causes of lymphadenopathy and its evaluation

In childhood, disorders of the blood or bone marrow often present with striking physical signs rather than complex symptomatology. The pallor of anaemia is the most common sign but abnormal bruising or bleeding, enlargement of the spleen or liver, or a propensity to infection can all reflect an underlying haematological problem.

PALLOR

It is easy to miss mild anaemia, especially in patients with pigmented skin. Pallor is best observed in the conjunctiva and palmar creases. Note that peripheral vasoconstriction also causes pallor, e.g. hypovolaemic shock.

Anaemia

The history and physical examination will often provide a good idea of the likely cause (Fig. 10.1). Few symptoms will occur with haemoglobin above 7–8 g/dL, except in acute blood loss.

Mean haemoglobin (g/dL) values in infancy and childhood are:

- 2 weeks   16.8 (13.0–20.0).
- 3 months to 6 years   12.0 (9.5–14.5).
- 7–12 years 13.0   (11.0–16.0).

History

This should include enquiry about:
- The presence of chronic diseases, (especially renal), or prematurity.
- Gastrointestinal symptoms.
- Dietary history: adequate iron intake?
- Family history: relatives with inherited disorders such as sickle cell disease, thalassaemia or hereditary spherocytosis.
- Place of birth: sickle cell screening has been part of the Guthrie test in the UK since 2002.

HINTS AND TIPS

It is sometimes difficult to elicit a family history of inherited anaemias. A family history of frequent blood transfusions is a useful pointer towards an inherited anaemia.

Examination

Age and ethnic group

Causes of anaemia are very age-dependent and inherited anaemias show a racial preponderance:
- Afro-Caribbean ancestry: sickle cell disease.
- Mediterranean and Asian ancestry: thalassaemia.

Associated signs

- Jaundice: suggests acute haemolysis.
- Petechiae or bruising: suggest marrow failure.
- Splenomegaly: suggests haemolysis, haemoglobinopathy or marrow failure.

Investigation

The most important initial investigation is a full blood count (FBC) to confirm reduced haemoglobin concentration and document red cell indices (Fig. 10.2). Additional valuable information from the FBC includes:

- Reticulocytes: an increase suggests haemolytic anaemia; a decrease suggests marrow aplasia.
- Pancytopenia: a reduction in all cell types suggests marrow failure or hypersplenism.
- A peripheral blood film can also reveal abnormal cells (blasts) commonly seen in leukaemias.

Depending on the initial results, further investigations to clarify the cause might include:

Fig. 10.1 Causes of anaemia in infants and children

Decreased red cell production	Reduced red cell lifespan (haemolytic anaemia)	Excessive blood loss
Iron deficiency anaemia: • Nutrition • Malabsorption, e.g. coeliac disease Marrow replacement: • Malignant disease, e.g. acute leukaemia • Marrow aplasia Chronic disease: • Renal failure • Inflammatory disorders	Intrinsic red cell defects: • Abnormal membrane, e.g. spherocytosis • Abnormal haemoglobin, e.g. sickle cell disease, thalassaemia • Enzyme deficiencies, e.g. G6PD (x-linked), pyruvate kinase Extrinsic disorders: • Immune mediated, e.g. ABO or rhesus incompatibility, autoimmune haemolysis • Malaria • Microangiopathy, e.g. haemolytic anaemic syndrome • Hypersplenism	GI: • Hookworm infestation • Meckel's diverticulum Iatrogenic, e.g. excessive venesection in babies Epistaxis Menorrhagia

- Iron studies: serum iron, ferritin and total iron-binding capacity.
- Direct antiglobulin test (DAT or Coombs' test): this is positive in immune-mediated haemolysis.
- Red cell folate, vitamin B_{12}.
- Haemoglobin electrophoresis.
- Red cell enzymes: glucose-6-phosphate dehydrogenase (G6PD), pyruvate kinase.
- Bone marrow aspiration.

BLEEDING DISORDERS

Normal haemostasis requires integrity of the coagulation factors, functional platelets and their interaction with the vessels. Disorders of the coagulation system may be hereditary or acquired. In the past, the coagulation cascade was thought to contain intrinsic and extrinsic pathways; however, it is now thought to comprise a common pathway involving tissue factor activation, with a central role for thrombin and membrane-associated complexes (Fig. 10.3).

Clinical evaluation

The history and examination aim to establish:

- Is there a generalized haemostatic problem?
- Is it inherited or acquired?
- What is the likely mechanism: vascular, platelets, coagulation or a combination?

Investigations will be required to establish the precise nature of the underlying abnormality.

Causes of bleeding disorders

The causes are set out in Fig. 10.4:

- The most common vascular problem is Henoch–Schönlein purpura.
- Bruising with thrombocytopenia in a well child is most commonly due to idiopathic thrombocytopenic purpura.
- Inherited coagulation disorders are uncommon but haemophilia must be considered in a male infant or child with a bleeding tendency.
- It is important to rule out bleeding disorders when considering bruising in the context of non-accidental injury.

Fig. 10.2 Red cell indices and film

MCV (mean corpuscular volume):
- Microcytic anaemia suggests iron deficiency, thalassaemia
- Macrocytic anaemia (normal in neonates) suggests folate, vitamin B_{12} deficiency (rare)

MCHC (mean corpuscular haemoglobin concentration):
- Hypochromic anaemia suggests iron deficiency, thalassaemia

The film may reveal:
- Sickle cells – sickle cell disease
- Microcytic, hypochromic cells – iron deficiency
- Spherocytes – hereditary spherocytosis
- Blast cells – malignancy

HINTS AND TIPS

Bruising – normal and abnormal:
- Mobile toddlers commonly have multiple bruises on shins but bruises in non-mobile infants need further evaluation.

Fig. 10.3 Coagulation cascade: tests and defects

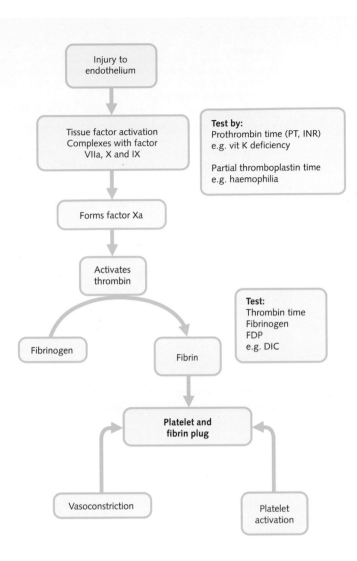

Examination

The commonest clinical manifestation is excessive bleeding into the skin but spontaneous bleeding into other sites such as nasal mucosa (epistaxis), gums, joints (haemarthrosis) and the genitourinary tract (haematuria) can also occur. Spontaneous bleeding from multiple sites suggests a generalized haemostatic disorder.

- Mongolian blue spots in infants can be mistaken for bruising.
- Newborns often have petechiae around the face and forehead.

History

- Age of onset: inherited disorders usually present in infancy but, if mild, may not be detected until adulthood.
- If the child has had a haemostatic challenge (e.g. tonsillectomy) without excessive bleeding then a bleeding disorder is unlikely.
- Family history: note that up to one-third of cases of haemophilia are from spontaneous mutation.

HINTS AND TIPS

- Bleeding into skin and mucous membranes: platelet or vascular disorder.
- Bleeding into muscles or joints: coagulation disorder.

Fig. 10.4 Bleeding disorders in childhood

Defect	Inherited	Acquired
Vascular defects	Hereditary haemorrhagic telangiectasia (rare) Ehlers–Danlos syndrome (rare)	Henoch–Schönlein purpura Scurvy (vitamin C deficiency) Cushing's disease Meningococcal septicaemia
Platelet defects: • Thrombocytopenia	Rare	Immune-mediated: • Idiopathic thrombocytopenic purpura (most common) Peripheral consumption: • Disseminated intravascular coagulation (DIC) • Haemolytic-uraemic syndrome Marrow failure: • Aplastic anaemia • Acute leukaemia
• Abnormal function	Rare	Drug-induced, e.g. aspirin, dipyridamole
Coagulation defects	Haemophilia A (factor VIII) Haemophilia B (factor IX, Christmas disease) von Willebrand disease	Vitamin K deficiency: • Haemorrhagic disease of newborn • Malabsorption • Liver disease Drugs – anticoagulant therapy with warfarin, heparin

Manifestations of bleeding into the skin

The terms used vary with the size of lesion. Test small lesions using a transparent glass to see if they blanch. Failure to blanch indicates extravasated blood.

- Petechiae: small red spots <3 mm.
- Purpura: confluent petechiae up to 1 cm.
- Ecchymosis: a large area of extravasated blood >1 cm (a synonym for a bruise).
- Haematoma: extravasated blood that has infiltrated subcutaneous tissue or muscle to produce a deformity.

An important differential diagnosis of excessive bruising is non-accidental injury.

HINTS AND TIPS

A petechial or purpuric rash in a febrile child should be treated as meningococcal sepsis until proved otherwise.

Investigations

Laboratory investigation of a suspected bleeding disorder initially includes:

- Blood film.
- Renal and liver function.
- Platelet count: normal is $150–450 \times 10^9$/L (spontaneous bleeding occurs at counts below 30×10^9/L).
- Coagulation screen: prothrombin time, activated thromboplastin time and thrombin time. Further

investigation for tissue factors should be done by a tertiary haematological centre.

SPLENOMEGALY

In neonates and very thin children, the tip of the spleen is often palpable. The spleen can enlarge during acute infections and in various haematological diseases. Hepatosplenomegaly suggests a different aetiology from that associated with isolated splenomegaly (Figs 10.5 and 10.6).

HINTS AND TIPS

Differential diagnosis of a left-sided abdominal mass:
- Splenomegaly.
- Renal masses: Wilms' tumour, hydronephrosis.
- Neoplasia: neuroblastoma (non-renal), lymphoma.

HINTS AND TIPS

In sickle cell disease:
- Splenomegaly is present in early life but splenic infarction subsequently reduces the spleen in size.
- A sudden increase in the size of the spleen suggests a sequestration crisis.

Fig. 10.5   Causes of splenomegaly

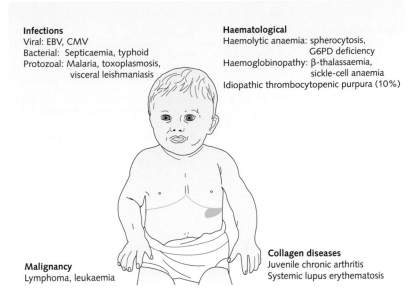

Infections
Viral: EBV, CMV
Bacterial: Septicaemia, typhoid
Protozoal: Malaria, toxoplasmosis,
            visceral leishmaniasis

Haematological
Haemolytic anaemia: spherocytosis,
                    G6PD deficiency
Haemoglobinopathy: β-thalassaemia,
                   sickle-cell anaemia
Idiopathic thrombocytopenic purpura (10%)

Malignancy
Lymphoma, leukaemia

Collagen diseases
Juvenile chronic arthritis
Systemic lupus erythematosis

Fig. 10.6   Causes of
hepatosplenomegaly

Infection
Congenital infections
Infectious mononucleosis
Hepatitis

Haematological
Haemoglobinopathy: β-thalassaemia

Liver disease
Portal hypertension

Malignancy
Lymphoma
Leukaemia

Storage disorders
Glycogen, lipid,
mucopolysaccharidosis

History

- Systems review: this might elicit symptoms related to the many infective causes.
- Family history: inherited anaemias, storage disorders, e.g. Gaucher's disease.

Examination

Note coexistent lymphadenopathy, hepatomegaly, pallor, fever or rash.

Investigations

- Haematological: FBC, blood film, reticulocyte count.
- Infections: serology (e.g. Epstein–Barr virus (EBV)), blood cultures, film for malaria parasites.
- Malignancy: bone marrow aspiration.
- Liver disease: liver function tests (LFTs), hepatitis serology.
- Abdominal ultrasound scan (USS).

LYMPHADENOPATHY

Lymph node enlargement, particularly in the cervical region, is a common clinical problem in children, and may be normal.

Local infection is the commonest cause of transient regional lymphadenopathy but uncommon sinister causes of persistent or progressive lymphadenopathy do exist (Figs 10.7–10.9).

History

The history should establish:

- Duration: less than 4 weeks in most infections; more than 1 year less likely to be neoplastic.
- Constitutional symptoms: e.g. weight loss, fever, night sweats.

Fig. 10.7 Causes of generalized lymphadenopathy

Cause	Example
Infection	Infectious mononucleosis Rubella Toxoplasmosis Cytomegalovirus HIV infection
Malignancy	Acute leukaemia Lymphoma
Immunological	Juvenile chronic arthritis (JCA) Sarcoidosis (rare) Kawasaki disease Atopic eczema

Fig. 10.8 Causes of cervical lymphadenopathy

Type	Features
Acute, short duration	Reactive and secondary to local infection in throat or scalp: Cervical adenitis – bacterial infection in gland
Persistent, non-inflamed	Reactive and secondary to local infection: • Tuberculous adenitis – tuberculosis, atypical mycobacteria • Neoplasia – lymphoma, neuroblastoma

Fig. 10.9 Features of worrying lymph nodes

Rapid growth
Skin ulceration
Fixation to skin or fascia
>3 cm with hard consistency
Greater than 3 cm for more than 6 weeks despite treatment

- Rash: associated rash suggests viral exanthemata.
- Pets: toxoplasmosis or cat scratch fever.
- Travel contacts and family history of tuberculosis (TB).
- Drugs: phenytoin, carbamazepine.

Examination

Palpate all nodal sites: look for regional or generalized lymphadenopathy. Examine the nodes:

- Size: more likely to be significant if large (>1 cm diameter), firm, or fixed.
- Erythema and tenderness: suggest bacterial adenitis.
- Drainage region: ear, nose and throat (ENT) and scalp for cervical nodes.
- Skin: infective lesions, atopic eczema and exanthemata.
- Abdomen: hepatosplenomegaly.

Also note systemic signs such as weight loss and pallor.

Investigations

The diagnosis is apparent in most children and further investigations are unnecessary in transient node enlargement with local infection, or in the context of diagnosed systemic illnesses such as Epstein–Barr virus, atopic eczema and Kawasaki disease.

By contrast, lymphadenopathy presenting in the following clinical contexts requires investigation to establish an underlying diagnosis:

Persistent significant cervical lymphadenopathy

Initial tests are:

- FBC: to determine infection.
- Chest X-ray: to check for TB, lymphoma.
- Tuberculin skin test: if positive this suggests myco-bacteria tuberculosis but weak false positives can be caused by non-tuberculous mycobacteria.

If malignancy is suspected, a lymph node biopsy might be indicated.

HINTS AND TIPS

Cervical nodes are quick to enlarge but are slow to resolve with local infection. Consider tuberculosis or malignancy in persistent and progressive cervical lymphadenopathy.

Generalized lymphadenopathy

Constitutional symptoms and hepatosplenomegaly might or might not be present.

Initial tests
- FBC plus differential.
- Monospot and Epstein–Barr IgM antibodies.
- Chest X-ray.
- Abdominal USS.
- Bone marrow aspiration should be considered.
- Lymph node biopsy should be considered.

Lymphadenitis

Acutely infected nodes are tender with associated red-ness and increased warmth. If untreated, they can form an abscess – indicated by the presence of fluctuance. An ultrasound of the node will help to identify an abscess which may need surgical drainage. Uncomplicated lymphadenitis is treated with antibiotics.

Short stature or developmental delay

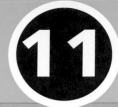

11

Objectives

At the end of this chapter, you should be able to:
- Understand the normal pattern of growth in children
- Take appropriate history and examine children with short stature
- Identify children with global and specific developmental delay

GROWTH

Four phases of growth are recognized:

1. Infantile phase (birth to 1 year): dependent on nutrition. Insulin and thyroxine also play a crucial role.
2. Childhood phase (1 year to 5 years): dependent on growth hormone and thyroxine.
3. Mid-childhood phase (5 years to puberty): increased levels of adrenal androgens influence growth.
4. Pubertal phase: growth spurt caused by increased levels of sex steroids.

Growth is assessed by measuring three specific parameters:

- Height (or length in children unable to stand).
- Weight.
- Head circumference.

Centile charts showing the normal range of values for these measurements from before birth to adulthood are available (see Part II). Problems with inadequate weight gain ('faltering growth') and abnormal head growth (microcephaly and macrocephaly) are considered elsewhere. An approach to the evaluation of 'short stature' is presented here. In preterm infants the corrected age (chronological age minus number of weeks preterm) should be used until 2 years of age.

Short stature

A pragmatic definition of short stature requiring further evaluation is:

- A height below the 0.4th centile for age.
- A predicted height less than the mid-parental target height.
- An abnormal growth velocity as indicated by the height changing by more than the width of one centile band over 1–2 years.

HINTS AND TIPS

Serial measurements of growth velocity for children with short stature form an integral part of their follow-up and assessment. A normal growth velocity for that child is reassuring and further investigation unnecessary.

The causes of short stature are shown in Fig. 11.1.

History

This should elicit information about:

- Early childhood illness and systemic disorders.
- Parental height: the genetic height potential is estimated by calculating the target centile range (TCR) from the mid-parental height (MPH).
- Family history: inherited skeletal dysplasias.

To estimate the adult height potential, calculate the mid-parental height (MPH):

- Father's height plus mother's height divided by 2.

Then adjust for the sex of the child:

- Boys: add 7 cm.
- Girls: subtract 7 cm.

Identify the mid-parental centile, i.e. the centile nearest to the MPH. The TCR is encompassed by MPH:

- ±10 cm in boys.
- ±8.5 cm in girls.

Examination

Examine the following:

- Height: measure accurately with a wall-mounted, calibrated stadiometer.
- Growth velocity: a minimum of two measurements, 6 months apart, is required. Adjust to cm/year and plot at midpoint in time.

> **Fig. 11.1** Causes of short stature
>
> Familial short stature
>
> Constitutional delay of pubertal growth spurt
>
> Endocrine disorders:
> • Growth hormone deficiency
> • Hypopituitarism
> • Hypothyroidism
> • Cushing syndrome/steroid excess
>
> Chromosomal disorders/syndromes:
> • Turner syndrome
> • Silver–Russell syndrome
>
> Skeletal dysplasias:
> • Achondroplasia
>
> Emotional/psychosocial deprivation
>
> Chronic illness:
> • Congenital heart disease
> • Cystic fibrosis
> • Cerebral palsy
> • Chronic renal failure

- Dysmorphic features: these might identify a syndrome (see Hints and tips box).
- Weight (see Hints and tips box).
- Visual fields and fundi: might indicate a pituitary tumour.
- Stage of puberty.

An approach to the evaluation of short stature is shown in Fig. 11.2.

Investigations

Investigations that might be of value include the following:

- Bone age: estimated from X-rays of the left wrist (delayed skeletal maturity in constitutional pubertal delay).
- Karyotype: chromosomal analysis to identify Turner syndrome (45, X0) in short girls.
- Skeletal survey: in disproportion (skeletal dysplasias).
- Endocrine investigations: thyroid function tests (T4, TSH) and growth hormone (secretion is pulsatile so a provocation test, e.g. exercise or insulin-induced hypoglycaemia, is necessary to identify deficiency).
- Computed tomography (CT) or magnetic resonance imaging (MRI): for suspected craniopharyngioma.
- MRI: looking at pituitary.

HINTS AND TIPS

Endocrine causes of short stature are often associated with increased weight, e.g.:
• Hypothyroidism.
• Growth hormone deficiency.
• Steroid excess.

Fig. 11.2 Short stature algorithm

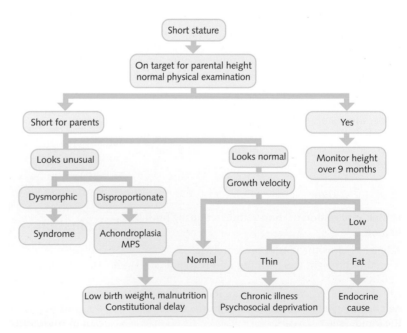

Syndromes associated with short stature:
- Turner syndrome: neck-webbing, wide-spaced nipples, low hairline in a girl.
- Prader–Willi syndrome: obesity, hypotonia and, in boys, small genitals.
- Skeletal dysplasias: disproportionate limbs and trunk – short limbs (achondroplasia) or short trunk (mucopolysaccharidosis; MPS).

Height should be monitored over 6–12 months in response to parental concern regardless of current centile.

DEVELOPMENTAL DELAY

Normal development depends on genetic potential and on the environment: nature and nurture. There is a wide variation in normal rates of development in all spheres. Delay can be global or specific; normal development is described in Chapter 2.

Delay can present through:
- Parental concern.
- Routine surveillance.
- Concern of teacher, health visitor, etc.

A list of warning signs shown in developmental delay by age is given in Fig. 11.3.

Development is assessed in four main areas:
- Gross motor.
- Vision and fine motor.
- Hearing and speech.
- Social behaviour.

Global delay

An intellectually impaired child is delayed in all aspects of development, but not all children with general delay are intellectually impaired; 40% will have a chromosomal abnormality, 5–10% will have developmental malformations and 4% will have a metabolic cause.

History

This should encompass:
- Birth history: details of pregnancy and birth including prematurity, hypoxia and significant perinatal events.

Fig. 11.3 Warning signs of developmental delay by age

Year	Sign
First 8 weeks	Not smiling in response Poor eye contact Head lag Silent baby – no coos, gurgles
8 months	Poor interaction Not sitting with support Not babbling
Second 18 months	Not recognizing own name Not walking three steps alone Not using first words
24 months	Not giving/receiving affection Unable to build a three-brick tower Not linking two words
Third	Unable to play Unsteady gait Not using more than 50 words

- Family history: of learning disability.
- Developmental milestones.
- Social history: risk factors, e.g. psychosocial deprivation.

Examination

You should examine the following:
- Developmental assessment.
- Appearance: dysmorphic features in syndromes associated with delay, e.g. Down syndrome, Williams syndrome, fragile X syndrome.
- Head circumference: microcephaly.

Investigations

These are directed towards identifying a specific aetiology (Fig. 11.4) and will include:
- Karyotype: Down syndrome, fragile X syndrome.
- Thyroid function tests.
- Congenital infection screen.
- Plasma and urine amino and organic acids.
- Brain imaging: MR spectroscopy.

It is important to distinguish developmental delay from actual regression. Loss of previously acquired skills suggests a serious inherited neurodegenerative disorder.

Specific developmental delay

Two common and important examples of delayed development in specific areas are walking and speech.

Fig. 11.4 Causes of global developmental delay

Type	Causes
Perinatal	Hypoxic-ischaemic Intracranial haemorrhage Teratogens
Metabolic	Hypothyroidism Inborn errors of metabolism
Infection	Meningitis Encephalitis
Genetic Neurodegenerative disease	Chromosome disorders Tay–Sachs syndrome Adrenoleucodystrophy

Fig. 11.5 Causes of late walking

Normal variants	Organic causes
Familial 'Bottom shuffler' 'Commando crawler'	Cerebral palsy Congenital dislocation of the hip Duchenne muscular dystrophy (boys)

Delayed walking

The percentage of children who are walking unsupported is:

- 50% by 12 months.
- 90% by 15 months.

Further assessment is indicated if a child is not walking unsupported by age 18 months. Many will be normal late walkers, especially if a 'bottom shuffler', but a small percentage will have an underlying problem (Fig. 11.5).

Examination

- Hips: signs of dislocation (waddling gait, leg length discrepancy, limited abduction).
- Tone, power, and tendon reflexes in all limbs.
- Locomotion: 'commando crawler' or 'bottom shuffler'?

Investigations

If indicated:

- Imaging of hips or spine.
- Creatine kinase for Duchenne muscular dystrophy.
- Vitamin D level and bone profile.

Speech and language delay

The development of normal speech and language requires:

- Adequate hearing.
- Cognitive development.
- Coordinated sound production.

Speech refers to the meaningful sounds that are made, whereas language encompasses the complex rules governing the use of these sounds for communication. Language can be further divided into language comprehension and language expression, and independent delays can occur in either aspect. As might be expected, the development of language is highly dependent on general intellectual development.

HINTS AND TIPS

Normal speech and language development:
- 6 months: babbles.
- 12 months: says 'mama' or 'dada', understands simple commands and responds to name.
- 18 months: single words with meaning.
- 2 years: speaks in phrases.
- 4 years: conversation.

The causes of delay in speech and language development include:

- Hearing impairment.
- Environmental factors: lack of stimulus.
- Global delay: the most common cause.
- Psychiatric disorders: autism.
- Familial.
- Bilingual household.

It is worth distinguishing between delay and actual disorders of speech and language such as stammering, dysarthria due to mechanical problems (e.g. cleft palate) or neuromuscular problems (e.g. cerebral palsy).

HINTS AND TIPS

Check the hearing in any child with delayed speech.

Neonatal problems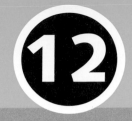

Objectives

At the end of this chapter, you should be able to:
- Understand the common feeding problems in newborns
- Define respiratory distress in newborns
- Identify the common causes of neonatal respiratory distress
- Identify fits in newborns
- Understand the common congenital malformations in newborns

Important presenting problems in the term newborn infant include:
- Feeding difficulties.
- Vomiting.
- Jaundice.
- Breathing difficulties.
- Seizures.
- Congenital malformations.
- Ambiguous genitalia.

FEEDING DIFFICULTIES

Difficulties in establishing feeding can occur with both breast- and bottle-fed newborn infants.

Weight gain in infants

All babies lose weight in the first week. Full term infants should regain their birth weight by day 7–10 and pre-term babies by day 14.

> **HINTS AND TIPS**
>
> Poor feeding in an infant (especially one who has previously fed normally) might indicate severe disease. It is important to note the quantity and frequency of feeds and plot the baby's weight on a centile chart.

Breast feeding

Breast feeding should be encouraged by antenatal education and then supported until it is established. Potential problems include:

- Latching on: chin forward and head tilted back. The areola should be in the baby's mouth as this encourages successful feeding and avoids damage to the nipple.
- Cracked nipples: occur commonly and are more likely if the baby does not latch on well.
- Breast engorgement: prevented by demand feeding and alleviated by expression after feeding.
- Intestinal hurry: frequent loose stools are common on day 4 or 5 when the supply of milk is plentiful. This is normal.

Bottle feeding

Problems that might occur include:

- Incorrect reconstitution: electrolyte abnormalities.
- Inadequate sterilization: gastroenteritis.
- Allergy to the cow's milk protein in formula.

Milks differ in composition and age-specific milks should be used.

VOMITING

Babies often regurgitate (posset) small amounts of milk during and between feeds. This is of no pathological significance and should not be confused with vomiting (the forceful expulsion of gastric contents through the mouth).

Vomiting in the newborn might reflect systemic disease or intestinal obstruction. It is important to establish whether the vomit is:

- Bile-stained.
- Blood-stained.

- Frothy, mucoid.
- Milk.

Important causes are listed in Fig. 12.1. Bile-stained vomit indicates intestinal obstruction until proven otherwise. Blood in the vomit might be of maternal or infant origin. Plain abdominal X-ray is the most useful investigation. Important findings include:

- Dilated loops in obstruction (atresias, malrotation) or ileus (e.g. sepsis).
- 'Double bubble' of duodenal atresia.
- Pneumatosis (gas in bowel wall) in necrotizing enterocolitis.
- Free air in perforation (may require lateral decubitus view).

HINTS AND TIPS

Bloodstained vomit in the newborn might be due to:
- Swallowed maternal blood – predelivery or from a cracked nipple.
- Trauma from a feeding tube.
- Haemorrhagic disease of the newborn – vitamin K deficiency.

JAUNDICE

Neonatal jaundice

Physiological jaundice occurs in most newborns, especially preterms. A combination of increased red cell breakdown and immaturity of the hepatic enzymes causes unconjugated hyperbilirubinaemia. It is exacerbated by dehydration, which can occur if establishment of feeding is delayed.

Onset of jaundice in the first 24 hours of life is always pathological; causes are listed in Fig. 12.2. Recognition and treatment of severe neonatal unconjugated hyperbilirubinaemia is important to avoid bilirubin encephalopathy or kernicterus (brain damage due to deposition of bilirubin in the basal ganglia). Early evaluation of conjugated hyperbilirubinaemia ($>20\,\mu mol/L$) is important to allow early (<6 weeks) diagnosis and treatment of biliary atresia. Jaundice persisting for >2 weeks also requires investigation.

Jaundice in the first 24 hours

This is always pathological. The most common cause is haemolysis, which can be due to:

Fig. 12.1 Vomiting in the newborn

Cause	Features/examples
Intestinal obstruction	Small bowel: • Duodenal atresia/stenosis (30% have Down syndrome) • Malrotation with volvulus • Meconium ileus (cystic fibrosis) Large bowel: • Hirschsprung's disease • Rectal atresia
Tracheo-oesophageal fistula	Frothy mucoid vomiting occurs if a feed is given
Infections: • Gastroenteritis • Urinary tract infection • Septicaemia • Meningitis	Often non-specific
Necrotizing enterocolitis	Preterm infants
Raised intracranial pressure	Bulging fontanelle
Congenital adrenal hyperplasia	Ambiguous genitalia in a female infant

Fig. 12.2 Causes of neonatal jaundice

Onset	Cause
Less than 24 hours old	Excess haemolysis: • Immune-mediated – rhesus or ABO incompatibility • Intrinsic red blood cell defects – G6PD, pyruvate kinase deficiency or hereditary spherocytosis Congenital infections
Between 24 hours and 2 weeks old	Physiological jaundice Breast milk jaundice Infection, e.g. urinary tract infection Excess haemolysis, bruising or polycythaemia
Persistent jaundice after 2 weeks old	Unconjugated: • Breast milk jaundice • Infections, e.g. urinary tract infection • Excess haemolysis, e.g. ABO incompatibility, G6PD deficiency • Hypothyroidism (screened for in newborn) • Galactosaemia Conjugated (>15% of total bilirubin): • Biliary atresia • Neonatal hepatitis

- Haemolytic disease of the newborn: rhesus or ABO incompatibility.
- Intrinsic red cell defects: spherocytosis, G6PD deficiency or pyruvate kinase deficiency.

Haemolytic disorders Isoimmune haemolysis is the destruction of fetal and neonatal red blood cells by maternal IgG antibodies that cross the placenta during pregnancy. Maternal sensitization is caused by fetal–maternal transfusion during current or previous pregnancies, or from mismatched blood transfusions.

The incidence of rhesus (Rh) haemolytic disease has fallen since the introduction of anti-D immune globulin, which is given to the Rh-negative mother immediately after birth of a Rh-positive infant, or after potentially sensitizing events, e.g. antepartum haemorrhage. Severe haemolysis may also occur antenatally causing anaemia and hydrops fetalis, which is treated by intrauterine blood transfusion.

ABO incompatibility is more common than Rh haemolytic disease. The usual combination is a group O mother with a group A, or less commonly group B, infant. The anti-A or anti-B haemolysins are comparatively weak. There is mild anaemia, no organomegaly, a weakly positive Coombs' test and mild jaundice peaking in the first few days. No prior sensitization is needed in ABO incompatibility.

Jaundice at 2 days to 2 weeks of age

The most common cause is physiological jaundice, due to the combination of liver enzyme immaturity and an increased load of bilirubin from red cell breakdown. Prematurity, bruising or polycythaemia (haematocrit >0.65) can exacerbate it. Physiological jaundice usually peaks on the third day of life.

Infection also causes unconjugated hyperbilirubinaemia at this time.

Prolonged jaundice (>2 weeks of age)

Prolonged jaundice (>2 weeks in term infants, >3 weeks in premature infants) is usually an unconjugated hyperbilirubinaemia, which can be due to:

- 'Breast milk' jaundice: affects 15% of healthy breast-fed infants. The cause is unknown. It usually resolves by 3–4 weeks of age.
- Infection: particularly of the urinary tract.
- Congenital hypothyroidism: this should have been detected on neonatal screening.

Investigations for babies presenting with prolonged jaundice include: measurement of conjugated fraction, full blood count (FBC), blood group (mother and baby) and direct antiglobulin test (DAT), urine culture and thyroid function if routine screening has not been performed.

Conjugated hyperbilirubinaemia is associated with dark urine and pale stools. Causes include neonatal hepatitis and biliary atresia. Early diagnosis of biliary atresia is important because delay in surgical treatment beyond 6 weeks of age compromises outcome.

Management of neonatal jaundice

Investigations are directed towards establishing the cause (see Chapter 28). Clinical estimation of the severity is unreliable and a transcutaneous or plasma bilirubin must be measured in any significantly jaundiced infant.

Bilirubin encephalopathy occurs when unconjugated bilirubin is deposited in the brain, especially in the basal ganglia and cerebellum. This presents initially with lethargy, rigidity, eye-rolling and seizures. The long-term sequelae include choreoathetoid cerebral palsy, sensorineural deafness and learning difficulties.

Many factors in addition to the bilirubin level influence this risk. These include:

- The infant's gestational age: risk increases for preterm infants.
- The postnatal age: risk decreases with increasing postnatal age.
- The serum albumin level: risk increases with hypoalbuminaemia.
- Coexistent asphyxia, acidosis or hypoglycaemia.

Consensus charts exist indicating levels at which treatment should be initiated, bearing those factors in mind. Treatment options are:

- Phototherapy.
- Exchange transfusion.

Phototherapy Blue light (not ultraviolet) of wavelength 450 nm converts the bilirubin in the skin and superficial capillaries into harmless water-soluble metabolites, which are excreted in urine and through the bowel. The eyes are covered to prevent discomfort and additional fluids are given to counteract increased losses from skin.

Exchange transfusion This is required if the bilirubin rises to levels considered dangerous despite phototherapy. It rapidly reduces the level of circulating bilirubin, and in isoimmune haemolytic disease also removes circulating antibodies and corrects anaemia. Techniques vary, but conventionally the exchange is done via umbilical artery and vein catheters. Aliquots of baby's blood (10–20 mL) are withdrawn, alternating with infusions of donor blood of the same volumes. Twice the infant's blood volume (i.e. 2×80 mL/kg) is exchanged over about 2 hours. It carries risks associated with transfusion, fluid overload, electrolyte imbalance and depletion of coagulation factors. In immune-mediated haemolysis administration of immunoglobulin is recommended as it may avoid the need for exchange transfusion.

HINTS AND TIPS

- Onset of jaundice in the first 24 hours of life is always pathological.
- Consider biliary atresia in an infant with persistent neonatal jaundice due to conjugated hyperbilirubinaemia and pale stools (rare but treatable).

HINTS AND TIPS

Definition of physiological jaundice:
- Onset after 24 hours of birth.
- Resolves within 2 weeks.
- Unconjugated.
- Total bilirubin <350 μmol/L.

BREATHING DIFFICULTIES

In the newborn, breathing difficulties are referred to as respiratory distress. The signs of respiratory distress are:

- Tachypnoea: respiratory rate over 60/min.
- Recession: subcostal or intercostal.
- Nasal flaring.
- Expiratory grunting.
- Cyanosis.

Common breathing difficulties

The most common cause of breathing difficulties in the newborn is the respiratory distress syndrome due to surfactant deficiency, a condition largely confined to preterm infants. The major causes of respiratory distress in term infants are shown in Fig. 12.3.

Fig. 12.3 Causes of respiratory distress in term infants

Pulmonary	Non-pulmonary
Transient tachypnoea of newborn	Septicaemia
Pneumonia	Severe anaemia
Meconium aspiration	Congenital cardiac disease
Respiratory diaphragmatic hernia	
Choanal atresia	
Pneumothorax	

Respiratory distress syndrome

Only 1% of cases of respiratory distress syndrome (RDS) occur in the term neonate. Such infants are often difficult to ventilate but do respond to surfactant therapy, in a similar manner to the preterm with RDS.

Transient tachypnoea of the newborn

Transient tachypnoea of the newborn (TTN) is a benign self-limiting condition believed to be caused by a delay in the normal reabsorption of the lung fluid at birth. It is more common after caesarean section and in infants of diabetic mothers. The chest X-ray (CXR) might show a streaky appearance with fluid in the horizontal fissure; it usually resolves within 48 hours.

Meconium aspiration

Approximately 10% of term neonates pass meconium before birth; it is rare in preterm babies. It is associated with fetal distress, e.g. hypoxic insult. Inhalation of meconium results in bronchial obstruction and collapse, chemical pneumonitis and secondary infection – all leading to respiratory distress. There is also a high incidence of air-leak (pneumothorax, pneumomediastinum) and pulmonary hypertension.

Pneumonia

Risk factors include premature labour and prolonged rupture of the membranes (over 24 hours). Group B streptococcal infection is an important cause of early onset pneumonia.

Pneumothorax

Spontaneous pneumothorax occurs in about 1% of term infants and does not usually require intervention. In ventilated babies it is commonly iatrogenic. Diagnosis is by CXR and transillumination of the chest.

Persistent pulmonary hypertension of the newborn

Pulmonary vascular resistance remains high after birth causing right to left shunting at both atrial and ductal levels with severe cyanosis. It can occur as a primary disorder but is more commonly a complication of perinatal asphyxia, meconium aspiration, severe sepsis or respiratory distress syndrome. A CXR might show pulmonary oligaemia. Diagnosis is suggested by differences in PaO_2 on pre- and postductal arterial blood gases (ABGs) and confirmed by echocardiography.

Diaphragmatic hernia

In this uncommon malformation (1:2000–4000 births), a hole in the diaphragm (usually on the left) allows the abdominal contents to herniate into the chest. Fortunately most are diagnosed on antenatal ultrasound scan, as this allows for appropriate early management: early intubation and nasogastric aspiration (to avoid inflation of the bowel). Surgical repair is then undertaken once the neonate is stable. If not antenatally diagnosed, it usually presents with failure to respond to resuscitation at birth. The apex beat and heart sounds are displaced to the right with poor air entry on the left. The relatively high mortality is accounted for by the inevitable pulmonary hypoplasia due to compression of the fetal lung.

Congenital malformations of the lung

Respiratory distress may arise from various congenital malformations including:

* Pulmonary hypoplasia: poor lung development may occur with oligohydramnios or neuromuscular abnormalities.
* Sequestration: development of a section of lung tissue not connected to the pulmonary vasculature.
* Cystic adenomatoid malformation of the lung: presence of a cystic, non-functioning area of lung (often a whole lobe).
* Congenital lobar emphysema.

Chylothorax

A rare cause of respiratory distress, due to accumulation of lymphatic fluid in the pleural cavity. Can be spontaneous (due to an anomaly of lymphatic drainage) or iatrogenic from birth trauma or thoracotomy.

NEONATAL SEIZURES

Seizures are more common in the neonatal period than at any other time of life because the neonatal brain is mostly excitatory. The manifestations of neonatal seizures are rather different from those in older children and it can be difficult to distinguish true seizures from normal baby movements.

HINTS AND TIPS

Neonatal episodes that are *not* seizures include:
* Jitteriness: the movement is a tremor – rhythmic movements of equal rate and amplitude (in seizures, clonic movements have a fast and slow component). There are no ocular phenomena. It is sensitive to external stimuli and is stopped by holding.
* Benign myoclonus: shock-like jerks when asleep.
* Stretching, sucking movements.

The main types of seizure are:
* Subtle seizures: eye deviation, apnoeas, autonomic phenomena and oral movements.
* Clonic seizures: seen as focal rhythmic and slow jerking; generalized clonic seizures are not seen in neonates.
* Myoclonic seizures: rapid isolated jerks.
* Tonic seizures: manifest as flexor or extensor posturing.

The perinatal and birth history together with clinical examination will often indicate the cause.

Initial investigations

* Blood glucose, electrolytes, Ca^{2+}, Mg^{2+}.
* Cerebrospinal fluid (CSF) analysis for infection.
* Cranial ultrasonography for haemorrhages.

As indicated:

* Inborn error of metabolism: blood ammonia, lactate and amino acids, urine amino acids, organic acids, IV pyridoxine test.
* Congenital infection screen.
* Cranial imaging: magnetic resonance imaging (MRI) or computed tomography (CT) may be appropriate. A detectable cause is present in the majority and varies with the time of onset (Fig. 12.4). The most common causes are hypoxic ischaemic encephalopathy, intracranial haemorrhage, CNS infection and congenital abnormality.

Fig. 12.4 Causes of neonatal seizures

Hypoxia	
Electrolyte and metabolic abnormalities	Hypoglycaemia Inborn errors of metabolism
CNS	Haemorrhage Infection Structural abnormality
Drug withdrawal	Opiates Benzodiazepines
Genetic disease	Neurocutaneous diseases
Hyperbilirubinaemia	Bilirubin encephalopathy

CONGENITAL MALFORMATIONS

Up to 70% of major congenital malformations can now be detected antenatally using ultrasound and can affect any of the major organ systems. Some of the most important are described below.

Craniofacial disorders

Cleft lip and palate

This affects about 1:1000 babies. It manifests as:

- Cleft lip alone: 35%.
- Cleft lip and palate: 25%.
- Cleft palate alone: 40%.

Aetiology remains unclear but is thought to be polygenic. Some drugs are specifically teratogenic, including anticonvulsants and methotrexate. Cleft lip is usually diagnosed at the 18–20-week scan but isolated cleft palates are difficult to diagnose antenatally. Some affected infants can be breast fed; others require special long teats or other feeding devices. Surgical repair is carried out at 6–12 months of age on the palate, and either early (first week) or late (3 months) on the lip.

Pierre Robin anomaly

This is an association of micrognathia, posterior displacement of the tongue and midline cleft of the soft palate. Prone positioning maintains airway patency until growth of the mandible is established. The cleft is surgically repaired.

Gastrointestinal disorders

Oesophageal atresia

The incidence is 1:3500 live births. A tracheo-oesophageal fistula (TOF) is usually present (Fig. 12.5). As the fetus is unable to swallow during intrauterine life, there is associated polyhydramnios. Diagnosis should be established before the first feed by attempting to pass a feeding tube into the stomach and checking its location by X-ray. Forty per cent of cases have other associated abnormalities, e.g. as part of the VACTERL association:

- Vertebral.
- Anorectal.
- Cardiac.
- Tracheo-oesophageal.
- Renal.
- Limb (radial).

Abdominal wall defects

Gastroschisis (1:5000)

The bowel protrudes without any covering sac through a defect in the anterior abdominal wall adjacent to the umbilicus. This is usually an isolated anomaly.

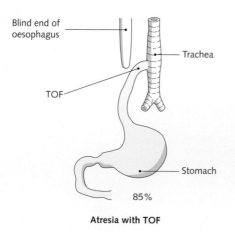
Atresia with TOF — 85%

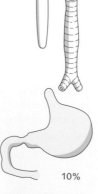
Atresia without TOF — 10%

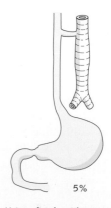
H-type fistula without atresia — 5%

Fig. 12.5 Oesophageal atresia and tracheo-oesophageal fistula (TOF)

Exomphalos (1:2500)

The abdominal contents herniate through the umbilical ring and are covered with a sac formed by the peritoneum and amniotic membrane. It is often associated with other major congenital abnormalities.

Neural tube defects

These arise from failure of fusion of the neural plate in the first 28 days after conception. The incidence in the UK has fallen dramatically since the 1970s because of improved maternal nutrition, folic acid supplementation and better antenatal screening.

> **HINTS AND TIPS**
>
> Folic acid supplements should ideally be taken pre-conception and all pregnant women are advised to take them during the first trimester.

The three main types are:

- Spina bifida occulta.
- Meningocele.
- Myelomeningocele.

They are usually in the lumbosacral region (Fig. 12.6). However neural tube defects also include:

- Encephalocoele: extrusion of the brain and meninges through a midline skull defect.
- Anencephaly: the cranium and brain fail to develop (detected on antenatal ultrasound and termination of pregnancy is usually offered).

Spina bifida occulta

The dorsal vertebral arch fails to fuse. There may be an overlying skin lesion such as a tuft of hair or small dermal sinus. Tethering of the cord (diastomyelia) can cause neurological deficits with growth.

Meningocele

This is uncommon (5% of cases). The smooth, intact, skin-covered cystic swelling is filled with CSF. There is no neurological deficit or hydrocephalus and excision and closure of the defect is undertaken after 3 months.

Myelomeningocele

This accounts for more than 90% of overt spina bifida. These are open with herniation of both the cord and meninges; there is commonly leaking of CSF. Neurological deficits are always present and can include:

- Motor and sensory loss in the lower limbs.
- Neuropathic bladder and bowel.

In addition, there is often scoliosis and associated hydrocephalus due to the Arnold–Chiari malformation (herniation of the cerebellar tonsils through the foramen magnum). Surgery prevents infection but does not restore neurological function.

Congenital talipes equinovarus (club foot)

The entire foot is fixed in an inverted and supinated position (Fig. 12.7). This should be distinguished from 'positional talipes', in which the deformity is mild and can be corrected with passive manipulation.

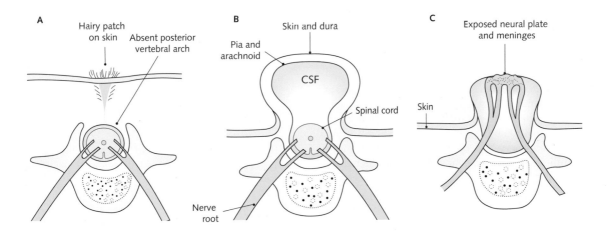

Fig. 12.6 Neural tube defects: (A) spina bifida occulta; (B) meningocele; (C) myelomeningocele

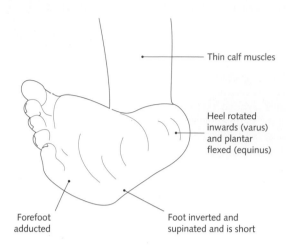

Fig. 12.7 Talipes equinovarus (club foot)

Referral should be made to orthopaedic surgeons and physiotherapy as early treatment (including serial casting where appropriate) is important to prevent disability.

HINTS AND TIPS

Features of talipes equinovarus:
- 1.5 per 1000 live births.
- Male to female ratio: 2:1.
- 50% bilateral.
- Multifactorial inheritance.
- Associated with oligohydramnios, congenital hip dislocation and neuromuscular disorders, e.g. spina bifida

COMPLEX GENITAL ANOMALY

Visible abnormalities of the external genitalia range from the common, e.g. hypospadias, to complex genital anomaly where the sex of the individual is unclear. Around 1 in 4500 infants have complex genital anomaly at birth. It is a very difficult area raising strong emotions in families and great care should be taken when discussing investigation and management. The most common cause of ambiguous external genitalia is congenital adrenal hyperplasia (CAH) leading to a virilized female (see Chapter 24).

HINTS AND TIPS

- Congenital adrenal hyperplasia (CAH) leading to virilization of a female infant is the most common cause of ambiguous genitalia.
- In two-thirds of children with CAH, a life-threatening, salt-losing adrenal crisis occurs at 1–3 weeks of age requiring urgent IV treatment with saline and glucose. This might be the first indication in boys.

COMMUNICATION

Establishing the definitive cause of ambiguous genitalia takes time and it is important not to attempt to guess the future sex of rearing. Parents also need to be reassured that the baby will be either male or female and not intersex, though it may take some time to determine that. Expert counselling is required.

Examination should include measurement of the blood pressure (adrenal problem). Investigations will include:

- Urgent chromosomal analysis: fluoresence in situ hybridization (FISH) for the sex-determining region of Y chromosome (SRY) and karyotype.
- Ultrasound imaging of pelvic organs and adrenal glands.
- Electrolyte and endocrine investigations (17-hydroxy-progesterone is increased in CAH).

The chromosomal sex does not necessarily determine the sex of rearing, The decision may include consideration of the ability to fashion external genitalia.

Further reading

World Health Organization (WHO) Genomics Resource Centre, Gender and genetics. www.who.int/genomics/gender/en/index.html.

National Institute for Health and Clinical Excellence (NICE), May 2010. Guidance on neonatal jaundice. http://www.nice.org.uk/CG98.

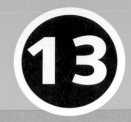
Objectives

At the end of this chapter you should be able to:
• Differentiate among the common viral exanthems
• Understand the common infectious diseases affecting children
• Identify the symptoms and signs of Kawasaki disease
• Know the common causes of immunodeficiency in children

Despite the spectacular successes achieved by public health measures and immunization programmes in preventing infectious diseases, these remain a major cause of mortality and morbidity in childhood:

• In the developing world, 12 million children under 5 years of age die each year from the combined effects of malnutrition and infections such as gastroenteritis, pneumonia, measles and malaria.

• In the developed world, major diseases such as diphtheria and polio have been effectively eliminated, and the infection rates of others such as invasive disease caused by *Haemophilus influenzae* type B, measles, mumps, rubella and pertussis are greatly reduced.

In the UK there has been a resurgence of some of these diseases, particularly measles due to a reduction in immunization coverage following adverse media reports on their safety. The worldwide resurgence of tuberculosis (TB), together with the growing impact of human immunodeficiency virus (HIV) infection in childhood, leaves no room for complacency.

VIRAL INFECTIONS

Viral exanthems

The term 'exanthem' is applied to diseases in which a rash is a prominent manifestation. Classically, six exanthems with similar rashes were described. They are numbered in the order in which they were described and are listed in Fig. 13.1. The second disease is, of course, bacterial in origin and the fourth disease is no longer recognized as an entity.

Measles ('first disease')

Incidence and aetiology

Measles is caused by infection with a single-stranded RNA virus of the *Morbillivirus* genus. The incidence in England and Wales declined dramatically after vaccination was introduced (1968), from a pattern of epidemics every 2 years, with up to 800 000 cases a year in the 1960s, to 50 000–100 000 cases a year in the 1980s. Following the introduction of the MMR (measles, mumps, rubella) vaccination in 1988, notifications fell further to just 10 000 cases in 1993. However, outbreaks are now being seen because the immunization rate fell after public concerns about the safety of MMR vaccination.

Clinical features

Fever, cough, coryza and conjunctivitis are followed (in some cases) by the pathognomonic Koplik's spots on the buccal mucosa and, after 3 or 4 days, by an erythematous maculopapular rash. The rash spreads downward from the hairline to the whole body, becomes blotchy and confluent and might desquamate in the second week.

Measles is highly infectious. Transmission is by droplet spread and the incubation period is about 10 days. Measles is very dangerous in immunocompromised children, such as those in remission from acute leukaemia or with HIV. These children are susceptible to giant cell pneumonia and encephalitis. In developing countries, malnutrition and particularly vitamin A deficiency impairs immunity and renders measles a more severe disease. A targeted immunization campaign has reduced deaths due to measles by 66% over the last 10 years.

Complications

Acute complications include febrile convulsions, otitis media, tracheobronchitis and pneumonia due either to the primary virus infection or bacterial superinfection (Fig. 13.2). Rarely, severe encephalitis occurs (1:5000 cases) about 8 days after onset of the illness. The mortality is 15% and severe neurological sequelae occur in 40% of survivors of encephalitis. (Subacute sclerosing panencephalitis, SSPE, is a very rare immune-mediated

Fig. 13.1 Viral exanthems

		Pathogen
First	Measles	Paramyxovirus
Second	Scarlet fever	Group A β-haemolytic streptococcus
Third	Rubella	Togavirus
Fourth	'Duke's disease'	–
Fifth	Erythema infectiosum	Parvovirus B19
Sixth	Roseola infantum	Human herpesvirus 6

Fig. 13.2 Complications of measles

Giant cell pneumonia
Conjunctivitis and keratitis
Middle ear infection
Secondary gastrointestinal infections
Encephalitis
Subacute sclerosing panencephalitis

neurodegenerative disease that can occur 7–10 years after measles.)

Diagnosis

Diagnosis can be made following a buccal swab analysis. Measles can also be confirmed by the detection of specific IgM in serum samples ideally taken from 3 days after the appearance of the rash. The disease is notifiable.

Management

Treatment is symptomatic.

COMMUNICATION

In February 1998, a single research paper authored by Dr Andrew Wakefield was published in *The Lancet* concerning links between MMR and autism. Further publications by Dr Wakefield ensued, criticizing the MMR vaccine, and as a result there was an unprecedented collapse in public confidence. In January 2010, Dr Wakefield was found guilty of three dozen charges and erased from the medical register. *The Lancet* also fully retracted the paper. Parents must therefore be reassured that there is no link to autism and the benefits of vaccination.

Rubella (German measles)

This mild childhood disease is caused by infection with the rubivirus. Its importance lies in the devastating effect maternal infection in early gestation has on the fetus.

Clinical features

Infection is subclinical in up to half of infected individuals. After an incubation period of 14–21 days, a low-grade fever is followed by a pink-red maculopapular rash, which starts on the face and spreads rapidly over the entire body. The rash is fleeting and might have gone entirely by the third day. Generalized lymphadenopathy, particularly affecting the suboccipital and postauricular nodes, is a prominent feature.

Complications

Complications are unusual in childhood but include arthritis (typically affecting the small joints of the hand), encephalitis and thrombocytopenia.

Diagnosis

Diagnosis is clinical and differentiation from other viral exanthems is often difficult. In circumstances in which it is important, detection of rubella-specific IgM in the saliva or serum is necessary to confirm the diagnosis.

Prevention (immunization)

A live, attenuated vaccine has been available for many years. Since 1988, this has been given as part of the MMR vaccine to all children at 13 months of age and a booster between 3 and 5 years of age. Vaccine failure is rare and, in most people, it provides lifelong protection. The presence of IgG, specific for rubella, indicates immunity as a result of prior infection or immunization.

Congenital rubella

Incidence and diagnosis

The risk and extent of fetal damage is mainly determined by the gestational age at the onset of maternal infection.

Maternal infection at up to 10 weeks' gestation confers a 90% risk of some degree of damage that is often severe and includes deafness, congenital heart disease and cataracts. Between 13 and 16 weeks' gestation, there is a 30% risk of hearing impairment. Beyond this gestation damage is unlikely. Although congenital rubella is now rare in the UK (14 cases notified in the period 1991–1994), the diagnosis is worth consideration in any growth-restricted newborn or child with unexplained sensorineural deafness.

Clinical features

Clinical features of congenital rubella are shown in Fig. 13.3.

Fig. 13.3 Clinical features of congenital rubella

Growth retardation
Hepatosplenomegaly
Congenital heart disease
• Patent ductus arteriosus
• Pulmonary stenosis
Eye
• Glaucoma
• Cataract
• Retinopathy
Ear
• Sensorineural deafness

Management

All pregnant women and women contemplating pregnancy should be screened for antirubella IgG. Immigrants to the UK from countries where rubella vaccination is not routine are at particular risk of not being immune. Women found to be seronegative on antenatal screening receive immunization after delivery.

Pregnant women exposed to rubella should be tested for antirubella IgG and IgM regardless of previous history or serological testing. A high likelihood of congenital rubella infection early in pregnancy is an indication for offering termination of the pregnancy.

Erythema infectiosum or slapped cheek disease ('fifth disease')

This is caused by infection with parvovirus B19, a small DNA virus that is the only parvovirus pathogenic to humans. Transmission can occur via respiratory secretions, from mother to fetus, and by transmission of contaminated blood products.

Clinical features

Asymptomatic infection is common. Erythema infectiosum describes the most common disease pattern of fever followed a week later by a characteristic rash. This starts as a red appearance on the face (hence the name 'slapped-cheek disease') and progresses to a symmetrical lacy rash on the extremities and trunk.

The virus suppresses erythropoiesis for up to 7 days. In children with haemolytic anaemia, such as sickle cell disease or hereditary spherocytosis, parvovirus infection can cause an aplastic crisis. Maternal infection during pregnancy can be transmitted to the fetus and causes hydrops fetalis (due to fetal anaemia and myocarditis), fetal death or spontaneous abortion.

Diagnosis and management

Diagnosis is clinical, but if confirmation is important (e.g. in pregnancy), specific IgM can be detected 2 weeks after exposure. Management is symptomatic.

'Sixth disease': roseola infantum

Roseola infantum is caused by infection with human herpesvirus (HHV)-6 or HHV-7.

Clinical features and diagnosis

Most children acquire the infection between the age of 3 months and 4 years; 65% are seropositive by 1 year of age. There is sudden onset of a high fever (>39 °C) with irritability lasting for 3–6 days. The fever then falls abruptly and a widespread maculopapular rash appears on the face, neck and trunk. Other common features include cervical lymphadenopathy, cough and coryza. Up to one-third of febrile convulsions in children <2 years of age are caused by HHV-6. Diagnosis is clinical.

Management

Management is supportive, paying attention to antipyretics for fever and fluid rehydration.

Rare complications include aseptic meningitis, encephalitis, hepatitis and massive lymphadenopathy.

Herpes infections

There are eight human herpesviruses. They cause a number of common and important diseases in children. The hallmark of these viruses is their capacity to become latent with subsequent recurrence, causing, for example, shingles (varicella zoster) and cold sores (HSV1).

The human herpesviruses and their corresponding diseases are shown in Fig. 13.4.

Herpes simplex virus 1 (HSV1, HHV-1)

Clinical features

Most primary infections with HSV1 are asymptomatic. The most common clinical manifestation in childhood is gingivostomatitis. The child (usually a toddler) presents with high fever, misery and vesicular lesions on the lips, gums, tongue and hard palate, which might progress to painful, extensive ulceration. The illness can last as long as 2 weeks.

Less commonly, infection can involve the:

• Eye: causing dendritic ulcers on the cornea.
• Skin: causing eczema herpeticum in children with eczema.
• Fingers: causing a herpetic whitlow.
• Brain: causing herpes simplex encephalitis (HSE).

Treatment

Occasionally, IV fluids will be required for gingivostomatitis but in this condition oral aciclovir has only a marginal effect. High-dose IV aciclovir is used in HSE.

The virus becomes latent in the dorsal root ganglion supplying the trigeminal nerve where subsequent reactivation (by UV light, stress or menstruation) can cause labial herpes (cold sores) in later life.

Fig. 13.4 Human herpesviruses (HHV) and their diseases

	Virus	Disease
HHV-1	Herpes simplex virus 1	Oral infection and encephalitis
HHV-2	Herpes simplex virus 2	Neonatal and genital infection
HHV-3	Varicella zoster	Chickenpox and shingles
HHV-4	Epstein–Barr virus	Glandular fever
HHV-5	Cytomegalovirus	Congenital infection and in immunosuppression
HHV-6/7		Roseola

Herpes simplex virus 2 (HSV2, HHV-2)

Transmission of HSV2 from the genital tract of a mother who is often asymptomatic can result in neonatal herpes infection. Neonatal herpes has high mortality and morbidity. It causes a generalized infection with pneumonia, hepatitis and encephalitis, with onset usually in the first week of life. Treatment is high-dose IV aciclovir and supportive care.

Elective caesarean section is indicated when a mother with active genital herpes goes into labour as this mode of delivery offers neonatal protection.

Varicella zoster (HHV-3, VZV)

Chickenpox is a common childhood disease caused by primary infection with the varicella zoster virus (VZV). It is highly infectious with transmission occurring by droplet infection (the respiratory route), direct contact or contact with soiled materials. The average incubation period is 14 days.

Clinical features
A brief coryzal period is followed by the eruption of an itchy, vesicular rash. This starts on the scalp or trunk and spreads centrifugally. Crops appear over 3–5 days and the mucous membranes might be involved.

Complications
Complications are unusual in immunocompetent children but can include secondary bacterial infection of the skin with staphylococci or streptococci and an encephalitis (often affecting the cerebellum), which appears 3–6 days after onset of the rash. Chickenpox can, however, be a very severe disease (mortality 20%) in the immunosuppressed child (children on systemic steroids) and in the newborn infant if the mother develops chickenpox just before delivery. Persisting fever after the typical chickenpox rash has erupted should prompt evaluation for secondary infection.

Diagnosis
Diagnosis is clinical but virus isolated from vesicular fluid can be identified by electron microscopy or culture. The period of infectivity is from 2 days before eruption of the rash until all the lesions are encrusted.

Treatment
Treatment is symptomatic. However, the exposed immunosuppressed child should be given varicella zoster immune globulin (VZIG) if known to be seronegative. VZIG should also be given to newborn babies if the mother develops varicella or herpes zoster in the 7 days before or after birth and to any exposed preterm infant. Aciclovir should be given in severe chickenpox or for clinical infection in an immunocompromised child or newborn infant. Antibiotics are also given concurrently to cover secondary skin infection.

A live, attenuated vaccine does exist but is not currently given in the UK.

Herpes zoster (shingles)

This is due to reactivation of latent varicella zoster and is uncommon in childhood. A vesicular eruption occurs in the distribution of a sensory dermatome, mainly in the cervical and sacral regions. In adults they tend to be thoracic and lumbar. Also, unlike adults, postherpetic neuralgia and malignant association are rare. Treatment with antivirals is not routinely indicated.

Epstein–Barr virus (HHV-4, EBV)

The Epstein–Barr virus (EBV) has a particular tropism for the epithelial cells of the oropharynx and nasopharynx, and for B lymphocytes. It is the major cause of infectious mononucleosis syndrome and is also involved in the pathogenesis of Burkitt's lymphoma and nasopharyngeal carcinoma.

Clinical features

Transmission occurs by droplet transmission or directly via saliva ('the kissing disease'). Most people are infected asymptomatically in childhood. Symptomatic infection (infectious mononucleosis or glandular fever) is most common in adolescents. The incubation period is 30–50 days.

Glandular fever is characterized by fever, malaise, pharyngitis (which may be exudative) and cervical lymphadenopathy. Petechiae might be seen on the palate and a sparse maculopapular rash might occur. Splenomegaly is present in 50% of cases and hepatomegaly with hepatitis (usually anicteric) in 10%. A florid rash might develop if amoxicillin is given. The infection can persist for up to 3 months.

Diagnosis

Diagnosis is usually clinical. The blood shows atypical lymphocytes (T cells) and a heterophile antibody, which is the basis of slide agglutination tests like Monospot and Paul–Bunnell tests. The latter appears only in the second week and might not be produced in young children. Specific EBV serology – IgM to viral capsid antigen (VCA) – is available and more reliable. The differential diagnosis is from other causes of infectious mononucleosis (cytomegalovirus, toxoplasmosis) and other causes of pharyngitis.

Management

Management is symptomatic. Rarely, massive pharyngeal swelling can compromise the airway. This is helped by corticosteroid treatment.

Cytomegalovirus (HHV-5, CMV)

Cytomegalovirus (CMV) is a common human pathogen. It is transmitted from mother to fetus via the placenta in utero, via the oral or genital routes, and by blood transfusion or organ transplantation.

> **HINTS AND TIPS**
>
> - CMV is a common congenital infection and can cause severe disease.
> - Congenital CMV infection is an important cause of sensorineural hearing loss.
> - CMV-negative blood must be used for transfusion in immunodeficient patients.

Incidence

In the UK, about half of all pregnant women are susceptible to CMV and about 1% of these will have a primary CMV infection during pregnancy. In almost half of these mothers, the infant will be infected, making CMV the most common congenital infection with an incidence of 3:1000 live births. However, many infants with congenital CMV are asymptomatic and develop normally.

Clinical features

Infection is mild or asymptomatic in adults or children with normal immunity. It can cause a mononucleosis syndrome with pharyngitis and lymphadenopathy. Severe congenital infection causes:

- Intrauterine growth restriction.
- Hepatosplenomegaly, jaundice and thrombocytopenia.
- Microcephaly, intracranial calcification and chorioretinitis.
- Long-term sequelae include cerebral palsy, epilepsy, learning disability and sensorineural hearing loss. Hearing loss might develop later in life without signs of infection in the newborn period.

In the immunocompromised host, CMV can cause severe disease including pneumonitis or encephalitis. It is a particularly important pathogen following organ transplantation.

Diagnosis and treatment

Diagnosis is made by viral isolation, especially from urine. To confirm congenital infection, specimens for viral isolation must be taken within 3 weeks of birth.

Treatment with ganciclovir might be effective in immunocompromised patients and can also be used to treat congenital CMV infection although the efficacy of this is still under investigation.

Mumps

Mumps is caused by infection with an RNA virus of the Paramyxoviridae family. Routine vaccination at 12–15 months, as a component of the MMR vaccine, has markedly reduced the incidence. Transmission is by droplet spread and the incubation period is 14–21 days.

Clinical features

The clinical manifestations include fever, malaise and parotitis. Pain and swelling of the parotid gland might initially be unilateral. Parotid gland enlargement is more easily seen than felt, between the angle of the mandible and sternomastoid – extending beneath the ear lobe, which is pushed upwards and outwards.

The swelling usually subsides within 7–10 days. Patients are infectious from a few days before the onset to up to 3 days after the enlargement subsides.

The central nervous system is commonly involved. Before vaccination was introduced, mumps was the commonest cause of aseptic meningitis. Up to 50% of patients have cerebrospinal fluid (CSF) lymphocytosis and 10% have signs of a meningoencephalitis.

Complications

Complications include pancreatitis (abdominal pain and raised serum amylase levels) and epididymo-orchitis. The latter is uncommon in prepubertal males and is usually unilateral. Even when it is bilateral, infertility is very rare. A postinfectious encephalomyelitis occurs in 1 out of 5000 cases.

Diagnosis and treatment

Diagnosis is usually clinical; treatment is symptomatic.

Enteroviruses

The human enteroviruses include:

- Coxsackie virus A and B.
- Echoviruses.
- Poliovirus.

Coxsackie viruses can cause aseptic meningitis, myocarditis, pericarditis, Bornholm disease (pleurodynia) and hand, foot and mouth disease.

Polio

Poliovirus is an enterovirus with antigenic types 1, 2 and 3. Immunization has rendered poliovirus infection uncommon in developed countries but it remains endemic in parts of the developing world such as Africa and the Indian subcontinent. Transmission is by the faecal–oral route with an incubation period of 7–21 days.

Clinical features

The clinical features vary:

- Over 90% of cases are asymptomatic.
- 5% have a 'minor illness' – fever, headache, malaise.
- 2% progress to CNS involvement – aseptic meningitis.
- In under 2%, 'paralytic polio' occurs due to the virus attacking the anterior horn cells of the spinal cord.

Diagnosis

Although imported infections and vaccine-associated infections are seen in the UK, they are rare. The differential diagnosis includes other causes of aseptic meningitis and acute paralytic disease such as Guillain–Barré syndrome. Polio is a notifiable disease.

Viral hepatitis

This can be caused by:

- Hepatitis virus A, B, C, D, E or G.
- Arbovirus-yellow fever.
- Cytomegalovirus, Epstein–Barr virus.

Hepatitis A virus (HAV)

This is an RNA virus spread by faecal–oral transmission. The incubation period is 2–6 weeks.

Clinical features

In infants and young children, many infections are asymptomatic or present as a non-specific febrile illness without jaundice. Older symptomatic children develop fever, malaise, anorexia, abdominal pain (from a tender enlarged liver) and jaundice. Dark urine (due to urobilinogen) may precede the jaundice.

Diagnosis

Diagnosis is often made on the combination of clinical features and history of exposure, but might be confirmed by measurement of IgM anti-HAV antibody. Serum transaminases and bilirubin levels are elevated.

Treatment

There is no specific treatment. The majority of children have a mild, self-limiting illness and recover within 2–4 weeks. The most serious but rare complication is fulminant hepatic failure.

Active immunization is available and is mostly used for frequent travellers. Close contacts should be given prophylaxis with intramuscular human normal immunoglobulin (HNIG).

Hepatitis B virus (HBV)

This is a DNA virus of the *Hepadnavirus* genus. It is a double-shelled particle with an inner core (HBc) and an outer lipoprotein coat comprising the hepatitis B surface antigen (HBsAg).

Transmission is parenteral via blood and other body fluids. In infants, the most important source of infection is vertical perinatal transmission from infected mothers. Most transmission occurs during or just after birth from exposure to maternal blood. The average incubation period is 20 days.

Incidence

HBV is an important cause of liver disease worldwide. The prevalence of infection in the population varies globally. In parts of Africa and Asia, up to 80% of children are infected by adolescence. In the UK, prevalence is under 2%.

Clinical features

In most children, infection is asymptomatic, although features of acute hepatitis might occur; fulminant hepatic failure occurs in 1% of cases. The most important consequence of infection is the risk of becoming a carrier with subsequent development of cirrhosis or hepatocellular carcinoma. The risk of developing carrier status rises with infection at a young age (reaching 90% in those infected perinatally). Between 30% and 50% of carrier children will develop chronic HBV liver disease.

Fig. 13.5 Serological markers of hepatitis B (HBV) infection

Serological markers of HBV infection				
	HBsAg	Anti-HBs	Anti-HBc IgM	Anti-HBc IgG
Acute HBV infection	+	−	+	+
HBV carrier	+	−	+ or −	+
Immune: previous infection	−	+ or −	−	+
Immune: immunization	−	+	−	−

Diagnosis

Diagnosis is dependent on serological testing for antibodies and antigens related to HBV. Acute HBV infection is associated with the presence of HBsAg and IgM antibodies to HBc antigen. Carrier status is defined as HBsAg persisting for more than 6 months. The presence of HBeAg correlates with high infectivity, whereas the presence of antibodies to HBeAg indicates low infectivity (Fig. 13.5).

Management

In the UK, there is no specific treatment for acute hepatitis B infection at any age. Interferon α and other antiviral drugs are currently used in the USA for treatment of hepatitis B infection.

Prevention

Effective immunization is available and is recommended:

- After perinatal exposure.
- For individuals at risk, e.g. doctors, dentists or intravenous drug abusers.
- Post-exposure, e.g. needlestick injury.

Perinatal exposure

All pregnant women should have antenatal screening for the HBsAg. All babies born to women known to be HBsAg positive should commence a course of hepatitis B vaccine within 24 hours of birth. Unless the mother is known to be anti-HBe positive, the baby should also receive hepatitis B specific immunoglobulin (HBIG).

BACTERIAL INFECTIONS

Staphylococcal infections

The coagulase-positive bacterium *Staphylococcus aureus* is the main pathogen but coagulase-negative bacteria, e.g. *Staphylococcus epidermidis*, are a major problem in intensive care units. Meticillin-resistant *Staphylococcus aureus* (MRSA), which lives harmlessly in the nose and skin of about one third of people, can cause infection in vulnerable individuals.

Staphylococcus epidermidis is part of the normal skin flora and *Staphylococcus aureus* is found in the nares and skin in up to 50% of children. Infections occur when defences are compromised. Many infections are therefore caused by the body's own bacteria, but transmission between individuals occurs with close contact.

Staphylococcus aureus most commonly causes superficial infection such as boils and impetigo, and occasionally deeper infections, e.g. of the bones, joints or lungs (Fig. 13.6). Toxin-producing *Staphylococcus aureus* causes scalded skin syndrome and toxic shock syndrome.

Impetigo

This highly contagious skin infection commonly occurs on the face in infants and young children – especially if there is pre-existing skin disease, e.g. eczema.

Clinical features

Erythematous macules develop into characteristic honey-coloured crusted lesions. Some cases are due to streptococcal infection.

Treatment

Topical antibiotics can be used for mild cases (e.g. mupirocin) but more severe infections require systemic antibiotics (e.g. flucloxacillin). Nasal carriage is an important source of reinfection and can be eradicated by nasal cream containing chlorhexidine and neomycin.

Fig. 13.6 Infections caused by *Staphylococcus aureus*

Direct infection	Toxin-mediated
Impetigo	Toxic shock syndrome
Folliculitis/boils	Scalded skin syndrome
Wound infections	Food poisoning
Abscess	
Pneumonia	
Osteomyelitis	
Septic arthritis	

Boils and abscesses

A boil (or furuncle) is an infection of a hair follicle or sweat gland and is usually caused by *Staphylococcus aureus.*

Clinical features

A painful, red, raised, hot lesion develops and usually discharges a purulent exudate heralding spontaneous resolution.

Treatment

Treatment is with systemic antibiotics. Deeper infection can lead to abscess formation in which case incision and drainage are usually required.

Osteomyelitis/septic arthritis

See Chapter 21.

Staphylococcal scalded skin syndrome

Staphylococcal scalded skin syndrome (SSSS) is a potentially life-threatening, toxin-mediated manifestation of localized skin infection.

Clinical features

SSSS results from the effect of epidermolytic toxins produced by certain phage types. They cause blistering by disrupting the epidermal granular cell layer. The lesions look like scalds.

Treatment

Management requires attention to fluid balance and treatment with intravenous flucloxacillin.

Streptococcal infections

Streptococci are Gram-positive cocci. Important pathogenic types include:

- Group A β-haemolytic streptococci (*Streptococcus pyogenes*).
- Group B streptococci.
- *Streptococcus pneumoniae* (pneumococcus).

These bacteria are responsible for a number of common and important paediatric diseases that can be caused by:

- Direct infection.
- Toxins.
- Postinfectious immune-mediated mechanisms (acute glomerulonephritis, rheumatic fever).

Infections caused by streptococci are shown in Fig. 13.7. Most of these are described elsewhere: tonsillitis (see Chapter 17), pneumonia (Chapter 17), meningitis (Chapter 20), glomerulonephritis (Chapter 19) and rheumatic fever (Chapter 16).

Fig. 13.7 Infections caused by *streptococci*

Organism	Disease caused
Group A streptococcus	Pharyngitis/tonsillitis Cellulitis Osteomyelitis Septicaemia Toxin-mediated: • Scarlet fever • Erysipelas • 'Toxic shock-like syndrome'
Streptococcus pneumoniae	Otitis media Pneumonia Meningitis Septicaemia
Group B streptococcus	Neonatal infection, e.g. pneumonia, meningitis, or septicaemia

Scarlet fever

This occurs in children who have streptococcal pharyngitis. The organism produces a toxin, which causes a characteristic rash.

Clinical features

The clinical features include:

- Tonsillitis.
- Strawberry tongue.
- Palatal petechiae.
- Rash: a widespread, erythematous rash starting on the trunk that becomes punctate and desquamates on resolution after 7–10 days (flushing of the face is often associated with circumoral pallor).
- Fever.

Diagnosis

Diagnosis is clinical, but can be confirmed by isolation of the streptococcus from a throat swab, and by elevated antistreptolysin O titres.

Treatment

Treatment is with penicillin (or erythromycin if the patient has penicillin allergy).

Erysipelas

This intradermal infection is caused by toxin-producing *Streptococcus pyogenes.*

Clinical features

The face or leg is the usual area affected. The skin is dusky and vesicles or bullae might develop.

Diagnosis and treatment

Skin swabs and blood cultures might be negative; treatment is with parenteral antibiotics.

Preseptal cellulitis

This presents as unilateral periorbital oedema in a young child, usually after an upper respiratory tract infection; fever might be present. The common pathogens are *Streptococcus* spp. and *Haemophilus influenzae* (more common in children under 3 years old).

It is important to distinguish this from the less common, but more serious orbital cellulitis, in which there is proptosis, limitation of ocular movement and impaired vision. It is imperative that all children with preseptal cellulitis have an ophthalmological review.

Treatment is with IV broad-spectrum antibiotics.

Tuberculosis

Incidence and aetiology

Tuberculosis (TB) remains a major global health problem, causing 3–5 million deaths annually. The increasing incidence in patients with HIV, combined with the emergence of multidrug-resistant strains of the causative organism, has generated new concern over this age-old public health problem.

Tuberculosis is more common among low socio-economic communities, especially in urban areas and the immunocompromised. Its incidence has been rising in the UK. It occurs in all racial groups but high rates are seen in children whose families have come from endemic areas such as:

- The Indian subcontinent (India, Pakistan and Bangladesh).
- Sub-Saharan Africa.

Tuberculosis is caused by infection with the acid-fast, slow-growing bacillus *Mycobacterium tuberculosis*. Children are usually infected by inhalation of infected droplet nuclei from an adult who is a regular or household contact. Children with the disease (even with active pulmonary disease) are almost always non-infectious. Therefore, once a child is identified as having TB, notification to public health is essential to identify the index case and contact trace.

Clinical features

The clinical features of TB (Fig. 13.8) reflect the wide variation in outcomes that follow inhalation of the tubercle bacillus or primary infection. Children under 4 years are at particularly high risk of disseminated disease, e.g. TB meningitis.

> **HINTS AND TIPS**
>
> TB contacts <4 years of age are at high risk of disseminated disease and should be evaluated promptly.

Tuberculous infection: asymptomatic infection

This is most common. A local inflammatory reaction limits disease progression and the disease becomes latent. Reactivation can occur subsequently.

Tuberculous disease: symptomatic infection

Multiplication within macrophages occurs at the peripheral alveolar site (the primary or Ghon focus) and the bacilli spread to the regional lymph nodes causing hilar lymphadenopathy. The peripheral lung lesion and nodes comprise the 'primary or Ghon complex'. Systemic symptoms can then develop, including fever, anorexia, weight loss and cough.

The pulmonary pathology can evolve in several different ways. Bronchial obstruction by enlarged lymph nodes might cause segmental collapse and consolidation. Rarer outcomes include development of a pleural effusion or progressive primary pulmonary TB with cavity formation (in adolescents and adults). Spread into the lymphoid system can result in cervical, supraclavicular or axillary lymphadenopathy.

Haematogenous dissemination

In addition to the above intrathoracic events, haematogenous spread probably occurs in most children, although dormant lesions rather than disease occur in these distant sites. Tubercle bacilli might spread to the bones (especially the vertebral column), joints, kidneys and meninges. Miliary TB is the most severe result of haematogenous spread. It occurs particularly in small infants or immunosuppressed individuals – lesions are found throughout the lungs, liver, spleen and bone marrow.

Diagnosis

This can be difficult and requires a high index of clinical suspicion. A history of close contact to an adult with smear-positive tuberculosis, symptoms (weight loss, night sweats, cough), clinical signs, tuberculin testing, chest X-ray (CXR) and examination of appropriate specimens by microscopy and culture (gastric washings) can suggest the diagnosis.

> **HINTS AND TIPS**
>
> Criteria for TB diagnosis include:
> - Adult TB contact.
> - Signs and symptoms.
> - CXR changes.
> - Positive Mantoux test.
> - Positive QuantiFERON blood test.
> - Positive cultures (gastric washings or other).

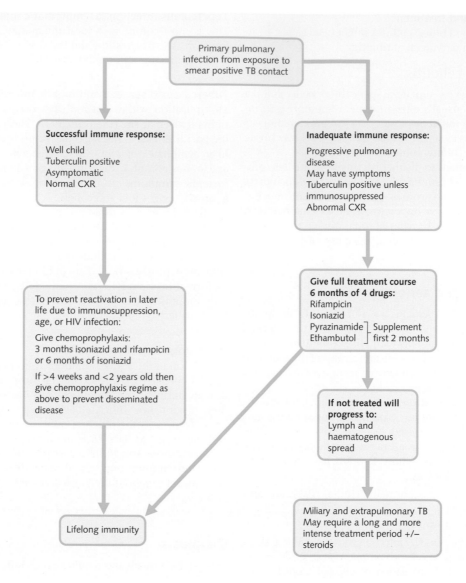

Fig. 13.8 Course of infection in tuberculosis

Tuberculin testing

A Mantoux is an intradermal injection of purified protein derivative (PPD) of tuberculin, e.g. 10 units (0.1 mL of 1:1000) is made on the volar aspect of the forearm. The site is read after 48–72 hours by measuring the transverse diameter of induration in millimetres. A 5 mm diameter reaction is considered positive, especially if risk factors are present. When previous BCG immunization has been carried out, a reaction of greater than 10 mm is indicative of infection. This remains the initial test of choice.

Interferon-gamma testing

This blood test exposes white blood cells in a sample to tuberculous antigens. If infection is present the white cells will secrete interferon-gamma. The amount secreted is measured to give the result. This test can be used in individuals with equivocal tuberculin results or those who have received BCG immunization for greater diagnostic accuracy.

Culture and histology

Isolation of *Mycobacterium tuberculosis* by culture is the 'gold standard' but positive cultures are obtained in a minority of children. Early-morning gastric washings on 3 successive days are the best specimens. It takes 6–8 weeks for the bacillus to grow. Microscopy is often negative but histological examination of a lymph node biopsy may reveal caseating granulomata and acid-fast bacilli.

Polymerase chain reaction (PCR) and T-SPOT.TB have been increasingly used in the diagnosis of tuberculosis.

Radiology

TB is suggested by hilar or mediastinal lymphadenopathy, especially if it is unilateral, or in combination with a 'wedge' of collapse or consolidation. Calcification also suggests TB.

Treatment and prevention

A 6-month regimen consisting of four drugs, isoniazid, rifampicin, pyrazinamide and ethambutol, for 2 months followed by isoniazid and rifampicin for a further 4 months is used in most instances, except in tuberculous meningitis where a 12 month regimen is appropriate. All children diagnosed with TB should be offered an HIV test. The treatment of contacts and latent TB is covered in the recent National Institute for Health and Clinical Excellence (NICE) guideline. The most important preventive measures are prompt and complete treatment of infectious cases and thorough contact tracing.

The BCG (bacille Calmette–Guerin) vaccine has been used in the UK since the 1950s to protect against TB, especially TB meningitis. Routine BCG immunization of all schoolchildren has been replaced by a more targeted approach since 2005. Currently in the UK, BCG is given to neonates in areas of high incidence or to neonates and children likely to be exposed to contacts.

> **COMMUNICATION**
>
> It is important to stress the importance of treatment – these children often become symptom-free after the first few weeks and the medication may be unpleasant. Compliance can be poor thereafter, which can lead to clinical infection later on. Parents should be made aware of the risks of inadequate treatment, including emergence of drug resistance.

Typhoid and paratyphoid fever

Typhoid fever is caused by *Salmonella typhi* and paratyphoid by *Salmonella paratyphi*. Both occur worldwide, but mostly in the developing world and the main reservoir is humans; they are invasive, systemic infections. Salmonellosis occurs after infection with *Salmonella enteritidis* or *Salmonella typhimurium*, which usually causes gastroenteritis (food poisoning) and is more common in the UK than typhoid fever – animals constitute the main reservoir for these strains and nearly half the human infections are transmitted by poultry products. Salmonellae are Gram-negative bacilli.

Transmission of typhoid fever, on the other hand, is by ingestion of food or water contaminated by faeces or urine from an infected person. The incubation period is 1–3 weeks.

Clinical features

The clinical presentation is similar in each case but paratyphoid fever is milder. Typhoid (enteric) fever is characterized by slow onset of fever, malaise, headache and tachypnoea. Signs include splenomegaly, and a characteristic rash of 'rose spots' on the trunk. Unlike adults, children do not usually develop a relative bradycardia. Paratyphoid is a milder illness but diarrhoea is more common.

Diagnosis

Diagnosis is made by culture of organisms from the blood (early in the disease) or from stool and urine (after the first week).

Management

If the child is systemically unwell, then a course of antibiotics is indicated for usually 14 days. Salmonella antibiotic resistance is a global concern that includes multidrug resistant strains. Traditional first-line antibiotic medications include ampicillin, chloramphenicol and trimethoprim-sulfamethoxazole but despite the increase in ciprofloxacin resistance, it is still considered the drug of choice. However, in the case of treatment failures, a third-generation cephalosporin can be used, e.g. ceftriaxone. Family and close contacts should be screened with stool cultures. Three consecutive negative stools signify clearance of infection. Long-term symptomless carriage can occur with a reservoir of infection in the gall bladder and excretion in the faeces.

PARASITIC INFECTIONS

Malaria

Incidence and aetiology

Malaria is a major global health problem with an annual mortality rate between 1.5 and 2.7 million. Although the majority of these are in the sub-Saharan Africa, imported malaria is increasingly reported from the UK.

Malaria is caused by infection with any of the four species of the protozoan parasite *Plasmodium*. Most of the 300 cases of childhood malaria imported to the UK each year are due to *Plasmodium falciparum*, which accounts for 85% of malaria seen in travellers to Africa. Half of these did not take chemoprophylaxis.

Fever in a child who has been to a malarious area is malaria until proven otherwise:

- Most cases are falciparum.
- *Plasmodium falciparum* requires treatment with quinine.

Transmission is vector-borne via the female anopheles mosquito. The onset is usually 7–10 days after inoculation but might be delayed by months or even years. The feeding female mosquito injects sporozoites, which pass to the liver via the bloodstream. After asexual multiplication in hepatocytes, these emerge as merozoites, which invade, multiply in and destroy the host's red blood cells. Some of the merozoites form gametocytes, which are sucked up by a feeding mosquito; the sexual phase of the life cycle then takes place in the mosquito with the formation of a new generation of sporozoites.

Clinical features

Malaria presents with fever and any child with a fever who has visited a malarious area in the preceding year should be considered to have malaria until proven otherwise. Non-specific symptoms include headache, rigors, abdominal and muscle pains, cough, diarrhoea and vomiting. Common misdiagnoses include viral influenza, gastroenteritis or hepatitis.

Apart from the fever, which is rarely periodic, there are no consistent clinical signs. Splenomegaly, anaemia and jaundice can all occur and a number of signs characterize the severe complication of algid malaria (shock), cerebral malaria (coma, fits) or blackwater fever (haemoglobinuria and renal failure).

Diagnosis

Diagnosis is made by the examination of thick and thin blood films. The former allows rapid scanning of a larger volume of blood per microscopic field. At least three films should be taken as one negative film does not exclude malaria. Both the species and the percentage of parasitaemia should be determined; parasitaemia >2% indicates moderately severe infection.

Management

Children with confirmed or suspected falciparum malaria require hospitalization and treatment with quinine or mefloquine (for those aged over 2 years). This is given orally in uncomplicated disease or intravenously if the parasite count is high or complications are present. In vivax infection, 2–3 weeks of primaquine is needed to clear dormant hypnozoite hepatic infection; falciparum does not have a dormant life cycle.

Travellers to endemic areas should seek advice about the most appropriate treatment for the area they plan to visit. Treatment is taken from 1 week before to 4 weeks after travel. Even with chemoprophylaxis efforts should be made to avoid mosquito bites by the use of nets and repellant.

Worms (nematodes)

Four important nematodes infect children:

- *Enterobius vermicularis* (pinworm or threadworm).
- *Ascaris lumbricoides* (roundworm).
- *Ancylostoma duodenale* (hookworm).
- *Toxocara canis.*

Threadworm

This is very common in preschool children. Transmission is via the faecal–oral route. Adult female worms lay their eggs in the perianal area at night. Scratching results in eggs being carried under the fingernails to the mouth and autoinfection.

Clinical features

Children present with perianal pruritus and vulvovaginitis but tissue invasion does not occur and systemic complications are uncommon. The worms appear like white cotton threads and might be visible at the anus.

Diagnosis

Diagnosis can be made by applying transparent adhesive tape to the perianal region in the morning and examining the tape for eggs with a magnifying glass 'the Sellotape test'.

Management

Treatment is with two doses of piperazine 2 weeks apart or a single dose of mebendazole (for children over 2 years). Reinfection is common and can be reduced by keeping fingernails short and wearing close-fitting pants. Family members should be treated even if asymptomatic.

Toxocariasis

Human toxocariasis is mainly caused by infection with *Toxocara canis,* a common gut parasite of dogs. Toxocara eggs are ingested when a child eats soil, play-pit sand or unwashed vegetables contaminated with infective dog or cat faeces.

Clinical features

There are two distinct forms of disease:

- Visceral larva migrans (VLM): characterized by fever, hepatomegaly, wheezing and eosinophilia.
- Ocular larva migrans: a granulomatous reaction in the retina causing a squint or reduced visual acuity.

Management

Treatment is with tiabendazole for VLM and steroids for the eye disease. Toxocara infection could be prevented by the regular de-worming of cats and dogs and by not allowing animals to defecate in public places, including sandpits.

KAWASAKI DISEASE

Kawasaki disease (KD), an uncommon systemic vasculitis. Early diagnosis and treatment might prevent lethal cardiac complications. It has replaced rheumatic fever as the most common cause of acquired heart disease in children.

HINTS AND TIPS

Early recognition and treatment of Kawasaki disease is vital to reduce the risk of cardiac complications:
- The signs may emerge sequentially and not be present all at once.
- Characteristically, the child is extremely miserable.
- Think of Kawasaki disease if a fever is present for more than 5 days in a row.

Incidence

First described in Japan in 1967, KD affects children mainly between the age of 6 months and 4 years (peak at 1 year). It is much more common in children of Asian origin. In the UK the incidence is 8 cases per 100 000.

Clinical features

The aetiology is unknown but the disease process is a vasculitis affecting the small and medium vessels including, most importantly, the coronary arteries leading to aneurysm formation. Subsequent scar formation causes vessel narrowing, myocardial ischaemia or even infarction, and – occasionally – sudden death.

Diagnosis

The diagnosis is based on clinical criteria, which emerge sequentially; five out of six are required to make a diagnosis (Fig. 13.9). Atypical disease is diagnosed if coronary aneurysms are present without all the criteria.

The differential diagnosis includes measles, scarlet fever, rubella, roseola and fifth disease. The following investigations are undertaken if KD is suspected:

- Full blood count (FBC), erythrocyte sedimentation rate (ESR).
- Urea and electrolytes (U&Es), liver function tests.
- Throat swab and antistreptolysin O titre (ASOT).

Fig. 13.9 Diagnostic criteria for Kawasaki disease

Fever for 5 days or more PLUS at least 4 out of the 5 following principal features:
Bilateral (non-purulent) conjunctival injection
Rash – polymorphous exanthem
Lips – red, dry, or cracked and strawberry tongue
Extremities:
- Reddening of palms and soles
- Indurative oedema of hands and feet
- Peeling of skin on hands and feet (convalescent phase)

Cervical lymphadenopathy (>1.5 cm) – often unilateral, non-purulent

---

- Blood cultures and viral titres.
- Echocardiography.
- Electrocardiogram (ECG).

Thrombocytosis, although common, is a late feature and therefore unhelpful in establishing the diagnosis.

Echocardiography is undertaken to detect coronary artery aneurysm formation. These occur in 30% of untreated cases and typically develop within the first 4–6 weeks of the illness. This investigation is repeated at intervals during the first year.

Treatment

The most effective treatment involves a single dose of IV immunoglobulin (2 g/kg). This reduces both the incidence and severity of coronary artery aneurysm formation if given within the first 10 days.

Aspirin is given concurrently to reduce the risk of thrombosis at a high dose initially (100 mg/kg/day in divided doses) until the pyrexia has resolved. A low dose (3–5 mg/kg/day) is continued for 6–8 weeks. Current evidence on steroid treatment is conflicting and their use is not routinely recommended.

COMMUNICATION

Immunoglobulin is a blood product and parents should be informed of the potential benefits (reduction in chance of aneurysm formation) and adverse effects (which can include anaphylaxis, infection).

IMMUNODEFICIENCY

This can be classified into:

- Primary: in which there is an inherited, intrinsic defect in the immune system.
- Secondary: in which a defect in the immune system has been acquired, as occurs in malnutrition,

infections (e.g. HIV, measles), immunosuppressive therapy (e.g. steroids, cytotoxic drugs), hyposplenism (e.g. sickle cell disease).

In acquired immunodeficiency, the cause is usually self-evident. Primary immunodeficiency should be suspected in the following clinical circumstances:

- An excess of infections: this is manifest by severe, unusual or persistent infections, or infections with unusual organisms (Fig. 13.10).
- Unexplained failure to thrive.
- Chronic diarrhoea.

HINTS AND TIPS

Suspect immunodeficiency in the following circumstances:
- Recurrent bacterial lower respiratory tract infections.
- Neonatal lymphocyte count less than 2.0×10^9/L.
- Failure to thrive.
  Unusual infection:
- Recurrent or chronic skin infection.
- Recurrent or chronic candidal infections.

Primary immunodeficiencies

These can be inherited as X-linked (affecting boys) or autosomal recessive disorders; 40% are diagnosed in first year of life. Examples are given below.

X-linked agammaglobulinaemia (Bruton's disease)

There is a failure of B cell development and immunoglobulin production. It presents with severe bacterial infections in the first 2 years of life.

Fig. 13.10 Immune defects and corresponding susceptibility	
Defect	Susceptibility
Antibody	Bacteria: *Pneumococcus, Staphylococcus, Streptococcus, Haemophilus influenzae* Viruses: Enteroviruses
Cell-mediated	Viruses: Herpes viruses, measles Fungi: *Candida, Aspergillus, Pneumocystis carinii* Bacteria: *Mycobacteria, Listeria*
Neutrophil function	Bacteria: Gram-positive, Gram-negative Fungi: *Candida, Aspergillus*

Severe combined immunodeficiency (SCID)

A heterogeneous group of disorders with profoundly defective cellular and humoral immunity (hence the name 'combined'). It presents in the first 6 months of life with failure to thrive, diarrhoea, candidal infections and recurrent, severe and unusual infections. A blood count often shows lymphopenia. Bone marrow transplantation is curative.

Common variable immunodeficiency (CVID)

This term encompasses a heterogeneous group of patients who have low levels of serum IgG and IgA. Usually present in late childhood with recurrent bacterial infection of sinuses or lungs.

Selective IgA deficiency

This is common (1:700 population). Most people with complete absence of IgA are asymptomatic. It is associated with autoimmune diseases in 40%, and also with IgG subclass deficiency. Children deficient in IgG2, the subclass providing immunity against polysaccharide antigens, might be susceptible to infection with encapsulated organisms (e.g. *Streptococcus pneumoniae, Haemophilus influenzae* type B).

Chronic granulomatous disease

An inherited disorder, usually X-linked, in which phagocytic cells fail to produce the superoxide anion. It presents with repeated bacterial and fungal infections involving the skin, lymph nodes, lungs, liver and bones. Granulomas and abscesses form in these sites. Diagnosis is confirmed by failure to reduce nitroblue tetrazolium (NBT test).

The management of primary immunodeficiency is outlined in Fig. 13.11.

Fig. 13.11 Management of primary immunodeficiency
The following treatment options are available:
- Antibiotic prophylaxis, e.g. co-trimoxazole, to prevent *Pneumocystis carinii* infection
- Vigorous antibiotic therapy for infections
- Immunoglobulin replacement therapy – regular IV immunoglobulin can be given for severe defects in antibody production
- Bone marrow transplantation
- Gene therapy – this has been successfully performed for severe combined immunodeficiency caused by adenosine deaminase deficiency

Secondary immunodeficiency

Immunosuppressive therapy

Therapeutic drugs, which cause immunosuppression, include:

- Cytotoxic agents.
- Steroids.

Cytotoxic chemotherapy for malignant disease (e.g. acute leukaemia) causes immunosuppression due to marrow suppression and neutropenia. Febrile children with neutrophil counts less than $0.5 \times 10^9/L$ are at risk for serious and potentially fatal bacterial and fungal infection.

Children on high-dose corticosteroids (e.g. for nephrotic syndrome) are particularly at risk for disseminated chickenpox infection. Children with organ transplants are prone to infection with cytomegalovirus.

Infection

Worldwide, the most important infection which causes immunodeficiency is HIV.

Paediatric HIV infection

Human immunodeficiency virus type 1 (HIV-1), the causative agent of acquired immunodeficiency syndrome (AIDS), is transmitted to infants and children by vertical transmission from HIV-infected women or by HIV-contaminated bodily fluids.

Incidence
The World Health Organization (WHO) estimates that 34 million people are living with HIV/AIDS and approximately 390 000 children are infected each year. The annual death rate due to AIDS is steadily falling but is still nearly 2 million people per year. With improvements in treatment HIV/AIDS is becoming a chronic disease to be managed rather than the terminal illness it once was. However, side-effects of antiretroviral therapy are a significant problem.

Transmission
The main route of transmission to children is vertically from mother to child: intrauterine, intrapartum or via breast feeding. Transmission rates vary with geographical area: lower in Europe and higher in Africa. With current management vertical transmission is now <1%.

Diagnosis
All newborns born to HIV-infected women will have circulating maternal HIV antibodies but only a proportion of these are infected with the virus. Passively acquired antibody disappears at 15–18 months of age so this is not a reliable test for infection under 18 months. HIV PCR is the usual test for infection in the infant.

Clinical manifestations: progression to AIDS
Changes in immune function are shown in Fig. 13.13, and the clinical manifestations in Figs 13.12 and 13.14.

Management
Mothers with HIV/AIDS should have an individualized birth plan specifying drug treatment after delivery based upon her viral loads and any drug resistance. After birth the antiretroviral therapy should be administered without delay. The primary immunization course should be given. BCG is not recommended but MMR should be deferred only if severely immunosuppressed.

Antiretroviral treatment is recommended when the child becomes symptomatic or there is a low or rapid fall in the CD4 count (<15%). This treatment comprises a combination of reverse transcriptase inhibitors with protease inhibitors.

Fig. 13.12 Clinical manifestations of HIV infection in children

Category	Severity	Manifestation
Category N	Asymptomatic	
Category A	Mild	Lymphadenopathy Hepatosplenomegaly Parotitis
Category B	Moderate	Severe bacterial infection Chronic diarrhoea Candidiasis Lymphocytic interstitial pneumonitis (LIP)
Category C	Severe (AIDS)	Wasting (severe failure to thrive) Opportunistic infections, e.g. *Pneumocystis carinii* pneumonia (PCP) Encephalopathy Severe bacterial infections Malignancy (rare)

Fig. 13.13 Immunological categories

	CD4 percentage
>25%	No evidence of suppression
15–25%	Moderate immunosuppression
<15%	Severe immunosuppression
Viral load	Unlike adults does not correlate well with disease course

Fig. 13.14 Non-infectious complications of AIDS

Neurological	Encephalopathy Motor defects Seizures
Gastrointestinal	Anorexia Nausea Diarrhoea Weight loss
Lymphoid hyperplasia syndrome	Lymphoid interstitial pneumonitis Polyglandular enlargement
Cutaneous	Kaposi's sarcoma

Coordinated psychological and social support for the whole family is a vital aspect of managing an HIV infected child. Issues include:

- Telling children the diagnosis.
- Retaining confidentiality.
- Two (mother and child) members of the family might be sick or dying at the same time.
- Social or cultural isolation.
- Stigma of diagnosis.

Prevention

Formula feeding and not breast feeding the infant plays a vital role in prevention in the developed world. Zidovudine, given to the mother in pregnancy and during delivery and to the neonate for the first 4 weeks of life, reduces the risk of vertical transmission of HIV. Caesarean section is recommended but if the maternal viral load is low then vaginal delivery appears to be possible as long as instrumentation or prolonged rupture of membranes does not occur. Antenatal HIV testing therefore confers potential benefits. Education campaigns can reduce but not eliminate the spread of HIV.

Further reading

The MMR research scandal. http://briandeer.com/mmr/lancet-summary.htm.

Other British Medical Journal reviews relating to the MMR scare.

http://www.bmj.com/content/342/bmj.c7452.full.

http://www.bmj.com/content/342/bmj.c5347.full.

http://www.bmj.com/content/342/bmj.c7001.full.

National Institute for Health and Clinical Excellence (NICE), March 2011. Clinical diagnosis and management of tuberculosis, and measures for its prevention and control. http://www.nice.org.uk/CG117.

Allergy and anaphylaxis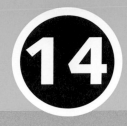

At the end of this chapter, you should be able to:
- Understand the natural history of allergies
- Take an appropriate history and perform relevant examination in a child with a suspected allergic reaction
- Understand the different tests used to diagnose allergies
- Understand the acute and long-term management of children with anaphylaxis

Allergy can be defined as a hypersensitive reaction initiated by immune mechanisms. Allergic reactions may be divided into IgE and non-IgE mediated forms. IgE reactions classically produce a biphasic response with an early and late component. They are associated with immediate reactions and cutaneous manifestations. The mechanism for non-IgE mediated allergy is less clear but thought to be T cell mediated and often causes more subacute reactions. Sensitization to allergens can lead to a more severe reaction at second exposure.

Typical allergic reactions include:

- Asthma.
- Food allergy.
- Allergic rhinoconjunctivitis.
- Atopic eczema.
- Anaphylaxis.

This chapter will cover mainly food allergy and anaphylaxis, as the others are discussed elsewhere.

EPIDEMIOLOGY

The increasing prevalence of allergy in children has led to an increased need for specialized services dealing in childhood allergy. Although part of the increase in cases of allergy stems from greater awareness and reporting, population-based studies have shown a significant rise in atopy and allergic diseases. There are several hypotheses for this major increase; however, there is no definitive evidence for any one theory:

- **Hygiene hypothesis**: excessive cleanliness and improved standard of living leads to less early exposure to infectious pathogens which may prevent switching of the immune system from a predominantly TH2-based system at birth to a TH1 system. This predisposes to hypersensitivity.

- **Delayed introduction of foods**: there is some evidence that late weaning and delay in exposure of the gut to allergens may increase likelihood of a reaction.
- **Food processing**: change in type of food to more highly processed forms may change the way antigens are presented from the gut.

Other theories include reduced antioxidants in the diet, change in types of fats ingested, vitamin D deficiency, and a possible role for *Staphylococcus aureus*-derived enterotoxins.

Approximately 6–8% of all children experience food allergy and 6% of all asthmatics have food-induced wheeze. In atopic eczema, approximately 60% will have a reaction to certain foods.

HINTS AND TIPS

Many allergies improve as the child grows older.

Different types of allergy tend to occur in different age groups (Fig. 14.1) as antigen exposure changes:

- Gastrointestinal (e.g. diarrhoea): in infancy, e.g. cow's milk protein allergy.
- Atopic dermatitis: peak incidence around 1 year.
- Wheeze: increasingly common through toddler years.
- Allergic rhinitis: rarely present in early childhood.

COMMUNICATION

Parents often want to know the likely outcome of food allergy – 85% of children outgrow cow's milk allergy at the age of 3 years but peanut allergy is often lifelong.

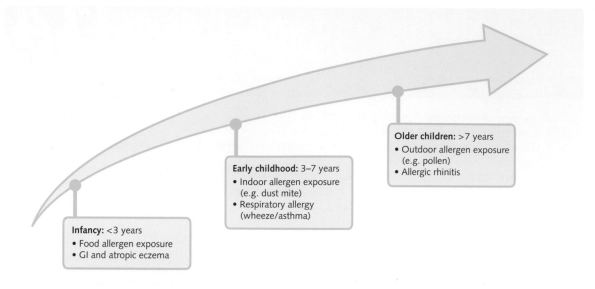

Infancy: <3 years
• Food allergen exposure
• GI and atropic eczema

Early childhood: 3–7 years
• Indoor allergen exposure
  (e.g. dust mite)
• Respiratory allergy
  (wheeze/asthma)

Older children: >7 years
• Outdoor allergen exposure
  (e.g. pollen)
• Allergic rhinitis

Fig. 14.1 The allergic march of childhood

CROSS-REACTION TO ALLERGENS

It is important to note that children sensitized to one allergen can develop reactions to another even though previous exposure has not occurred. This is because certain allergens share the same binding site (epitope) to IgE and one mimics the other. Examples are:

• Grass and peanut.
• Peanuts, soy beans and lentils.
• Latex and banana.

It is rare to have IgE-mediated reactions to more than three foods and allergy testing results that show cross-reaction should be confirmed by food challenge.

CLINICAL ASPECTS OF ALLERGY

Diagnosis

Investigations for allergy can be difficult to interpret. The history is critical to their interpretation and diagnosis. The aim is to distinguish true allergy from more common non-allergic reactions (e.g. 90% of cases of reported reactions to penicillin reaction are non-allergic). It should also try to distinguish IgE mediated from non-IgE mediated allergy.

The history should include:

• Personal or family history of atopy.
• Age of onset.

• Temporal relationship: speed of onset, new exposures, duration of reaction.
• Frequency and reproducibility of reaction.
• Feeding history.

Features helping to distinguish IgE from non-IgE mediated allergy are outlined in Fig. 14.2.

Examination of the child should focus on eliciting signs of allergy (Fig. 14.3), co-morbid atopic features (e.g. asthma, allergic rhinitis) and on growth/nutritional status.

Allergy testing is indicated where there is suspicion of a IgE mediated reaction and evidence from the history of the potential allergen. So-called 'fishing expeditions', using tests to multiple possible allergens with no correlation in the history, are not helpful. The main options for IgE mediated allergies are skin-prick testing or specific serum IgE assays. There is no equivalent test available at present for non-IgE mediated allergy and the only option is a trial of elimination and reintroduction. A blinded food challenge is the gold standard and is used when doubts remain about the role of particular allergens.

Fig. 14.2 Features helping to distinguish IgE from non-IgE mediated allergy

Non Ig E mediated allergy	IgE mediated allergy
Atopic eczema	Urticaria
Gastro-oesophageal reflux	Angioedema
Blood/mucus in stool	Vomiting
Food aversion	Wheeze
	Rhinitis

Fig. 14.3	Examining a child for allergy
Respiratory	Asthma/wheeze Stridor and angio-oedema Hoarseness Rhinoconjunctivitis
Gastrointestinal	Nausea, vomiting and diarrhoea Abdominal distension Failure to thrive
Cardiovascular	Hypotension and shock Dizziness
Skin	Pruritus Urticaria Atopic dermatitis Angio-oedema

Food challenge

This is the gold standard, used where there is diagnostic uncertainty, particularly where non-IgE mechanisms are suspected. This is the only investigation that can predict the severity of reaction following allergen exposure.

> **HINTS AND TIPS**
>
> Allergen challenging is useful but can cause anaphylaxis. It should only be done in the hospital setting, and informed consent must be taken from parents.

MANAGEMENT OF ALLERGY

Children with suspected food allergy should be assessed by a paediatrician with expertise in allergy and with support from a dietician. The education of both family and school plays an important part.

A major consideration in management is the anxiety that affects both child and carers. Avoidance of the allergen might be difficult. It is often hard for parents to identify suitable foods; the help of a dietician is essential. Inhaled allergen avoidance is extremely difficult and the effectiveness of allergen avoidance in these cases is controversial. Pharmacological treatment remains standard for asthma and eczema. Antihistamines can be useful and immunotherapy might play a greater role in the future.

> **HINTS AND TIPS**
>
> - Skin-prick testing is useful in all ages but not over areas of eczema.
> - Size of skin-prick reaction and IgE levels are poor predictors of severity of reaction.
> - Food challenge is indicated in cases of doubt.

Skin-prick testing

This is the most common test because it is cheap, quick and has a good safety profile. Small amounts of allergen are injected subcutaneously (along with saline and histamine controls) and the amount of wheal and flare observed. Reactions must be interpreted with a good clinical history because a positive test gives only a 50–60% chance that the child will react to the allergen. If there is a strong history of food reaction and a positive skin-prick test then a food challenge is not needed to confirm the allergen responsible for symptoms.

Skin-prick testing should only be performed in places equipped to deal with anaphylaxis.

Serum-specific IgE

This may take the form of RAST (radioallergosorbent test) testing, although other assays are increasingly used. They measure levels of IgE that are food specific and are useful where skin-prick testing is unsuitable (e.g. active eczema, patients on steroids or antihistamines and the drug cannot be stopped) or unavailable. Like skin-prick tests, a negative result is good for ruling out allergens but a positive result is useful only in the context of a positive history.

ANAPHYLAXIS

Anaphylaxis is a severe hypersensitivity reaction that manifests with respiratory difficulty (wheeze or upper airway swelling and obstruction) and/or cardiovascular symptoms (shock and hypotension). As with other forms of allergy the prevalence is increasing.

It is caused by rapid degranulation of mast cells and basophils, with systemic release of inflammatory mediators, capillary leak, mucosal oedema and smooth muscle contraction.

Anaphylaxis may be:

- Immunologic: mediated by IgE or immune complexes/complement.
- Non-immunologic: systemic mast cell/basophil degranulation not mediated by immunoglobulins.

The term 'anaphylactoid' is no longer used.

In children the most common cause of anaphylaxis is food, in adults this is superseded by drugs.

Foods

Peanuts are the most common food triggering anaphylaxis, followed by tree nuts, cow's milk and shellfish.

Insect venom

Anaphylaxis to venom is rare in children but it is associated with the greatest anxiety.

Latex

Anaphylaxis to latex is rare in children and is usually found in those who have had numerous surgical procedures. It important to advise latex allergic adolescents of the potential reaction from latex condoms. Note cross-reaction with banana.

Drugs

Vaccines and penicillins account for the majority of reactions, but are rare. Parents can be concerned about giving vaccinations in children with egg allergy. The measles, mumps and rubella (MMR) vaccination no longer contains any egg as it is grown on chick fibroblasts. It can be safely given to children with egg allergy. Where there has been a previous severe anaphylactic reaction to egg, discussion with an expert is advised about location of immunization (e.g. in hospital). Influenza and yellow fever vaccines should not be given to children with egg allergy.

> **HINTS AND TIPS**
>
> When taking a history of drug allergy it is important to identify the type of reaction as true allergy is uncommon.

Recognition

Early recognition and treatment of anaphylaxis is life-saving. The diagnosis is highly likely when there is a combination of mucosal involvement (hives, pruritis, flushing, swelling of lips tongue and uvula) with one or more of the following:

- Respiratory compromise (dyspnoea, wheeze, stridor, hypoxia).
- Cardiovascular compromise (hypotension, tachycardia, syncope).
- Gastrointestinal involvement (crampy abdominal pain, diarrhoea, vomiting).

Respiratory difficulty is more common than cardiovascular collapse. Initial symptoms can be subtle and progression rapid.

> **Fig. 14.4**   How to use an adrenaline (epinephrine) autoinjector
>
> To use an adrenaline (epinephrine) autoinjector:
> - Remove lid and check expiry date
> - Form a fist around the pen – **do not put your finger over the end**
> - Hold alongside outer thigh with injecting side facing towards body
> - Inject firmly into outer thigh
> - Do not inject into buttocks as this may be ineffective
> - **Attend hospital immediately after injection**

Treatment

Anaphylaxis is an emergency treated promptly with an ABC approach (airway, breathing, circulation). The mainstay of drug treatment is adrenaline (epinephrine) which both acts as a bronchodilator and supports the cardiovascular system through inotropic effects and peripheral vasoconstriction:

- Remove allergen where possible.
- Intramuscular adrenaline (epinephrine) (1 microgram/kg 1:1000); out of hospital an adrenaline (epinephrine) autoinjector should be used.
- IV hydrocortisone and antihistamine (chlorphenamine): to dampen ongoing response.

Prevention

Allergen avoidance is the only preventive measure and all children with suspected anaphylaxis should be referred for allergy testing. The use of an adrenaline (epinephrine) autoinjector which allows intramuscular administration of adrenaline (epinephrine) can be life-saving but it is essential that carers are trained in its use (Fig. 14.4). Only 32% of parents were able to correctly demonstrate correct use in one study. The adrenaline (epinephrine) autoinjector is only one part of managing severe allergic reactions. Management should also include:

- Identifying causes.
- Education on allergen avoidance.
- Treatment plan.
- Training of carers and school.
- Annual reinforcement.

> **HINTS AND TIPS**
>
> Adrenaline autoinjectors in anaphylaxis are useful if carers are trained in their use.

Further reading

National Institute for Health and Clinical Excellence (NICE), February 2011. Food allergy in children and young people (CG116). http://guidance.nice.org.uk/CG116.

Sicherer, S.H., Wood, R.A., American Academy of Pediatrics Section on Allergy and Immunology, 2012. Allergy testing in childhood: using allergen-specific IgE tests. Pediatrics 129, 193–197.

National Institute for Health and Clinical Excellence (NICE), December 2011. Anaphylaxis: assessment to confirm an anaphylactic reaction and the decision to refer after emergency treatment for a suspected anaphylactic episode (CG134). http://www.nice.org.uk/nicemedia/live/13626/57474/57474.pdf.

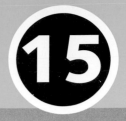
At the end of this chapter, you should be able to:
- Describe the different types of eczema and understand its management
- Identify some of the common fungal skin infections
- Understand the management of common infestations like scabies and head lice

ECZEMA (DERMATITIS)

Eczema also known as dermatitis is a chronic inflammatory skin condition that usually starts in childhood. Three main varieties occur in infants and children:

- Infantile seborrhoeic eczema.
- Atopic eczema.
- Napkin dermatitis.

Infantile seborrhoeic eczema

This mild condition presents in the first 2 months of life with a scaly, non-itchy rash initially on the scalp ('cradle cap'); this might spread to involve the face, flexures and napkin area (Fig. 15.1). Treatment is with emollients and mild topical steroids.

Atopic eczema

Atopic eczema is very common and affects 10–20% of children. There is often a family history of atopic disorders (eczema, asthma and allergic rhinitis), reflecting a genetic predisposition that confers an abnormal immune response to environmental allergens. Eczema is often the first manifestation of the 'allergic march' that may continue with allergic rhinitis and asthma.

Clinical features

It is usually an episodic condition though may be continuous in severe cases. A dry, red itchy rash occurs that usually starts on, the extensor surfaces and face in infants and young children, and the flexures (the antecubital and popliteal fossae) in older children (Fig. 15.2). However, the skin appearance can vary from an acute, weeping papulovesicular eruption to the chronic, dry, scaly, thickened (lichenified) skin that develops in older

children. Itching is the most important and troublesome symptom.

Diagnosis

The diagnosis is clinical although total IgE is likely to be raised. Food and environmental allergens play a role and identifying these using exclusion diets or RAST and skin prick tests may be helpful.

Management

The mainstay of treatment is the use of emollients even when the eczema is under control. In addition to this a step wise approach should be used dependant on eczema control (Fig. 15.3).

- Eradication of triggers.
- Stepwise medical treatment
- Treatment of secondary infection.

If treatment with emollients and topical steroids alone is not sufficient newer topical therapies such as tacrolimus and pimecrolimus may be used (topical calcineurin

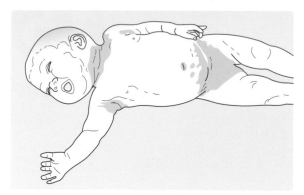

Fig. 15.1 Distribution of infantile seborrhoeic eczema

inhibitors). Systemic therapy with immunosuppressive agents is required for a small number of children with severe eczema.

HINTS AND TIPS

Topical steroids:
• Potency tailored to severity to eczema and site.
• Should not replace emollients during flares.
• Used on affected skin only.

Complications

The most important is secondary infection with either viruses or bacteria. Infection with herpes simplex (eczema herpeticum) is potentially serious and should be treated with aciclovir. Bacterial superinfection is usually caused by staphylococci or streptococci and requires antibiotic treatment.

Napkin dermatitis

Rashes in the napkin area are common and can be due to:
• An irritant contact dermatitis (nappy rash).
• Candidiasis.
• Seborrhoeic dermatitis.

Clinical features

Nappy rash
Ordinary nappy rash is due to the prolonged contact of urine and faeces with skin. Particular causes include skin wetness and ammonia from the breakdown of urine by faecal enzymes. The skin is red, moist and might ulcerate. The inguinal folds are spared.

Nappy rash can be prevented by frequent nappy changes and barrier creams. Exposure to air can hasten recovery but it is often impractical to implement this at home.

Candidiasis
Candidiasis is also common and is distinguished by bright red skin with satellite lesions and involvement of the skin folds. Candidal infection can be treated with a topical and oral preparation antifungal such as nystatin.

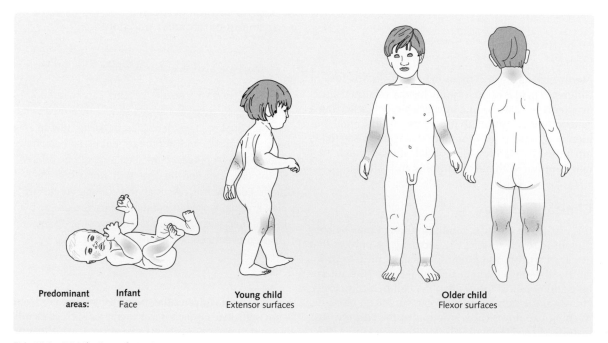

| Predominant areas: | Infant Face | Young child Extensor surfaces | Older child Flexor surfaces |

Fig. 15.2 Distribution of atopic eczema

Fig. 15.3 Stepwise treatment of atopic eczema

Mild	Moderate	Severe
Emollients	Emollients	Emollients
Mild topical steroids	Moderate topical steroids	Potent topical steroids
	Topical calcineurin inhibitors	Topical calcineurin inhibitors
	Wet wraps	Wet wraps
		Phototherapy
		Systemic therapy

INFECTIONS

Bacterial

Bacterial infections of the skin in children include common and important entities such as:

- Impetigo.
- Boils and furuncles.
- Staphylococcal scalded skin syndrome.
- Erysipelas.

These are considered in Chapter 13.

VIRAL

Viral warts

Hands and feet
The human papilloma virus (HPV) causes viral warts. Two types are seen:

- Skin warts are common on the fingers and soles in school-age children.
- Plantar warts (verrucae) are flat, hyperkeratotic lesions on the soles of the feet.

Most viral warts resolve within a year when immunity develops. Treatment options include:

- Salicylic and lactic acid paint.
- Cryotherapy with liquid nitrogen.

Repeat treatments over many weeks are required.

Other sites
Viral warts also occur in other locations:

- Laryngeal papillomas are found on the vocal cords.
- Genital warts (condylomata acuminata) are papular or frond-like growths in the perineal area.

These can be a sign of sexual abuse in young children.

Molluscum contagiosum

This common eruption in children is caused by the mollusci poxvirus.

Clinical features
Smooth, pearly papules with an obvious central dimple arise in crops (often on the trunk). They are not irritating and are of low infectivity.

Management
The papules resolve spontaneously without scarring usually within 6 months to 2 years and treatment is not required, although cryotherapy can be used if rapid removal is required.

Fungal

These include the dermatophytosis (ringworm) and candidiasis (thrush).

Dermatophytoses (tinea capitis, corporis, pedis and unguium)

Dermatophytes are filamentous fungi that infect the outer layer of the skin and also the hair and nails. They also affect some animal species (e.g. cattle and cats).

Clinical features

Clinical features vary with the site of infection.

Tinea capitis (scalp ringworm)
On the scalp, tinea causes patchy alopecia and occasionally a boggy inflammatory mass called a kerion.

Tinea corporis (body ringworm)
On the trunk, tinea appears as annular lesions with central clearing and a palpable, erythematous border.

Tinea pedis (athlete's foot)
This presents as itchy, scaling and cracking of the skin of the feet, especially between the toes.

Diagnosis

Examination under ultraviolet light (Wood's) shows a green–yellow fluorescence of infected hairs with certain fungal species. Diagnosis can be made by microscopic examination of skin scrapings for fungal hyphae. Culture of the organism is definitive.

Treatment

This varies with the severity of infection:

- Mild infections are treated with topical antifungal preparations such as clotrimazole or miconazole.
- Severe infections require systemic treatment with griseofulvin for several weeks.

Candidiasis (thrush, moniliasis)

Candida albicans, a yeast (budding, unicellular organism), is the most common pathogen. The organism colonizes the skin and mucous membranes. Transmission is via person-to-person contact, contaminated feeding bottles, etc.

Clinical features

In infants, candidal infections frequently involve the oral cavity (thrush) or the napkin area. It is acquired from the mother's vaginal flora. It can also affect the nipples of breastfeeding mothers.

Diagnosis

Diagnosis is clinical:

- Oral thrush presents as white plaques on the tongue and buccal mucosa.
- Monilial dermatitis: localized shiny redness typically affecting moist areas and *not* sparing flexural skin creases (this may occur in the absence of oral thrush).

Management

Topical nystatin is first-line therapy. Oral treatment should be given as well as direct treatment to lesions in perineal disease.

Prevention requires good hygiene and rigorous disinfection of feeding bottles and dummies.

Chronic or recurrent mucocutaneous candidiasis should raise the suspicion of immunodeficiency.

INFESTATIONS

Papular urticaria

This term describes crops of itchy, erythematous papules or small blisters. They are caused by insect bites, most commonly by the fleas or mites from domestic dogs or cats; bedbugs can also be the culprits. Secondary infection might occur.

Scabies

Scabies is caused by the mite *Sarcoptes scabiei*. It is transmitted by prolonged skin-to-skin contact. In the first infestation, the incubation period can be up to 8 weeks. The fertilized adult female mite burrows deep in the stratum corneum laying two or three eggs a day until she dies after about 5 weeks. The eggs hatch after a few days and larvae move on to the skin surface, maturing into adults in 10–14 days.

Clinical features

The first symptom is pruritus (this is worse at night), which is related to hypersensitivity to the mite or its faeces. The presence of burrows is pathognomonic. Common sites for burrows are the interdigital webs and the anterior aspects of the wrists. In infants, the soles of the feet, head and neck are commonly affected.

The rash consists of vesicles, weals and papules, which may become excoriated and secondarily infected.

Diagnosis

Diagnosis is clinical and can be confirmed by identification of mites or ova in scrapings from burrows or vesicles.

> **HINTS AND TIPS**
>
> Suspect scabies when:
> - There is itching in the family.
> - Itchy papules or blisters are present on the soles of the feet.

Treatment

Treatment is permethrin cream 5%. This is given twice, one week apart, to the body from the neck down. In infants, the scalp and face should be included. It can take several weeks for the pruritus to subside after successful treatment as hypersensitivity persists. This can be managed with oral antihistamines and topical steroids.

> **HINTS AND TIPS**
>
> It is important to treat all contacts. Parents should also be advised to wash all clothes and bedding to prevent reinfection.

Head lice (Pediculosis capitis)

Pediculosis capitis is a blood-sucking arthropod that infests the scalps of up to 10% of schoolchildren in some urban areas. Transmission is by head-to-head contact. The head louse prefers clean hair.

Clinical features and diagnosis

The louse egg is attached to the base of the scalp hair and is visible as a small, white, grain-like particle. Eggs hatch after a week and the louse lives for 2–3 months. Many infestations are asymptomatic but the most common manifestation is severe itching of the scalp often accompanied by enlarged cervical lymph nodes. Nits are the egg cases and only finding a louse is diagnostic.

Treatment

Treatment is with dimeticone which should be applied twice, a week apart. All the family should be treated. Wet combing with a nit comb can also control lice but needs to be done regularly.

OTHER CHILDHOOD SKIN DISEASES

Pityriasis rosea

This common, acute, benign and self-limiting condition is thought to be of viral origin. It begins with a 'herald patch', an oval or round, scaly, erythematous macule on the trunk, neck or proximal part of limbs. This is followed within 1–3 days by a shower of smaller dull pink macules on the trunk in a so-called 'Christmas tree' pattern following the lines of the ribs. Spontaneous resolution occurs within 6–8 weeks. No treatment is required.

Acne vulgaris

This is a chronic inflammatory disorder of the sebaceous glands and probably reflects an abnormal response to circulating androgens. It is an almost universal problem of adolescence, peaking in severity at age 16–18 years.

Clinical features

A variety of lesions occur on the face and upper trunk. Characteristically, comedones occur: plugs of keratin and sebum within the dilated orifice of a hair follicle. These can be open (blackheads) or closed (whiteheads). They progress to papules and pustules (bacterial superinfection) and in severe cases to cystic and nodular lesions, which can cause scarring.

Treatment

Treatment options include:

- Topical treatment with keratolytic agents, e.g. benzoyl peroxide.
- Ultraviolet light therapy: exposure to natural sunlight should be encouraged.
- Oral antibiotics: low-dose therapy with minocycline, oxytetracycline (>12 years age) or erythromycin is useful for moderate to severe pustular acne. Antibiotics are given for at least 3 months.
- The vitamin A analogue, 13-*cis*-retinoic acid: for severe acne that has not responded to conventional treatment. This should be prescribed only by a dermatologist.

Urticaria (hives)

Urticaria is a transient, itchy, erythematous rash characterized by the presence of raised weals (hives). It is induced by mast cell degranulation, in which histamine and other vasoactive mediators are released causing vasodilatation and an increase in capillary permeability. Most cases are caused by viral infections but an allergy history is needed to exclude allergic causes.

Clinical features

Urticaria can be accompanied by oedema of the lips and eyes (angioedema). Involvement of the lips and tongue is an emergency because there is a risk of respiratory obstruction. Chronic urticaria can occur and usually clears spontaneously in about 6 months.

Management

Acute urticaria usually resolves spontaneously within a few hours. If itchy, it can be treated with an antihistamine, e.g. chlorphenamine maleate. Precipitating factors should be avoided.

HINTS AND TIPS

Causes of an 'itchy' rash:
- Atopic eczema.
- Scabies.
- Papular urticaria.
- Urticaria (hives).
- Chickenpox.

Further reading

National Institute for Health and Clinical Excellence (NICE), December 2007. Atopic eczema in children (CG57). http://www.nice.org.uk/CG57.

Cardiovascular disorders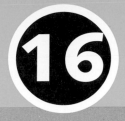

Objectives

At the end of this chapter, you should be able to:

- Distinguish between cyanotic and acyanotic congenital heart disease
- Understand the pathology and clinical features of common congenital heart disease
- Understand the common inflammatory conditions affecting the heart

In developed countries, congenital heart disease (CHD) accounts for the majority of cardiovascular problems in infants and children. With improved cardiac surgery, 80–85% of children with congenital cardiac disease survive into adulthood. In contrast to its incidence in adults, ischaemic heart disease is rare in children although it can occur in Kawasaki disease. Arrhythmias are very rare, with the exception of supraventricular tachycardias (SVTs). Important infections that affect the cardiovascular system (CVS) are infective endocarditis and viral myocarditis.

CONGENITAL HEART DISEASE

CHD comprises the most common group of structural malformations, affecting 6–8 out of 1000 liveborn infants. A number of important causative factors are recognized (Fig. 16.1) but, in the majority of cases, the cause is unknown. CHD presents or might be diagnosed in a limited number of ways. These include:

- Antenatal diagnosis by ultrasound.
- Heart murmur.
- Cyanosis.
- Shock: low cardiac output.
- Cardiac failure (see Chapter 5).

Although there are over 100 different cardiac malformations, a small number account for the majority of cases (Fig. 16.2). These are conveniently classified into:

- Acyanotic forms.
- Cyanotic forms.

Initial evaluation should include a chest X-ray (CXR) and electrocardiogram (ECG), although these investigations do not usually provide a lesion diagnosis. Diagnosis is usually achieved by a combination of echocardiography and Doppler ultrasound. Common investigations are shown in Fig. 16.3.

Acyanotic congenital heart disease

These conditions are caused by lesions that allow blood to shunt from the left to the right side of the circulation, or which obstruct the flow of blood by narrowing a valve or vessel.

Left to right shunts (L to R)

Atrial septal defect (ASD)

There are two types of ASD:

- The most common ASD (6 in 10000 live births) is an ostium secundum defect, high in the atrial septum. It is more common in girls (F:M = 2:1) and accounts for 6% of all cases of CHD.
- Much less common is the ostium primum type, which occurs lower in the atrial septum (often associated with mitral regurgitation), and is a common defect in Down syndrome.

Secundum defects are usually asymptomatic in childhood. The left to right shunt develops very slowly and pulmonary hypertension is extremely uncommon. It is important to distinguish ASDs from patent foramen ovale (PFO), which is present in one-quarter of all children. The patent foramen opens only in conditions of raised atrial pressure or volumes, whereas ASDs are large and always open.

Clinical features   The clinical features include:

- Abnormal right ventricular impulse.
- Widely split and fixed second sound (S2).
- Tricuspid flow murmur: rumbling mid-diastolic murmur at the left sternal edge.
- Pulmonary flow murmur: soft, ejection systolic murmur in the pulmonary area.

No murmur is generated by the low velocity flow across the ASD. A significant left to right shunt generates flow murmurs at the tricuspid and pulmonary valves.

Fig. 16.1 Causes of congenital heart disease

Genetic chromosomal disorders
Down syndrome, e.g. atrioventricular septal defect
Turner syndrome, e.g. aortic stenosis, coarctation of aorta
Williams syndrome, e.g. supravalvular aortic stenosis

Teratogens
Congenital rubella, e.g. patent ductus arteriosus,
   pulmonary stenosis
Alcohol, e.g. atrial septal defect, ventricular septal defect

Fig. 16.2 Common forms of congenital heart disease

Type	Name	Abbreviation	% of CHD
Acyanotic	Ventricular septal defect	VSD	32
	Patent ductus arteriosus	PDA	12
	Pulmonary stenosis	PS	8
	Atrial septal defect	ASD	6
	Coarctation of the aorta	COA	6
	Aortic stenosis	AS	5
Cyanotic	Tetralogy of Fallot	–	6
	Transposition of the great arteries	TGA	5

Fig. 16.3 Investigations in congenital heart disease

Investigation	Demonstrates
Chest X-ray	Cardiac shadow – may be enlarged or abnormal Lung fields – pulmonary vascular markings may be: Increased (plethora): significant L to R shunt, e.g. ventricular septal defect Decreased (oligaemia): reduced pulmonary blood flow, e.g. pulmonary stenosis
Electrocardiogram	Rate and rhythm of heart Mean QRS axis Hypertrophy of either ventricle
Echocardiogram	Precise anatomical abnormality
Cardiac catheter	Physiological/haemodynamic status rather than anatomy

Diagnosis   The CXR shows pulmonary plethora and the ECG shows right ventricular hypertrophy with incomplete right bundle branch block. Echocardiography is diagnostic without cardiac catheterization.

Management   Treatment is surgical and aims to prevent cardiac failure and arrhythmias in later life. Transcatheter closure of ASDs is now established practice at most cardiac centres with successful implantation rates of more than 96% and this is best done at 3–5 years of age.

Ventricular septal defect (VSD)
Most are single, although multiple defects do occur and other heart defects coexist in about one-third of affected children. The natural history and prognosis depends on the:

- Size and position of the defect.
- Development of changes due to blood shunting from left to right through the defect. This includes narrowing of the right ventricular outflow tract and progressive pulmonary hypertension, both of which reduce the size of the shunt.

> **HINTS AND TIPS**
>
> A ventricular septal defect is the most common variety of congenital heart disease. It accounts for one-third of all cases.

The clinical features, treatment and outcome are best considered separately for the different sizes of defect.

Small VSD (maladie de Roger)
The child is asymptomatic and the murmur is often first noted on routine examination. The only abnormality is a pansystolic murmur (sometimes with a palpable thrill) at the lower left sternal border.

Spontaneous closure might occur but if the murmur persists at 12 months then an echocardiogram is warranted to look for any associated complications.

Medium VSD
These usually present with symptoms during infancy including slow weight gain, difficulty with feeding and recurrent chest infections. In time, symptoms might actually disappear due to relative or actual closure of the defect.

On examination, there may be:

- An increased cardiac impulse.
- Palpable thrill.
- Harsh pansystolic murmur, loudest in the third and fourth left intercostal spaces.

If the pulmonary blood flow is high, a mid-diastolic murmur occurs due to blood flow across the normal mitral valve.

A CXR will show moderate cardiac enlargement, a prominent pulmonary artery and increased vascularity of the lungs. Echocardiography will show the position of the defect. The shunt is measured by Doppler studies.

Heart failure, if present, should be treated with diuretics and angiotensin-converting enzyme (ACE) inhibitors. Spontaneous improvement occurs in many childhood cases and surgical correction can be avoided. The decision to operate should be made on a case by case basis taking into account several factors, e.g. severity of cardiac failure and likely progression of cardiovascular disease.

Large VSD

Heart failure develops early on, especially if a chest infection occurs. The cardiac signs are similar to those of a medium VSD but it is worth noting that the systolic murmur might be soft in a very large defect. The defect tends to be larger than the cross-sectional area of the aortic valve.

Initial medical treatment of the heart failure is required and surgical closure under cardiopulmonary bypass is usually necessary. In young infants with multiple defects, banding of the pulmonary artery allows a temporary respite until the child is big enough for definitive correction. An example of a VSD is shown in Fig. 16.4.

Patent ductus arteriosus (PDA)

The ductus arteriosus connects the aorta to the left pulmonary artery and usually closes by the fourth day of life. A PDA is diagnosed if the duct does not close after 1 month of life. Risk factors include preterm infants, Down syndrome and high altitudes. PDA seen in preterm infants is a distinct clinical entity from congenital PDA in term infants.

Clinical features   A shunt develops between the aorta and pulmonary artery. The clinical features include:

- 'Bounding' pulses: wide pulse pressure.
- Murmur: initially 'systolic'. As pulmonary vascular resistance falls a continuous run-off from the aorta to the pulmonary artery occurs with a continuous 'machinery' murmur.

The PDA is commonly asymptomatic. If the duct is large, a significant left to right shunt develops as pulmonary vascular resistance falls and cardiac failure occurs.

Diagnosis   CXR and ECG changes with a large symptomatic PDA are similar to those seen in a patient with a large VSD. The CXR is usually normal but in large PDAs increased pulmonary markings are seen.

A PDA can be directly visualized by two-dimensional echocardiography and the ductal shunt can be confirmed by Doppler ultrasound.

Management   The duct can be closed in the cardiac catheter laboratory at 1 year of age but, if large, it might need surgical closure at 1–3 months.

Fig. 16.4 Ventricular septal defect and chest X-ray changes

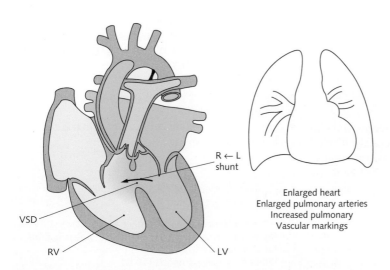

R ← L shunt

Enlarged heart
Enlarged pulmonary arteries
Increased pulmonary
Vascular markings

VSD

RV

LV

Ventricular septal defect

Obstructive lesions

Coarctation of the aorta (COA)

This accounts for about 6% of CHDs and has a male preponderance (M:F = 2:1). There is a narrowing of the aorta, which can be preductal or postductal. The site and severity of the coarctation determines the clinical features, which range from a severely ill newborn to an asymptomatic child, or adult, with hypertension.

> **HINTS AND TIPS**
>
> The key to clinical diagnosis of coarctation of the aorta is weak or absent femoral pulses.

Preductal coarctation: symptomatic infants

The abnormal circulation is often diagnosed antenatally but after birth it presents as a sick neonate with absent femoral pulses. While the ductus arteriosus is open the right ventricle can maintain adequate cardiac output to the systemic circulation. There is usually no murmur and cardiac failure occurs when the duct closes.

On diagnosis, prostaglandin infusion to maintain ductal patency and transfer to a cardiac centre for surgery is indicated.

Postductal coarctation: asymptomatic children

Although usually asymptomatic, there might be leg pains or headache. On examination, there is hypertension in the arm and weak or absent femoral pulses. There might be an ejection click (due to an associated bicuspid aortic valve) and a systolic ejection murmur audible in the left interscapular area.

Surgical correction is required. Options include:

- Balloon dilatation.
- Resection of the coarcted segment with end-to-end anastomosis.

Aortic stenosis (AS)

This accounts for 5% of all CHDs and has a male preponderance (M:F = 4:1). Symptoms and signs depend on the severity of the stenosis:

- Children with mild or moderate stenosis present with an asymptomatic murmur and a thrill often conducted to the aorta and the suprasternal notch.
- Severe stenosis can present with heart failure in the infant or with chest pain on exertion and syncope in older children.

Sustained, strenuous exercise should be avoided in children with moderate to severe AS. Surgical treatment depends on the severity and site of the stenosis. Options include balloon or surgical valvotomy. Aortic valve replacement is often required for neonates and children with a significant stenosis requiring early treatment.

Pulmonary stenosis (PS)

This accounts for about 8% of CHD and might be valvular (90%), subvalvular (infundibular) or supravalvular. Infundibular PS occurs in association with a large VSD as part of the tetralogy of Fallot.

Most cases are mild and asymptomatic. The clinical features include:

- Widely split S2, with soft pulmonary component (P2).
- Systolic ejection click (valvular PS).
- A systolic ejection murmur maximal at the upper left sternal border, radiating to the back.

Treatment options include transvenous balloon dilatation or pulmonary valvotomy.

Cyanotic congenital heart disease

There are two principal pathophysiological mechanisms for cyanosis in congenital heart disease:

- Decreased pulmonary blood flow with shunting of deoxygenated blood from the right side of the circulation to the left (systemic circulation), e.g. tetralogy of Fallot.
- Abnormal mixing of systemic and pulmonary venous return, usually associated with an increased pulmonary blood flow, e.g. transposition of great arteries (TGA).

Tetralogy of Fallot

This represents 6–10% of all CHDs and is the most common cause of cyanotic CHDs presenting beyond infancy. The four cardinal anatomical features are shown in Fig. 16.5.

Clinical features

Most patients present with cyanosis in the first 1–2 months of life. Hypoxic (hypercyanotic) spells are a characteristic feature, as is squatting on exercise which develops in late infancy.

Clinical signs include:

- Cyanosis with or without clubbing.
- Loud and single S2.
- Loud ejection systolic murmur maximal at the third, left intercostal space.

Fig. 16.5 The four cardinal anatomical features of tetralogy of Fallot

- A large ventricular septal defect
- Right ventricular outflow tract (RVOT) obstruction:
  Infundibular stenosis (50%)
  Pulmonary valve stenosis (10%)
  Combination of above (30%)
- Aorta overriding the ventricular septum
- Right ventricular hypertrophy

Diagnosis

The ECG shows right axis deviation and right ventricular hypertrophy but normal at birth. The CXR shows a characteristic 'boot-shaped' heart caused by right ventricular hypertrophy and a concavity on the left heart border where the main pulmonary artery and RV outflow tract normally create a convexity (Fig. 16.6). Pulmonary vascular markings are diminished. Congestive cardiac failure does not occur in tetralogy of Fallot.

Management

Prolonged hypercyanotic spells require treatment with:

- Morphine – relieves pain and abolishes hyperpnoea.
- Sodium bicarbonate (IV) to correct acidosis.
- Propranolol to cause peripheral vasoconstriction and relieve infundibular spasm. Oral propranolol can prevent hypoxic spells.

Definitive treatment is surgical. Palliative procedures might be required in infants with severe cyanosis or uncontrollable hypoxic spells. Pulmonary blood flow is increased by creating a shunt between the subclavian and the pulmonary arteries. Corrective total repair can now be carried out from 4–6 months of age. This involves patch closure of the VSD and widening of the right ventricular outflow tract.

Transposition of the great arteries

This accounts for about 5% of CHDs and is more common in males (M:F = 3:1). In complete or D-transposition:

- The aorta arises anteriorly from the right ventricle.
- The pulmonary artery arises posteriorly from the left ventricle (Fig. 16.7).

Clearly, if completely separate, two such parallel circulations would be incompatible with life, but defects allowing mixing of the two circulations coexist. These include ASD, VSD or PDA.

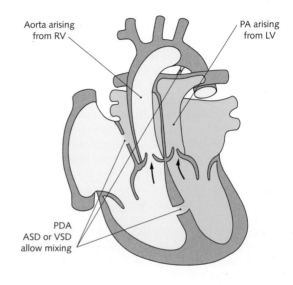

Fig. 16.7   Transposition of the great arteries

Fig. 16.6   Tetralogy of Fallot and chest X-ray changes

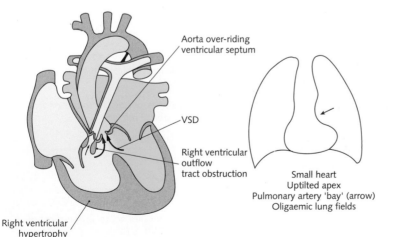

Clinical features

Most cases present with severe cyanosis, often within the first day or two of life. Spontaneous closure of the ductus arteriosus reduces mixing of the systemic and pulmonary circulations. Arterial hypoxaemia is often profound (PaO_2 1–3 kPa) and unresponsive to O_2 inhalation.

The second sound is single and loud. If the ventricular septum is intact, no heart murmur is audible. The systolic murmur of a VSD or PDA might be present.

Management

The immediate aim is to improve mixing of saturated and unsaturated blood. In the sick, cyanosed newborn, an infusion of prostaglandin (PG) E1 is started to reopen the ductus arteriosus. Emergency cardiac catheterization and therapeutic balloon atrial septostomy (Rashkind procedure) is a lifesaving palliative procedure. Definitive repair is usually achieved with an arterial switch procedure, which can be performed at a few weeks of age. The pulmonary artery and aorta are transected and switched over.

HINTS AND TIPS

Mixing of blood from left and right sides in cyanotic congenital cardiac disease is essential and might be done through a patent ductus arteriosus. A prostaglandin infusion can open the ductus, allowing mixing.

RHEUMATIC FEVER

Acute rheumatic fever is a sequela of group A β-haemolytic streptococcal infection, usually a tonsillo-pharyngitis. It is caused by an abnormal immune response that occurs in less than 1% of patients with streptococcal infection. Although the disease has largely been eradicated in developed countries with improved sanitation and the use of antibiotics for tonsillitis, it remains the most common cause of cardiac valvular disease worldwide. It mainly affects children aged between 5 and 15 years.

Clinical features

Polyarthritis, fever and malaise develop 2–6 weeks after the pharyngeal infection. The arthritis is 'fleeting', lasting less than a week in individual joints and commonly affects the large joints such as the knees and ankles.

There is a pancarditis in 50% of patients:

- Pericarditis can cause a friction rub and pericardial effusion.
- Myocarditis can cause heart failure.
- Endocarditis commonly affects the left-sided valves leading to murmurs, e.g. of mitral incompetence.

Erythema marginatum – pink macules on the trunk and limbs – is an uncommon painless, early manifestation. Hard subcutaneous nodules occur on the extensor surfaces in a minority of cases.

Sydenham's chorea is a late manifestation occurring 2–6 months after streptococcal infection in 10% of patients. There is emotional lability followed by involuntary, random, jerky movements lasting 2–3 months. Recovery is usually complete.

Diagnosis

The diagnosis is clinical and is based on a modified version of the Duckett Jones criteria (Fig. 16.8).

Diagnosis requires evidence of a preceding streptococcal infection together with two major criteria or one major and two minor criteria. The former is usually done serologically by finding an increase in antibodies to various streptococcal antigens, e.g. antistreptolysin O titre. Throat swab is often negative at the time of presentation.

Laboratory investigations in a suspected case include:

- Erythrocyte sedimentation rate (ESR), C-reactive protein (CRP): elevated.
- Antistreptolysin O titre: might be elevated.
- Throat swab: usually negative at time of presentation.
- ECG: prolonged P-R interval.
- Echocardiography: might show evidence of carditis.

Management

The acute episode is treated by:

- Bed rest (depending upon severity of disease and joint involvement).
- High-dose aspirin to suppress fever and arthritis.
- Steroids for severe carditis.

Fig. 16.8 Modified Duckett Jones criteria for diagnosis of rheumatic fever

Modified Duckett Jones criteria (2 major or 1 major and 2 minor)	
Major	Minor
Carditis	Fever
Polyarthritis	Arthralgia
Chorea	Previous rheumatic fever
Erythema marginatum	Positive acute-phase reactant (ESR, CRP) Leucocytosis
Subcutaneous nodules	Prolonged P-R interval on ECG

- Diuretics and ACE inhibitors for heart failure.
- Antibiotics if there is evidence of persisting streptococcal infection.

Recurrent attacks should be prevented by prophylactic penicillin (given either orally or as monthly intramuscular injections of benzathine penicillin). Lifelong prophylaxis has been advocated.

Complications

Rheumatic valvular disease is the most common form of long-term damage, its severity increasing with the number of acute episodes. There is scarring and fibrosis of valve tissue, most commonly affecting the mitral valve.

CARDIAC INFECTIONS

These are uncommon and include:

- Infective endocarditis.
- Myocarditis.

Infective endocarditis

This may be defined as infection of the endocardium or endothelium of the great vessels. It is a cause of great morbidity and prevention in high-risk groups by using prophylactic antibiotics is essential.

HINTS AND TIPS

Children at risk of bacterial endocarditis include those with:
- Acquired valvular heart disease with stenosis or regurgitation.
- Valve replacement.
- Structural congenital heart disease, including surgically corrected or palliated structural conditions, but excluding isolated atrial septal defect, fully repaired ventricular septal defect or fully repaired patent ductus arteriosus, and closure devices that are judged to be endothelialized.
- Hypertrophic cardiomyopathy.
- Previous infective endocarditis.

Clinical features

Endocarditis should be suspected in any child with fever and a significant cardiac murmur. The clinical features are caused by:

- Bacteraemia: fever, malaise.
- Valvulitis: cardiac failure and murmurs.

- Immunological causes: glomerulonephritis.
- Embolic causes: CNS abscess, splinter haemorrhages.

Non-cardiac manifestations are less common in children than in adults.

Diagnosis

It is important to stress that endocarditis is a clinical and laboratory diagnosis.

- Blood cultures: at least three should be obtained in the first 24 hours of hospitalization. The causative organism – most commonly *Streptococcus viridans* (α-haemolytic streptococcus) – is identified in 90% of cases.
- Cross-sectional echocardiography: although this might confirm the diagnosis by the identification of vegetations, it cannot exclude it. Vegetations might persist after successful antibiotic treatment has been completed.
- Acute-phase reactants: elevated.

Management

Treatment comprises 4–6 weeks of intravenous antibiotics, e.g. high-dose ampicillin with an aminoglycoside. Surgical removal of infected prosthetic material might be required.

HINTS AND TIPS

Antibiotics have previously been offered routinely as a preventative measure to children at risk of infective endocarditis undergoing interventional procedures. However, there is little evidence to support this practice. Antibiotic prophylaxis has not been proven to be effective and there is no clear association between episodes of infective endocarditis and interventional procedures (please refer to NICE guidance in Further reading).

Myocarditis

This uncommon disease primarily affects infants and neonates. Coxsackie and echoviruses, as well as rubella, have been associated with myocarditis. It can present acutely with cardiovascular collapse or slowly with a gradual onset of congestive cardiac failure.

Treatment is supportive. Most children recover but some develop a chronic dilated cardiomyopathy.

Kawasaki disease

Kawasaki disease is the most common cause of acquired cardiac disease in children. The underlying aetiological agent is at present unknown. It can result in coronary artery aneurysms. It is covered more fully in Chapter 13.

CARDIAC ARRHYTHMIAS

Sinus arrhythmia is more pronounced in children and shows as an increase in heart rate during inspiration and slowing during expiration. Normal sinus rhythm can be up to 210 beats/min and premature atrial and ventricular contractions are common and benign.

Supraventricular tachycardia

The child has a heart rate >220 beats/min and often is asymptomatic, although infants can develop cardiac failure. An accessory connection can be present in up to 95% of all young children and infants.

Clinical features

Infants might present with signs of cardiac failure, such as poor feeding, sweating and irritability. Older children often feel unwell, describing palpitations, and may complain of chest pain, difficulty breathing and dizziness.

Diagnosis

The ECG usually shows a narrow complex tachycardia with P waves discernible after the QRS complex. In sinus rhythm, the Wolff–Parkinson–White syndrome might be evident if there is an accessory bundle allowing premature activation of the ventricles. The PR interval is short and there is a wide QRS with slurred upstroke (delta wave).

Management

An acute episode can be terminated and sinus rhythm restored by:

- Vagal stimulation: applying an ice-cold compress to the face or carotid sinus massage.
- Intravenous adenosine: safe and effective.
- Synchronized DC cardioversion: if the above fail.

The prognosis is good in the majority of cases. Ninety per cent of children will have no further episodes after infancy (over 1 year old). Radio-frequency ablation of the bypass tract has been used for those with persistent, frequently recurring paroxysms.

Further reading

National Institute for Health and Clinical Excellence (NICE), March 2008. Prophylaxis against infective endocarditis (CG64). http://www.nice.org.uk/CG64.

Management of isolated ventricular septal defects in infants and children. February 2012. UptoDate. http://www.uptodate.com/home/clinicians/index.html.

Rushani, D., Kaufman, J.S., Ionescu-Ittu, R., et al., 2012. Cumulative risk of infective endocarditis in children with congenital heart disease – a population-based study. J. Am. Coll. Cardiol. 59 (13s1), E819–E819. doi:10.1016/S0735-1097 (12)60820 1.

Disorders of the respiratory system

At the end of this chapter, you should be able to:
- Understand the common upper respiratory tract infections in children
- Understand the aetiology, clinical features and management of pneumonia in children
- Identify the clinical features of bronchiolitis
- Understand the aetiology, clinical features and management of chronic asthma
- Outline the management of acute severe asthma in children
- Understand the aetiology and clinical features of cystic fibrosis in children

Respiratory tract infections are the most common infections of childhood and range from trivial to life-threatening illnesses; 90% of these infections are caused by viruses. They are classified into upper respiratory tract infections (URTIs) and lower respiratory tract infections (LRTIs). The other common and important diseases of this system are asthma and cystic fibrosis.

Children are more susceptible to the effects of respiratory tract infections than adults for many reasons:

- Chest wall is more compliant than that of an adult.
- Fatiguability of respiratory muscles.
- Increased mucous gland concentration.
- Poor collateral ventilation.
- Low chest wall elastic recoil.

HINTS AND TIPS

Parental smoking should be discouraged because passive smoking worsens symptoms of all respiratory disease.

UPPER RESPIRATORY TRACT INFECTIONS

The upper respiratory tract comprises the ears, nose, throat, tonsils, pharynx and sinuses, together with the extrathoracic airways.

The common cold (acute nasopharyngitis)

This is a viral infection causing a clear or mucopurulent nasal discharge (coryza), cough, fever and malaise. Although over 200 viral types are known, 25–40% of colds are caused by rhinoviruses. Symptomatic treatment (e.g. paracetamol) is all that is required for this self-limiting illness as no known treatment affects clinical outcome. Young infants, who are obligate nose-breathers, might experience feeding difficulties.

Sore throat (pharyngitis and tonsillitis)

These are commonly viral, especially in children under 3 years, but might also be caused by group A β-haemolytic streptococci. Children present with a sore throat, fever and constitutional upset. It is very difficult to distinguish viral and bacterial infection clinically. However, a purulent exudate, lymphadenopathy and severe pain suggest a bacterial cause.

Treatment

Analgesia is the mainstay of treatment to enable drinking. Antibiotics are given to prevent complications but the number needed to treat is approximately 3000 for rheumatic fever.

Complications

These include:

- Retropharyngeal abscess.
- Peritonsillar abscess (quinsy).
- Poststreptococcal glomerulonephritis or rheumatic fever.

Tonsillectomy is now less commonly performed than it used to be. Indications include recurrent tonsillitis, quinsy or obstructive sleep apnoea.

Acute otitis media

The cause of this can be viral – e.g. respiratory syncytial virus (RSV) influenza – or bacterial (*Pneumococcus* species, *Haemophilus influenzae*, group B streptococci, *Moraxella catarrhalis*). It is very common in preschool children, who present with fever, vomiting and distress. It is important to examine the eardrums in any ill and febrile toddler, as only older children will localize the pain to the ear.

Clinical features

Examination reveals a red eardrum with loss of the light reflex. The eardrum might bulge and perforation might occur, with a purulent discharge.

Management

Symptomatic treatment is usually all that is needed; antibiotics can reduce symptoms but not complications.

Recurrent infections are associated with otitis media with effusion. Mastoiditis and meningitis are now uncommon complications of acute otitis media.

Otitis media with effusion (OME, secretory otitis media, glue ear)

In young children who are prone to recurrent upper respiratory tract infections, it is common for the middle ear fluid to persist (an effusion), causing a conductive hearing loss and an increased susceptibility to reinfection. An effusion can also occur without a history of acute infections and is probably due to poor Eustachian tube ventilation due to enlarged adenoids or allergy. The effusion and resulting hearing impairment is often transient but, if it is persistent, it can be an indication for surgical drainage of the middle ear with grommet insertion. A grommet is a hollow plastic tube that ventilates the middle ear and remains effective only while patent. However, there is little evidence for the long-term benefits of grommets on hearing and speech development.

Obstructive sleep apnoea

Obstructive sleep apnoea (OSA) is covered in Chapter 5.

Croup

Croup, or viral laryngotracheobronchitis, is most commonly caused by the parainfluenza virus. It has a peak incidence in winter in the second year of life.

Clinical features

Symptoms of upper respiratory tract infection (coryza, fever) are usually present for a day or two before the onset of a characteristic barking ('sea lion') cough and stridor (which is caused by subglottic inflammation and oedema). Symptoms typically start, and are worse, at night.

Management

Most children are mildly affected and improve spontaneously within 24 hours. Management at home is symptomatic and duration of symptoms 3 days. About 1 in 10 children require hospitalization because of:

- More severe illness.
- Young age (under 12 months).
- Signs of fatigue or respiratory failure.

Croup can be categorized into mild, moderate and severe disease based upon the Westley scoring system. There is evidence that a single dose of dexamethasone 0.15 mg/kg or nebulized budesonide 2 mg has a beneficial effect in mild, moderate and severe croup. Humidifiers and steam therapy are ineffective and the latter should also be avoided due to the risk of accidental burns.

Nebulized adrenaline (epinephrine) provides transient improvement by constricting local blood vessels and reducing swelling and oedema. It should be given only under close supervision in hospital where it can provide rapid, if transient, relief of airway obstruction, allowing time for transfer to the intensive therapy unit (ITU) and intubation in a child with severe airway obstruction.

Diphtheria

This potentially fatal and highly infectious disease is caused by a toxin produced by *Corynebacterium diphtheriae* that usually affects the mucous membranes of the nose and throat. Diphtheria typically causes a sore throat, fever, lymphadenopathy and respiratory distress (stridor). The hallmark sign is a thick, grey material covering the back of the throat. In the UK, this scourge of childhood has been eliminated by an effective immunization programme, but it remains endemic in some countries and imported cases occur.

Acute epiglottitis

Acute bacterial epiglottitis is an uncommon life-threatening emergency caused by infection with *Haemophilus influenzae* type B. It has become rare since the introduction of Hib immunization. It is most common in children aged 1–6 years.

Clinical features

The onset is rapid over a few hours with the development of an intensely painful throat. The characteristic picture is of an ill, toxic, febrile child who is unable to speak or swallow, with a muffled voice and soft inspiratory stridor. The child tends to sit upright with an open mouth to maximize the airway, and might drool saliva.

Management

It is vital to distinguish this illness from viral croup because the management is different:

- The child should be managed in the resuscitation room.
- A senior paediatrician, ear, nose and throat (ENT) surgeon and anaesthetist should be present.
- No attempt should be made to lie the child down, to examine the throat with a spatula or to take blood, as these manoeuvres can precipitate total airway obstruction and death.

Examination under anaesthetic should be arranged without delay to allow confirmation of the diagnosis, followed by intubation. Once the airway is secured, blood should be taken for culture and intravenous antibiotics started using a third-generation cephalosporin, e.g. cefuroxime. Intubation is not usually required for longer than 48 hours.

Bacterial tracheitis

This is an uncommon infectious disease in children but is more prevalent than acute epiglottitis. The usual pathogens are *Staphylococcus aureus*, *Haemophilus influenzae*, streptococci, and *Neisseria* spp.

Clinical features

Children are often systemically unwell with high fever and respiratory distress. Stridor and hoarse voice are the predominant features but in contrast to acute epiglottis, there is no drooling.

Management

The management is very similar to that of acute epiglottitis, i.e. securing the airway followed by blood cultures and broad-spectrum intravenous antibiotics.

HINTS AND TIPS

Do not examine the throat if epiglottitis is suspected: complete airway obstruction might be provoked.

LOWER RESPIRATORY TRACT INFECTIONS

A minority of infections involve the lower respiratory tract, but these are more likely to be serious than infections of the upper respiratory tract and are more common in infants. Causative agents include viruses and bacteria. They vary with the child's age and the site of infection. Infection can occur by direct spread from airway epithelium or via the bloodstream.

A number of well-defined clinical syndromes (determined by the predominant anatomical site of inflammation) are recognized (e.g. bronchiolitis and pneumonia) and often provide a clue to the likely pathogen. The term 'chest infection' should be avoided. The hallmarks of a lower respiratory tract infection are apparent on inspection (Fig. 17.1).

Pneumonia

Pneumonia is characterized by inflammation of the lung parenchyma with consolidation of alveoli. It can be caused by a wide range of pathogens and different organisms affect different age groups (Fig. 17.2).

Clinical features

Usually, following an URTI the patient develops worsening fever, cough and breathlessness. Tachypnoea is a key sign. The classic signs of consolidation (dullness to percussion, decreased breath sounds and bronchial breathing) might be present but they are difficult to detect in infants; crackles might also be present. In bacterial pneumonia, pleural inflammation causing chest (or abdominal) pain and an effusion more commonly develops.

Diagnosis

Diagnosis is largely clinical and a chest X-ray (CXR) is only indicated when there is a failure to respond to treatment or if complications are suspected. A full blood count (FBC), C-reactive protein, blood culture and nasopharyngeal aspirate (NPA) for viral isolation and PCR should be carried out in hospitalized children. Blood cultures are positive in just 10% of cases; addition of NPA for culture and PCR increase yield of causative organisms up to 30%.

It is often difficult to distinguish between viral and bacterial infections clinically. Young children and babies are not good providers of sputum and definitive diagnosis of bacterial infection remains difficult. However, the following all suggest bacterial pneumonia:

- Polymorphonuclear leucocytosis.
- Lobar consolidation.
- Pleural effusion.

Fig. 17.1 Signs of lower respiratory tract infection in the infant

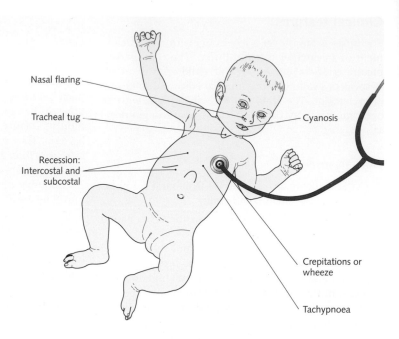

Nasal flaring

Tracheal tug

Recession: Intercostal and subcostal

Cyanosis

Crepitations or wheeze

Tachypnoea

Fig. 17.2 Pathogens causing pneumonia in infants and children

Age	Pathogens
Neonates (<1 month)	Group B streptococci
	Escherichia coli
	Chlamydia trachomatis *Listeria monocytogenes*
Infants	Respiratory viruses, e.g. RSV, adenovirus
	Streptococcus pneumoniae *Haemophilus influenzae* *Bordetella pertussis*
Children	*Streptococcus pneumoniae* *Haemophilus influenzae* Group A streptococci
	Mycoplasma pneumonia (>5 years of age)

Mycoplasma infection can be diagnosed reliably by acute and convalescent serology or by demonstration of cold agglutinins.

Management

Antibiotics are usually given if a diagnosis of bacterial pneumonia is made, the choice is dictated by the child's age and the severity of illness (e.g. toxic or requires O_2):

- Penicillin is first line in most children.
- Cefuroxime and flucloxacillin is indicated in severe illness.
- If mycoplasma is suspected, a macrolide antibiotic should be given.

Rarely, pneumonia can be complicated by empyema; this should be evaluated by ultrasound and initially needs drainage via a small bore chest drain or, if necessary, may require surgery. Recurrent or persistent pneumonia should raise the possibility of an inhaled foreign object or congenital abnormality of the lung, cystic fibrosis or tuberculosis.

Bronchiolitis

This common condition is caused by a viral infection, mainly RSV. Annual winter epidemics occur in infants and many will be hospitalized. The infection causes an inflammatory response, predominantly in the bronchioles, hence the name.

HINTS AND TIPS

Bronchiolitis is a common and severe infection in infants in the winter months.
- Oxygen and feeding support are the most important elements of management of bronchiolitis. Little evidence exists for drug or nebulized therapy.
- Infants at high risk of developing severe bronchiolitis include those with chronic lung disease, congenital heart disease, trisomy 21 and infants less than 6 weeks of age.

Clinical features

Coryzal symptoms are followed by a cough with increasing breathlessness and associated difficulty in breathing. Small infants might develop apnoeic episodes. Examination reveals:

- Tachypnoea.
- Subcostal and intercostal recession.
- Chest hyperinflation.
- Bilateral fine crackles.
- Wheeze on auscultation.

Diagnosis

The CXR, if taken, usually shows hyperinflation of the lungs. The virus can be detected by immunofluorescence and cultured on a nasopharyngeal aspirate.

Management

Management is supportive with attention to treating hypoxia and maintaining hydration (Fig. 17.3). Respiratory rate, heart rate and oxygen saturation are monitored. Oxygen is the mainstay of treatment and is given via nasal cannulae or humidified via a headbox. Some infants might be well enough to continue oral feeds but most require fluids to be given either by nasogastric tube or intravenously. A minority of hospitalized infants require assisted ventilation (only 1–2%). Secondary bacterial infection might occur, in which case antibiotic therapy is appropriate.

Fig. 17.3	Management of bronchiolitis
Mild	Feeding well Respiratory rate <40/min Minimal intercostal recession S_pO_2 >92% in air Manage at home – regular review
Moderate	Difficulty feeding Moderate tachypnoea – rate >40/min Marked intercostal recession S_pO_2 <92% in air Admit to hospital O_2 via nasal cannulae or head box Fluids intravenously or nasogastrically
Severe	Tachypnoea – rate >60/min Recurrent apnoea Severe recession Hypoxia in air – saturation <92% Admit to ICU or high-dependency area High inspired O_2 Intubation and assistive ventilation for respiratory failure or recurrent severe apnoea IV fluids

For high-risk infants, a monoclonal antibody (palivizumab) can be given in the winter months to prevent RSV infection but does not protect against the many other viruses.

Complications

Although most infants make a full recovery within 2 weeks, some have recurrent episodes of cough and wheeze over the subsequent few years. It is known that a subset of these infants will develop asthma.

Whooping cough (pertussis)

Whooping cough or pertussis is a highly contagious clinical syndrome caused by a number of pathogens, most commonly *Bordetella pertussis*. It is endemic, with epidemics occurring every 4 years. An effective vaccine exists and is a component of the routine triple vaccine containing diphtheria, tetanus and pertussis (DTP).

Whooping cough is spread by droplet infection and has an incubation period of 7–10 days. A case is infectious from 7 days after exposure to 3 weeks after the onset of the paroxysmal cough.

> **HINTS AND TIPS**
>
> - Whooping cough is most dangerous to very young infants.
> - Vaccination is given early to confer protection on this vulnerable group.

Clinical features

The clinical course can be divided into catarrhal, paroxysmal and convalescent stages.

During paroxysms of coughing (which are often worse at night) the child might go blue and vomit. The inspiratory whoop can be absent in infants. Nosebleeds and subconjunctival haemorrhage can occur after vigorous coughing. Symptoms can persist for 3 months (the '100-day' cough).

Diagnosis

A marked lymphocytosis ($>15.0 \times 10^9$/L) is characteristic and the organism can be cultured from a pernasal swab or PCR early in the disease.

Treatment

Erythromycin given early in the disease eradicates the organism and reduces infectivity but does not shorten the duration of the disease.

Complications

Complications, including pneumonia, convulsions, apnoea, bronchiectasis and death, are more common in infants under 6 months of age.

ASTHMA

Asthma is a chronic inflammatory disorder of the airways associated with widespread variable airflow obstruction and an increase in airways resistance in response to a variety of stimuli. The symptoms are reversible spontaneously or with treatment.

Asthma is the most common chronic respiratory disorder of childhood with a prevalence of approximately 10% in the UK. It has increased in prevalence in the last decade and is twice as common in boys as girls.

Aetiology

Asthma is associated with a number of risk factors:

- Family history or coexistent atopy.
- Male sex.
- Parental smoking.

Pathophysiology

The pathophysiology of airway narrowing in asthma includes chronic inflammation of the bronchial mucosa associated with mucosal oedema, secretions and the constriction of airway smooth muscle (Fig. 17.4).

In children there are many different patterns of asthma. In the infant age group there are many infants with recurrent wheeze due to having underlying small airways, their symptoms improving as the airway grows. There is an association of small airways with exposure to antenatal smoking. These infants may not have the typical inflammatory changes we associate with asthma and often wheeze just with viral infections.

History

Enquiry should be made concerning the pattern of symptoms (episodic or persistent), a family history of asthma, trigger factors and those features that allow the clinical evaluation of severity (exercise tolerance, night-time disturbance, school absence). A full history should cover the differential diagnosis, e.g. growth, infections, gastrointestinal symptoms.

There are distinct patterns of asthma in childhood (Fig. 17.5).

Fig. 17.4 Factors in the pathogenesis of asthma

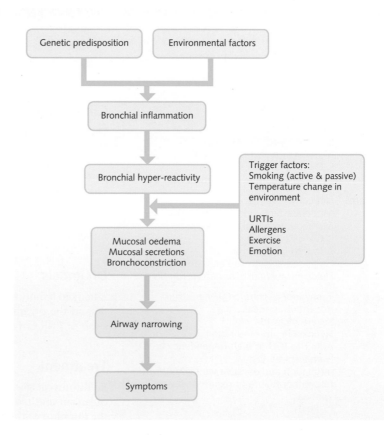

Fig. 17.5 Asthma: patterns

Pattern	Infrequent episodic	Frequent episodic	Persistent episodic
Proportion affected	Most common: 75% of all asthmatics	20%	5%
Clinical features	Triggered by viral URTIs Normal lung function and examination	Exacerbations more severe but mild interval symptoms, especially exercise-induced	Daily symptoms and use of bronchodilators Abnormal lung function
		Abnormal lung function when symptomatic	
Management step	Treat with intermittent bronchodilators and short course of oral steroids for severe exacerbations Step 1	Treat with inhaled steroids ± add on therapy Step 2–3	Treat with inhaled steroid with add on therapy Need specialist advice (Step 4–5)
Prognosis	40% will remain symptomatic in adulthood	70% remain symptomatic in adulthood	90% remain symptomatic in adulthood

Examination

Auscultation of the chest is usually normal between attacks. Chronic, severe asthma is associated with thoracic deformity:

- Hyperexpansion.
- Pigeon chest (pectus carinatum).
- Harrison sulcus.

Diagnosis

A working practical definition is a child with recurrent cough and wheeze in a clinical setting where asthma is likely (e.g. atopy, family history of asthma) and in whom other rarer causes (e.g. suppurative lung disease) have been excluded.

In most children, a careful history and examination should distinguish those with asthma. Not all that wheezes is asthma and some important conditions that need to be distinguished from asthma are shown in Fig. 17.6.

Investigations

A plain CXR can be useful at initial presentation. In children aged over 5 years, the peak expiratory flow rate (PEFR) can aid diagnosis if the child can carry this out reliably. Significant diurnal variability or decrease after exercise suggests bronchial hyperreactivity. Spirometry in older children might demonstrate reversible airway obstruction. However, in the majority of children a diagnosis is made without lung function testing because this is too difficult to measure in young

Fig. 17.6 Differential diagnosis of asthma

	Clues
Cystic fibrosis	Failure to thrive, productive cough and finger clubbing
Gastro-oesophageal reflux	Excessive vomiting
Central airways disease	Inspiratory stridor with wheeze
Laryngeal problems	Abnormal voice
Inhaled foreign body	Sudden onset
Postviral wheeze	Recent respiratory infection in children under 2 years age

children; instead, an assessment of the child's response to a treatment is performed.

Allergy tests might indicate evidence of atopy, which is associated with asthma, but 50% of asthmatics are non-atopic.

Management

The aim of asthma treatment is to have:

- No daytime symptoms or waking at night due to asthma.
- No exacerbations.

- No need for reliever therapy.
- No limitations on activity.
- Normal lung function.
- Minimal side-effects of therapy.

Important ways of achieving these goals are:

- An education and management plan for child and carers (the Asthma UK website is a useful source of information).
- Establishing the minimal effective dose of preventer medication, especially steroids.
- An age-appropriate delivery device.
- Accurate diagnosis and assessment of severity, with regular review.
- Avoiding triggers.

Triggers of asthma

Although the evidence for allergy avoidance is poor, skin-prick testing or specific IgE might identify allergens and a trial of avoidance may be indicated.

HINTS AND TIPS

The single most effective modification is eradication of exposure to cigarette smoke. Other measures directed at removing house dust mite are of limited use. Food allergy is uncommon as a trigger in asthma but anaphylaxis in an asthmatic child is more likely to be fatal.

Medication

The drugs used in the management of asthma in children can be classified into 'preventers' and 'relievers'.

HINTS AND TIPS

There is a colour code for asthma drug inhaler devices:
- 'Preventers' are mostly brown, e.g. inhaled steroid. Other colours are purple, red, green and orange.
- 'Relievers' are blue, e.g. inhaled salbutamol.

A stepwise approach to treatment has been devised (British Guidelines for Asthma Management) and is summarized in Fig. 17.7. Patients should start treatment at the step most appropriate to the initial severity. Once control is achieved, treatment can be stepped down. A rescue course of oral prednisolone might be needed at any step (under 1 year old: 1–2 mg/kg/day; 1–5 years: 20 mg/day; maximum dose 40 mg/day). In children with marked seasonal variation in asthma severity, the treatment should be varied according to the season.

Fig. 17.7 Stepwise management of chronic asthma in children

Step 1	All asthmatic children should have an inhaled β_2 bronchodilator
Step 2 If requiring 2–3 times daily inhaled β_2 agonists	Add low-dose inhaled steroids
Step 3	Try adding on long-acting β agonists or leukotriene receptor antagonists before increasing steroid dose
Step 4 If increasing steroid dose ineffective	Consider: • Leukotriene receptor antagonists • Oral theophylline • High-dose inhaled steroids
Step 5	Alternate day oral steroids

Inhalation therapy is central to most asthma treatment. The basic systems available are considered in Figs 17.8 and 17.9.

The mode of action, indications for use and side-effects of the most commonly used bronchodilator drugs are outlined in Fig. 17.10.

Fig. 17.8 Administration of medication by inhalation

	Advantages	Disadvantages
Metered dose inhaler (MDI) with spacer	Coordination not required Usable at all ages Effective for acute asthma unless needing oxygen	Bulky
Dry powder inhaler (DPI)	Coordination unimportant Small and portable Easy to operate	Requires rapid inspiration Unsuitable for children <5 years
Nebulizer	Coordination unimportant Usable at all ages Effective in severe attack	Expensive, noisy, cumbersome Treatment takes a long time, >5 min May not prompt and hence, delay hospital attention Frightens some infants

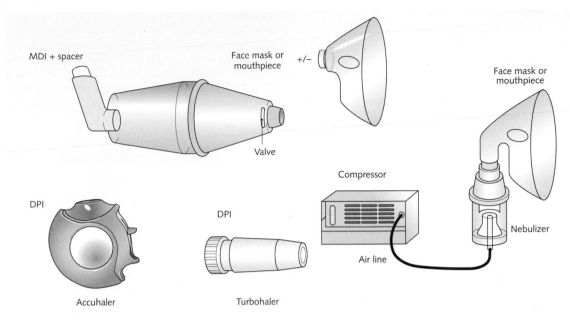

Fig. 17.9 Inhaler devices

Fig. 17.10 Asthma drug therapy: mode of action, indications and side-effects of bronchodilators			
Relievers (bronchodilators)	**Mode of action**	**Use**	**Side-effects**
Short-acting β_2 agonists, e.g. salbutamol, terbutaline	Smooth muscle relaxation	Relief of bronchospasm	Tachycardia Hypokalaemia Restlessness
Long-acting β_2 agonists, e.g. salmeterol	Smooth muscle relaxation	Nocturnal asthma, exercise-induced asthma Trial alternative to high-dose inhaled steroids	
Theophylline	Phosphodiesterase inhibition	Oral theophylline for nocturnal asthma IV aminophylline in acute severe asthma	Restlessness Diuresis Cardiac arrhythmias
Anticholinergics, e.g. ipratropium bromide	Inhibit cholinergic bronchoconstriction; add on to β_2 agonists in acute attack	First-line bronchodilator in infants	Dry mouth Urinary retention

Steroid therapy in asthma

Glucocorticoids are key drugs in the management of asthma, both in prophylaxis and the treatment of acute attacks. They can be given:

- By inhalation.
- Orally.
- Intravenously: in acute asthma.

HINTS AND TIPS

Which inhaler device for which patient?
- MDI (metered dose inhaler): suitable only for competent older children (breath-activated MDIs are available and do not require such a high level of coordination).
- MDI and spacer: beneficial in all children and as effective as nebulizers if used correctly.
- DPI (dry powder inhaler): children from age 5 years.

Inhaled steroids

Inhaled steroids are now the 'preventers' of choice in the management of childhood asthma. The lowest dose that achieves control should be used. They are indicated in frequent interval symptoms, nocturnal asthma, poor lung function tests and if using bronchodilator more than 3 times a week as rescue treatment. Inhaled steroids:

- Inhibit synthesis of inflammatory mediators (cytokines, leukotrienes and prostaglandins).
- Reduce airway hyperresponsiveness.
- Reduce both the symptoms and frequency of attacks.
- Prevent irreversible airway narrowing.

Local side-effects, such as oral thrush or dysphonia, are uncommon. Ninety per cent of the dose is deposited in the mouth and pharynx, but this can be reduced by the use of a spacer (with MDIs) and mouth washing (with DPIs). High doses (>800 micrograms) are associated with decreased growth and adrenal suppression, and children taking inhaled steroids must have their height monitored closely.

COMMUNICATION

Parents, and sometimes children, are anxious about the adverse effects of long-term inhaled steroids. Since the dose is low and is targeted at the lungs, systemic absorption is less and therefore systemic adverse effects are rare. While transient growth failure can occur, there is good evidence that the final height is not affected. In addition, asthma itself can lead to growth failure, which is probably worse than that due to steroids. Steroids can cause adrenal failure, but this is again rare unless high doses are used.

Long-acting β_2 agonists

This class of inhaled drug can be used as an add-on therapy in children over 4 years if control is poor with low-dose inhaled steroids. New combination inhaled steroid and long-acting β_2 agonists are available.

Leukotriene receptor antagonists

This class of oral drug, e.g. montelukast, acts by inhibiting leukotrienes which are released from mast cells, eosinophils and basophils that lead to increased inflammation, secretions and airway narrowing. They can be used in children under 5 years who cannot take an inhaled steroid or in children where a steroid inhaler has not controlled symptoms.

Theophylline

This oral drug can be used in difficult to treat asthma but its use is limited by side-effects.

Oral steroids

Prednisolone as a single daily dose is the drug of choice. Short courses (3 days) are indicated for acute exacerbations. Regular oral steroids are indicated only for the most severe asthma that cannot be controlled with high-dose inhaled steroids and regular bronchodilators. Alternative day dosage is preferred to reduce systemic side-effects.

Anti IgE monoclonal antibody and immunosuppressant therapies

More recent treatments include anti IgE monoclonal antibodies, e.g. omalizumab, which binds to circulating IgE, markedly reducing levels of free serum IgE. In children over 6 years of age, it is licensed in the UK for patients on high-dose inhaled steroids and long-acting $\beta2$ agonists who have impaired lung function, are symptomatic with frequent exacerbations and have allergy as an important cause of their asthma. Omalizumab is given as a subcutaneous injection every 2–4 weeks depending on dose. Omalizumab as add-on therapy to inhaled corticosteroids has been studied in children 6–12 years of age with moderate to severe asthma and has been shown to significantly reduce clinically significant exacerbations over a period of 52 weeks.

Immunosuppressants (e.g. methotrexate, ciclosporin and oral gold) may be given as a 3-month trial, once other drug treatments have proved unsuccessful and their risks and benefits should be discussed with the patient and family. Treatment and monitoring should be supervised in a specialist centre experienced in immunosuppressant medication.

Acute severe asthma

This is considered in more detail in Chapter 29. Features of acute severe asthma include:

- Respiratory rate >50 breaths/min.
- Pulse >140 beats/min.
- Use of accessory muscles.
- Too breathless to talk.

Life-threatening features include:

- Cyanosis.
- Silent chest (insufficient airflow to generate wheeze).
- Exhaustion, poor respiratory effort.
- Agitation, diminished consciousness (indicate hypoxia).

Immediate management

- High-flow O_2 via facemask.
- Salbutamol (2.5–5.0 mg) and ipratropium bromide 250 micrograms via an oxygen-driven nebulizer.

- Prednisolone orally (20–40 mg) or IV hydrocortisone (4 mg/kg).
- Pulse oximetry: O_2 saturation <92% in air indicates need for hospitalization.

If life-threatening features (or poor response):

- IV salbutamol bolus (15 micrograms/kg) followed by a salbutamol infusion (1–2 micrograms/kg/h).
- Intravenous magnesium sulphate as adjunct therapy.
- Consider IV aminophylline.
- Discuss with paediatric ITU.

Prognosis of asthma

Most children with asthma improve as they get older (see Fig. 17.5). Prognosis is better with earlier age at diagnosis. Children with poor pulmonary function testing and frequent wheezy episodes are associated with recurrent wheeze in adulthood.

CYSTIC FIBROSIS

Incidence and aetiology

Cystic fibrosis (CF) is the most common lethal genetic disease in Caucasian people. It has a carrier rate of 1:25 and incidence of 1:2500 live births. CF is an autosomal recessive disease arising from mutations in a gene on chromosome 7 that encodes an ATP-binding cassette (ABC) transporter, the cystic fibrosis transmembrane regulator (CFTR) protein. The most common mutation is a three base-pair deletion that removes the phenylalanine at position 508 (ΔF508). This is found in 90% of disease chromosomes, but 1200 mutations have now been identified so far.

The mutations in the CFTR result in defective chloride ion transport across epithelial cells and increased viscosity of secretions, especially in the respiratory tract and exocrine pancreas. This predisposes to recurrent chest infections and pancreatic insufficiency. In addition, abnormal transport in sweat gland epithelium results in high concentrations of sodium and chloride in sweat, which form the basis of the most useful diagnostic test, the sweat test.

Clinical features

Cystic fibrosis should be considered in any child with recurrent chest infection and failure to thrive. Viscid mucus in the small airways predisposes to infection with *Staphylococcus aureus*, *Haemophilus influenzae* and *Pseudomonas* species. Repeated infection leads to bronchial wall damage with bronchiectasis and abscess formation.

There is a cough productive of purulent sputum and on examination there might be:

- Hyperinflation.
- Crackles.
- Wheeze.
- Finger clubbing.

An example of typical chest X-ray changes is shown in Fig. 17.11.

In most children, deficiency of pancreatic enzymes (protease, amylase and lipase) results in malabsorption, steatorrhoea and failure to thrive. Stools are pale, greasy and offensive. About 10% of infants with CF present with 'meconium ileus' in the neonatal period, in which inspissated meconium causes internal obstruction.

Diagnosis

Screening for CF is performed as part of the newborn blood spot test using immunoreactive trypsinogen (IRT) with the aim of early diagnosis to preserve lung function. The gold standard diagnostic test is the sweat test, using pilocarpine iontophoresis. Failure of the normal reabsorption of sodium and chloride by the sweat duct epithelium leads to abnormally salty sweat: chloride concentrations of 60–125 mmol/L are found (the normal value is <15 mmol/L). Two sweat tests showing a chloride of >60 mmol/L confirm CF.

A CF genotype using DNA analysis is also available for the more common mutations and can help confirm a diagnosis.

Management

Cystic fibrosis is a multisystem disease (Fig. 17.12) and management requires a multidisciplinary approach,

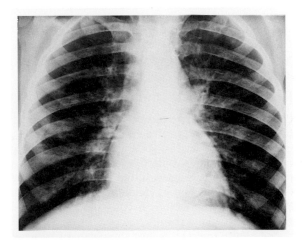

Fig. 17.11 Typical chest X-ray of a child with cystic fibrosis, showing bilateral severe lung pathology: hyperinflated lungs with bronchial wall thickening

Fig. 17.12 Multisystem aspects of cystic fibrosis

Non-pulmonary aspects of cystic fibrosis	
Airway	Nasal polyps
Gastrointestinal	Distal ileal obstruction syndrome
Pancreas/endocrine	Cystic fibrosis and diabetes Poor growth Osteoporosis
Reproductive	Infertility in males from absent vas deferens
Joints	Arthropathy
Vascular	Vasculitis
Hepatic Psychological	Portal hypertension

which is delivered most effectively by a specialist centre. The main aims are to:

- Prevent progression of lung disease.
- Promote adequate nutrition and growth.

A team approach is required, involving paediatricians with an interest in CF, physiotherapists, dieticians, CF nurses, community nurses, psychologists, the primary care team and the child's parents or carers. The Cystic Fibrosis Trust plays an extremely important role in supporting families.

> **HINTS AND TIPS**
>
> Cornerstones of CF treatment are:
> - Prevention of colonization and infection of the lungs.
> - Effective mucociliary clearance.
> - Nutritional support.

Respiratory management

Physiotherapy (chest percussion with postural drainage, breathing exercises, positive expiratory pressure (PEP) masks and flutter devices) is the mainstay of respiratory management. Many centres recommend continuous prophylactic antibiotics with oral flucloxacillin in the first 2 years of life and, if children are colonized with *Pseudomonas*, antipseudomonal nebulized antibiotics. Acute exacerbations require vigorous treatment, with IV antibiotics directed against the common bacterial pathogens (*Haemophilus influenzae*, *Staphylococcus aureus* and *Pseudomonas aeruginosa*) and guided by recent sputum culture results if available. Use of indwelling vascular devices (e.g. Port-A-Cath) aid regular intravenous antibiotic courses.

Mucolytics such as nebulized DNase or hypertonic saline to reduce sputum viscosity can help mucociliary clearance.

Nutritional management

The combined threats of malabsorption due to pancreatic insufficiency, poor appetite, increased metabolism due to chronic infection and increased respiratory work render nutritional management of vital importance in CF. The following supplements can be given:

- A high-calorie diet with vitamin supplements, especially fat-soluble vitamins A, D, E and K. Oral high calorie diet alone may be inadequate in many children and enteral feeding via a gastrostomy is often needed in older patients.
- Pancreatic enzyme supplementation using enteric-coated microspheres in gelatin-coated capsules (e.g. Creon), which contain amylase, lipase and protease. This usually has a marked effect on steatorrhoea and allows 'catch-up' growth.

Prognosis

Half of the present CF population are expected to live beyond 40 years and this will hopefully improve in the future. CF-associated severe lung disease may warrant referral to a lung transplantation centre and the child's local CF care team involved may discuss this option with the patient and family. Lung transplantation for some patients is an option but lack of donors means its role is limited. As many as 90% of patients with CF are alive 1 year after transplantation and 50% are alive after 5 years.

Further reading

British Guideline on the Management of Asthma (British Thoracic Society (BTS)/Scottish Intercollegiate Guidelines Network (SIGN)), May 2008 (revised January 2012): http://www.brit-thoracic.org.uk/guidelines/asthma-guidelines.aspx.

British Thoracic Society Community Acquired Pneumonia in Children Guideline Group, 2011. Guidelines for the management of community acquired pneumonia in children (update 2011). http://www.brit-thoracic.org.uk/guidelines/pneumonia-guidelines.aspx.

National Institute for Health and Clinical Excellence (NICE), July 2008. Respiratory tract infections – antibiotic prescribing. http://www.nice.org.uk/CG69.

Scottish Intercollegiate Guidelines Network (SIGN), November 2006. Bronchiolitis in children: a national clinical guideline. http://www.sign.ac.uk/pdf/sign91.pdf.

Newborn bloodspot screening programme. http://newbornbloodspot.screening.nhs.uk/cf.

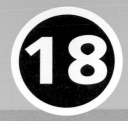
Objectives

At the end of this chapter, you should be able to:
- Identify the common causes of vomiting in children
- Recognize dehydration in a child with diarrhoeal illness and calculate the fluid requirements
- Understand some of the common surgical conditions involving the gastrointestinal tract
- Understand the pathology and clinical features of inflammatory bowel disease

Both medical and surgical disorders of the gastrointestinal tract are common in paediatric practice. Over 2 million children die each year from diarrhoeal diseases worldwide.

The range of pathological processes affecting the gastrointestinal tract is broad. It includes:
- Congenital abnormalities
- Infection
- Immune-mediated allergy or inflammation

INFANTILE COLIC

This is a common syndrome characterized by recurrent inconsolable crying often accompanied by drawing up of the legs. It usually occurs from around 2 weeks until about 4 months of age. It can occur several times a day, particularly in the evening.

Diagnosis

The differential diagnosis of inconsolable screaming includes some important conditions which should be considered before a diagnosis of colic is made.

HINTS AND TIPS

Inconsolable crying in an infant, consider:
- Colic.
- Gastro-oesophageal reflux.
- Cow's milk protein allergy.
- Otitis media.
- Incarcerated hernia.
- Urinary tract infection.
- Intussusception.

Treatment and prognosis

The condition is benign and has a good prognosis, although it is a cause of great concern to parents and can be a risk factor for non-accidental injury. A sympathetic explanation of the condition is helpful but there is no evidence for medication.

GASTRO-OESOPHAGEAL REFLUX

The involuntary passage of gastric contents into the oesophagus is a common problem, especially in babies during the first year of life. More frequent relaxation of the lower oesophageal sphincter, liquid milk rather than solid feeds and a supine posture are all contributory factors. It is a physiological finding in infancy.

Clinical features

Symptoms are usually mild (regurgitation/posseting) and no treatment is required. In a minority, however, symptoms are severe and complications such as failure to thrive, oesophagitis or recurrent aspiration pneumonia might occur.

Infants at risk of severe gastro-oesophageal reflux include:

- Preterm infants: especially those with chronic lung disease.
- Children with cerebral palsy.
- Infants with congenital oesophageal anomalies, e.g. after repair of a tracheo-oesophageal fistula.

The main symptom is recurrent regurgitation or vomiting. About 10% of infants with symptomatic reflux develop complications. Oesophagitis might be manifested by:

- Irritability.
- Features of pain after feeding.

- Blood in the vomit.
- Iron-deficiency anaemia.

Reflux can cause recurrent aspiration pneumonia, failure to thrive, cough, bronchospasm (with wheezing) and bronchiectasis.

Diagnosis

Most reflux can be diagnosed clinically but several techniques are available for confirming the diagnosis and assessing the severity:

- Twenty-four-hour oesophageal pH monitoring in older children or impedance studies in infants.
- Barium studies: might be required to exclude underlying anatomical abnormalities.
- Endoscopy: indicated in patients with suspected oesophagitis.

In the majority of mildly affected infants, reassurance is all that is required and 95% will resolve by the age of 18 months. More troublesome reflux might respond to thickening the feed with inert carob-based agents.

The following drugs can be used in more severe reflux:

- Prokinetic drugs such as domperidone: these speed gastric emptying and increase lower oesophageal sphincter pressure.
- Drugs to reduce gastric acid secretion (H2 antagonists or proton pump inhibitors): especially if there is evidence of oesophagitis.

Surgery is required for very severe cases with complications. The most commonly used procedure is Nissen fundoplication in which the fundus of the stomach is wrapped around the lower oesophagus.

GASTROENTERITIS

Gastroenteritis is an infection of the gastrointestinal tract which presents with a combination of diarrhoea and vomiting (D&V).

Incidence and aetiology

In developed countries it is usually mild and self-limiting (affecting 1 in 10 children under the age of 2 years) but in the developing world approximately 2 million children under 5 years old die from gastroenteritis each year.

Viruses cause the majority of cases in the UK with rotavirus being the most common. Other causes include:

- Bacteria, including *Shigellae*, *Salmonellae* and *Campylobacter* species and *Escherichia coli*.
- Parasites: *Entamoeba histolytica*, *Giardia lamblia* and *Cryptosporidium* species.

Clinical features

Viral infection can cause a prodromal illness followed by vomiting and diarrhoea:

- The vomiting might precede diarrhoea and is not usually stained with bile or blood.
- Abdominal pain and blood or mucus in the stool suggests an invasive bacterial pathogen.
- If the child appears toxic with high fever a viral aetiology is unlikely.

Examination is necessary to assess the presence or absence of dehydration and shock; clinical features are outlined in Fig. 18.1.

Diagnosis

The differential diagnosis includes at least two important surgical conditions:

- In young infants, especially boys (aged 2–12 weeks), vomiting might be due to pyloric stenosis. Visible peristalsis and a palpable pyloric mass might be evident.
- In older infants and toddlers (aged 1–2 years) intussusception presents with vomiting. Paroxysmal abdominal pain and the eventual passage of 'redcurrant jelly' stools should raise suspicion of this condition, which is fatal if overlooked.

Fig. 18.1 Clinical features of dehydration

No dehydration	Clinical dehydration	Clinical shock
Alert and responsive	Altered responsiveness	Decreased level of consciousness
Normal urine output	Decreased urine output	Decreased or absent urine output
Skin colour normal	Skin colour normal	Mottled skin
Warm peripheries	Warm peripheries	Cold peripheries
Moist mucous membranes	Dry mucous membranes	Dry mucous membranes
Normal heart and respiratory rate	Raised heart and respiratory rate	Raised heart and respiratory rate
Normal blood pressure and capillary refill time	Normal blood pressure and capillary refill time	Low blood pressure and prolonged capillary refill time

Most children will not require investigations. Plasma urea, electrolytes and glucose should be measured if IV therapy is used or hypernatraemic dehydration suspected. Stool culture is indicated if the stool is bloody or the child is septic or immunocompromised.

Management

Rehydration

The key to management is rehydration with correction of the fluid and electrolyte imbalance. The strategy depends on the severity of dehydration.

If the child shows no signs of dehydration (wet nappies, normal observations, moist mucous membranes) then encourage parents to continue with normal fluid intake with oral rehydration salts (ORS) as supplemental fluid if the condition worsens.

If there is evidence of clinical dehydration (decreased urine output, tachycardia, tachypnoea, dry mucous membranes) give 50 mL/kg ORS over 4 hours in addition to maintenance fluids as ORS.

If there is evidence of shock (decreased conscious level, poor perfusion, hypotension) give 20 mL/kg 0.9% saline rapidly and repeat if necessary. Then continue IV rehydration with 0.9% saline adding 100 mL/kg to maintenance requirements.

To calculate maintenance fluids:
- 100 mL/kg/24 h for 0–10 kg bodyweight.
- 50 mL/kg/24 h for 10–20 kg bodyweight.
- 20 mL/kg/24 h for >20 kg bodyweight.

If diarrhoea continues give an additional 5 mL/kg ORS for each large watery stool.

Medication

There is no role for antidiarrhoeal medication in gastroenteritis. Antibiotics are rarely indicated except for specific bacterial infections, such as invasive salmonellosis or severe *Campylobacter* infection, and amoebiasis or giardiasis.

PYLORIC STENOSIS

Pyloric stenosis is due to hypertrophy of the smooth muscle of the pylorus and is an important cause of vomiting in babies.

Incidence

The incidence of pyloric stenosis is 1–5 per 1000 live births.

Clinical features

It presents with persistent, projectile non-bilious vomiting usually between 2 and 8 weeks of age. The infant remains hungry and eager to feed after vomiting. Weight loss, constipation, mild jaundice and dehydration develop after a few days.

Diagnosis

Diagnosis is clinical and made by palpation of the hypertrophied pylorus during a test feed. Peristaltic waves might be visible.

Ultrasound of the abdomen can confirm diagnosis, demonstrating the hypertrophied pylorus. In addition, a characteristic electrolyte disturbance develops with a hypochloraemic hypokalaemic metabolic alkalosis (serum HCO_3^- elevated to 25–35 mEq/L). This is due to the loss of acidic gastric contents and the kidneys retaining hydrogen ions at the expense of potassium.

Management

Medical

Correction of fluid and electrolyte abnormalities is vital prior to surgical correction.

Surgical

The definitive treatment is the Ramstedt's procedure, in which the hypertrophied pyloric musculature is divided.

INTUSSUSCEPTION

Intussusception is a condition in which one segment of bowel telescopes into an adjacent distal part of the bowel. The peak age is between 6 and 9 months. It most commonly begins just proximal to the ileocaecal valve (ileum invaginates into caecum-ileocolic). The lead point is believed to be Peyer's patches that have been enlarged by a preceding viral infection. An anatomical lead point, such as a Meckel's diverticulum or polyp, is more likely to be present in an older child.

Clinical features

The classical presenting 'triad' is:

- Colicky abdominal pain.
- Vomiting.
- An abdominal mass.

The typical history is of episodes of screaming during which the infant draws up the legs and becomes pale. Vomiting occurs and the vomit might be bile-stained. As the blood supply to the bowel becomes progressively compromised, the characteristic 'redcurrant jelly' stool will be passed. This is a late sign.

HINTS AND TIPS

Suspect intussusception if there is:
- An infant aged 6–9 months.
- Paroxysmal severe colicky abdominal pain.
- Vomiting.
- 'Redcurrant jelly' stool.
- A 'sausage-shaped' mass in right upper quadrant.

Examination might reveal a 'sausage-shaped' mass formed by the intussusceptum, which is usually palpable in the right upper quadrant. Signs of intestinal obstruction and shock develop over 24–48 hours. Ultrasound is the imaging modality of choice.

Management

Intussusception is a life-threatening condition and can easily be misdiagnosed as gastroenteritis or colic by the unwary. If suspected, an immediate diagnostic enema using air or contrast material (barium or gastrograffin) should be carried out.

In most cases, reduction by air enema is possible; however if this is unsuccessful, operative reduction is necessary.

MECKEL'S DIVERTICULUM

This remnant of the fetal vitello-intestinal duct occurs in 2% of the population. It is usually 2 inches (5 cm) long and found 2 feet (60 cm) proximal to the ileocaecal valve (the rule of 2 s). It contains ectopic gastric mucosa. Diagnosis is by a technetium scan. The majority are asymptomatic but the most typical presentation is painless, severe rectal bleeding due to peptic ulceration. Treatment is surgical.

ACUTE APPENDICITIS

This important cause of acute abdominal pain occurs when the appendix becomes obstructed (usually by a faecolith) or inflamed by lymphatic hyperplasia. It occurs at any age, although it is rare in infants when the lumen of the appendix is wider and well drained.

Clinical features

The classic symptoms are a central abdominal pain that moves to the right iliac fossa (RIF) over a period of hours. The pain is of increasing severity and aggravated by movement (as the peritoneum is exquisitely pain sensitive).

HINTS AND TIPS

Atypical presentations with poorly localized pain are common in young children (<5 years) or when the inflamed appendix is retrocaecal or pelvic.

Anorexia is usual and often associated with nausea and vomiting. Constipation might be a feature. Clinical signs include:

- Mild fever.
- Tachycardia.
- Dehydration.
- RIF tenderness.
- Guarding in a toxic child.

The differential diagnosis is shown in Fig. 18.2.

Fig. 18.2	The differential diagnosis of acute abdominal pain
Surgical	**Medical**
Appendicitis	Mesenteric adenitis
Intussusception	Gastroenteritis
Volvulus	Constipation
Meckel's diverticulum	Urinary tract infection
Strangulated hernia	Lower lobe pneumonia
Ovarian torsion	Diabetic ketoacidosis
	Henoch–Schönlein
	purpura
	Sickle cell crisis

Diagnosis

The diagnosis is usually made clinically. If there is diagnostic uncertainty, useful investigations include:

- Urine: microscopy and culture.
- Full blood count (FBC).
- Chest X-ray (CXR): pneumonia can mimic appendicitis.
- Abdominal ultrasound.

Management

A short period of observation can be undertaken before appendectomy when there is uncertainty, although progression to peritonitis can occur within a few hours in young children.

Other complications include septicaemia, appendix abscess and appendix mass. An abscess requires surgical drainage. Conservative management is given for an appendix mass with elective appendectomy carried out 6 weeks later.

MESENTERIC ADENITIS

This non-specific inflammation of mesenteric lymph nodes is thought to provoke a peritoneal reaction causing acute abdominal pain that mimics appendicitis.

Clinical features

It occurs commonly in children and is often associated with other systemic symptoms and signs including fever, headache, pharyngitis and cervical lymphadenopathy. It is likely to be viral in origin.

Diagnosis and management

Observation in hospital is often required due to the difficult diagnosis. Management is conservative, as the symptoms are self-limiting, although persisting right iliac fossa tenderness warrants surgical exploration to identify appendicitis.

COELIAC DISEASE

Incidence and aetiology

Coeliac disease is a state of heightened immunological response to ingested gluten in genetically susceptible people which causes damage to the mucosa of the proximal small intestine with subsequent atrophy of the villi and loss of the absorptive surface. The incidence varies between 0.5% and 3% in children.

There is a familial predisposition with approximately 10% of first-degree relatives affected. HLA DQ2 is found in 95% of affected individuals.

Clinical features

The classic presentation of faltering growth, steatorrhoea and abdominal distension is less common and features may be more subtle. They include:

- Diarrhoea.
- Abdominal pain.
- Constipation.
- Fatigue.
- Iron or folate deficiency anaemia.
- Amenorrhoea.
- Short stature.

Diagnosis

IgA tissue transglutaminase (tTGA) is the serological test of choice. If this is positive a definitive diagnosis requires the demonstration of a flat mucosa on jejunal biopsy followed by clinical improvement on dietary gluten withdrawal. A third biopsy on gluten challenge should be then taken to confirm the diagnosis but is commonly omitted in children.

Management

A diet free of gluten-containing products should be adhered to for life. Multidisciplinary care is required with support from a dietician.

Coeliac disease is associated with a variety of autoimmune disorders, including thyroid disease and pernicious anaemia, an increased risk of small bowel malignancy (especially lymphoma) and osteoporosis. Lifelong follow-up is required to monitor for these conditions. A strict gluten-free diet reduces the malignancy risk.

FOOD INTOLERANCE

Adverse reactions to specific foods or food ingredients are not uncommon and can be transitory or permanent. The majority are immune-mediated reactions, usually to proteins, and are properly referred to as food allergies. However, non-immune mediated intolerance also occurs, e.g. lactose intolerance due to intestinal disaccharidase deficiency.

Lactose intolerance

Lactose is the predominant disaccharide in milk and requires the intestinal brush-border enzyme lactase for its digestion. Lactase deficiency is most commonly encountered as a secondary and transient phenomenon after gastroenteritis. Congenital lactase deficiency is rare; hereditary late-onset lactose intolerance is predominantly seen in Afro-Caribbean and oriental people.

Clinical features

Accumulation of intestinal sugar results in watery diarrhoea and bacterial production of organic acids, which lowers stool pH and causes excoriation of the perianal region.

Diagnosis

Lactose is a reducing sugar and may therefore be detected in the stool by the Clinitest method.

Treatment

Treatment is with a diet free of products containing lactose.

INFLAMMATORY BOWEL DISEASE

Up to one-quarter of cases of inflammatory bowel disease have their onset during childhood or adolescence (Fig. 18.3).

Crohn's disease

Crohn's disease is a transmural and focal inflammatory process that can affect any portion of the gastrointestinal tract from the mouth to the anus; the distal ileum or the colon are most frequently involved. The cause is unknown, although there is a clear genetic predisposition. Affected intestine is thickened and non-caseating epithelioid cell granulomata are found on histology.

Fig. 18.3 Comparison of Crohn's disease with ulcerative colitis

Feature	Crohn's disease	Ulcerative colitis
Colonic disease	50–75%	100%
Transmural involvement	Common	Unusual
Skip lesions	Common	Not present
Rectal bleeding	Sometimes	Common
Abdominal pain	Common	Variable
Growth failure	Common	Variable
Perianal disease	Sometimes	Unusual
Mouth ulceration	Common	Unusual

Ulcerative colitis

Ulcerative colitis is a chronic, recurrent inflammatory disease involving the mucous membrane of the colon. The disease process is restricted to the mucosa and begins in the rectum, extending proximally.

Clinical features of inflammatory bowel disease

It may present with:

- Cramping lower abdominal pain.
- Bloody diarrhoea.
- Weight loss/faltering growth.
- Perianal disease (abscess or fistula formation).

Extra-intestinal features might be present, including delayed puberty, arthritis, spondylitis and erythema nodosum.

Management

Crohn's disease is managed initially with an elemental diet with steroids for active relapse. Immunosuppressive agents such as azathioprine are the next line followed by anti-TNF antibodies such as infliximab. Surgery remains an option for failure of medical treatment.

Ulcerative colitis is treated with aminosalicylates with steroids reserved for active disease. Surgery may be used when medical treatment has failed.

HIRSCHSPRUNG'S DISEASE (CONGENITAL AGANGLIONIC MEGACOLON)

This is a rare genetic disorder of bowel innervation. There is an absence of ganglion cells in the myenteric and submucosal plexuses for a variable segment of bowel extending from the anus to the colon. The aganglionic segment is narrow and contracted. It ends proximally in a normally innervated and dilated colon. It is more common in males.

Clinical features

Infants with the disease usually present in the neonatal period with:

- Delayed passage of meconium (>48 h of life).
- Subsequent intestinal obstruction with bilious vomiting and abdominal distension.

Enterocolitis is a severe, life-threatening complication. Older children present with:

- Chronic, severe constipation present from birth.
- Abdominal distension.
- An absence of faeces in the narrow rectum.

Diagnosis and management

A barium enema might demonstrate a transition zone where the bowel lumen changes in diameter. Confirmation of the diagnosis is made by demonstrating the absence of ganglion cells on a suction biopsy of the rectum. Surgical resection of the involved colon is required. An initial colostomy is usually followed by a definitive pull-through procedure to anastomose normally innervated bowel to the anus.

BILE DUCT OBSTRUCTION

Obstruction of bile flow due to biliary atresia or a choledochal cyst are rare, but treatable, causes of persistent neonatal jaundice. Early recognition and diagnosis of these liver diseases is important.

Biliary atresia

This is a rare disorder of unknown aetiology in which there is either destruction or absence of the extrahepatic biliary tree. It represents a rare but important cause of persistent neonatal jaundice (Fig. 18.4).

Clinical features

The jaundice persists from the second day after birth and is distinguished by being due to a predominantly conjugated hyperbilirubinaemia accompanied by dark urine and pale stools. As the disease progresses there is failure to thrive due to:

- Malabsorption.
- Enlargement of the liver and spleen.

A bleeding tendency might develop due to vitamin K deficiency.

Diagnosis

Abdominal ultrasound, liver biopsy and intraoperative cholangiography might be required to clarify the diagnosis.

Fig. 18.4 Liver disease presenting in the newborn period: causes of conjugated hyperbilirubinaemia

Bile duct obstruction	Biliary atresia Choledochal cyst
Neonatal hepatitis	Congenital infection Inborn errors: α_1 antitrypsin deficiency Galactosaemia

Treatment

Treatment consists of the Kasai procedure (hepatoportoenterostomy), which should ideally be carried out before the age of 6 weeks. Liver transplantation is needed if this fails or if presentation is late.

CONSTIPATION

Constipation is common. It is the delay or difficulty in defecation for greater than 2 weeks. The majority is idiopathic but history and examination should be targeted at identifying any underlying causes.

> **HINTS AND TIPS**
>
> Red flag signs and symptoms of constipation:
> - Starts in first few weeks of life.
> - Meconium passed >24 hours.
> - Faltering growth.
> - Delayed walking or lower limb neurology.
> - Abdominal distension or vomiting.
> - Child protection concerns.

Management is with laxatives and re-establishing a regular bowel habit. Treatment is often prolonged and in some cases requires psychological support.

Further reading

National Institute for Health and Clinical Excellence (NICE), April 2009. CG84 Diarrhoea and vomiting in children under 5. http://www.nice.org.uk/CG84.

National Institute for Health and Clinical Excellence (NICE), May 2009. CG86 Recognition and assessment of coeliac disease. http://www.nice.org.uk/CG86.

National Institute for Health and Clinical Excellence (NICE), May 2010. CG99 Constipation in children and young people. http://www.nice.org.uk/guidance/CG99.

Renal and genitourinary disorders

Objectives

At the end of this chapter, you should be able to:
- Know the common developmental anomalies of the urinary tract
- Recognize common inguinoscrotal conditions such as undescended testes and inguinal hernia
- Know the pathogenesis and clinical features of urinary tract infection (UTI) in children
- Outline the investigations for a child with UTI
- Distinguish between acute nephritis and nephrotic syndrome

Structural abnormalities of the kidney and urinary tract are common and many are now identified on antenatal ultrasound screening. The most common disease encountered in this system is urinary tract infection (UTI), which has special significance because of its potential to damage the growing kidneys, leading to hypertension and chronic renal failure.

HINTS AND TIPS

Presentation of urinary tract anomalies:
- Urinary tract infection.
- Recurrent abdominal pain.
- Palpable mass.
- Haematuria.
- Failure to thrive

URINARY TRACT ANOMALIES

Congenital abnormalities of the kidneys and urinary tract can be identified in about 1 in 400 fetuses. They might be detected on antenatal ultrasound screening or present with a variety of symptoms and signs in infancy or later childhood.

Congenital anomalies of the urinary tract include:
- Renal anomalies.
- Obstructive lesions of the urinary tract.
- Vesicoureteric reflux.

Renal anomalies

Anomalies of the renal parenchyma include a wide range of abnormalities, e.g.:
- Complete bilateral renal agenesis.

- Abnormalities of ascent and rotation.
- Duplex kidney (Fig. 19.1).
- Horseshoe kidney (Fig. 19.1).
- Cystic disease of the kidney.
- Renal dysplasia.

Absence of both kidneys (renal agenesis) results in Potter syndrome in which oligohydramnios (caused by lack of fetal urine) leads to lung hypoplasia and postural deformities. Ectopia of the kidney is common and pain arising from an ectopic kidney can be misleading on account of its site.

Duplex systems are commonly associated with other abnormalities such as renal dysplasia and vesicoureteric reflux. The upper pole ureter might be ectopic (draining into the urethra or vagina) and the lower pole ureter often refluxes.

There are many conditions associated with cystic kidneys including:

- Autosomal recessive polycystic kidney disease (infantile form).
- Autosomal dominant polycystic kidney disease (adult-type).
- Tuberous sclerosis (see Chapter 20).

Obstructive lesions of the urinary tract

The site of obstruction may be at the pelviureteric (PU) junction, the vesicoureteric (VU) junction, the bladder or the urethra (Fig. 19.2). If undetected before birth, the patient can present with:

- A urinary tract infection.
- Abdominal or loin pain.
- Haematuria.
- A palpable bladder or kidney.

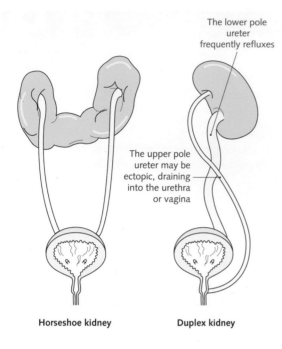

The lower pole ureter frequently refluxes

The upper pole ureter may be ectopic, draining into the urethra or vagina

Horseshoe kidney   Duplex kidney

Fig. 19.1 Urinary tract anomalies

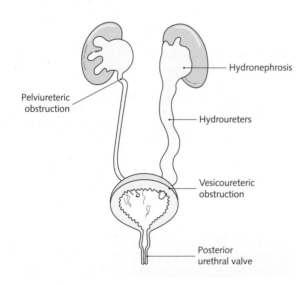

Pelviureteric obstruction

Hydronephrosis

Hydroureters

Vesicoureteric obstruction

Posterior urethral valve

Fig. 19.2 Sites of urinary tract obstruction and dilatation

Pelviureteric obstruction

Obstruction is caused by a narrow lumen or compression by a fibrous band or blood vessel, and can vary in degree from partial to almost complete obstruction (with gross hydronephrosis and minimal remaining renal tissue).

Mild degrees of obstruction can resolve spontaneously but severe obstruction requires surgical treatment with conservation of renal tissue wherever possible.

Vesicoureteric obstruction

Obstruction can be due to stenosis, kinking or dilatation of the lower part of the ureter (ureterocoele) and can be unilateral or bilateral. There is a combination of hydroureter and hydronephrosis.

Posterior urethral valves

These are abnormal folds of the urethral mucous membrane, which occur in males in the region of the verumontanum (where the seminal ducts enter the urethra). They are often diagnosed antenatally. They impede the flow of urine with back-pressure on the bladder, ureters and kidneys. The degree of obstruction varies from very severe (with Potter syndrome or renal failure leading to death) to less severe presentations (urinary tract infections, poor stream and renal insufficiency). Temporary drainage and stabilization is followed by definitive surgical management.

Vesicoureteric reflux

This is a condition in which urine refluxes up the ureter during voiding, predisposing to infection and exposing the kidneys to bacteria and high pressure. This can lead to scarring (reflux nephropathy) and if severe results in hypertension and chronic renal failure.

Primary vesicoureteric reflux (VUR) is caused by a developmental anomaly of the vesicoureteric junction. The ureters usually enter the bladder at an angle, with a large section of ureter within the muscular wall; this is compressed with bladder contraction. In primary VUR the ureters enter perpendicularly, hence the segment of ureter within the bladder wall is abnormally short and there is inadequate ureter closure during voiding. There is a spectrum of severity which is graded I–V (Fig. 19.3).

Clinical features

VUR is often associated with other genitourinary anomalies and may be secondary to bladder pathology, e.g. neuropathic bladder. It is often asymptomatic, picked

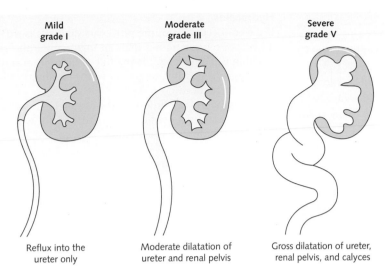

Mild
grade I

Moderate
grade III

Severe
grade V

Fig. 19.3 Grades of vesicoureteric reflux

Reflux into the
ureter only

Moderate dilatation of
ureter and renal pelvis

Gross dilatation of ureter,
renal pelvis, and calyces

up on ultrasound scan (may be antenatally diagnosed) but may present with recurrent urinary tract infections or pyelonephritis.

Diagnosis

VUR is diagnosed by a micturating cystourethrogram (MCUG).

Management

Mild VUR resolves spontaneously (10% each year) but prophylactic antibiotics (e.g. trimethoprim) may be given to prevent infection in more serious cases.

Surgery is indicated if there are recurrent UTIs or grade IV–V VUR. The siblings of children should be investigated as there is a strong genetic component.

GENITALIA

Inguinoscrotal disorders

Inguinoscrotal disorders include:

* Undescended testis.
* Inguinal hernia and hydrocele.
* The acute scrotum.

Undescended testis

The testes develop intra-abdominally and migrate through the inguinal canal to the scrotum in the third trimester. The testes are therefore normally in the scrotum in term neonates, but are frequently undescended in preterm infants. Undescended testes are the most common congenital genitourinary anomaly.

Clinical features and examination

A testis that has not reached the scrotum might be:

* Retractile: normally descended with exaggerated cremasteric reflex. Can be coaxed into scrotum; may become 'ascended' and require monitoring until puberty.
* Maldescended:
    * Arrested descent: found along the normal pathway.
    * Ectopic (<1%): deviated from normal pathway.

The testes are examined during routine surveillance in the newborn and at 6–8 weeks. Referral to a surgeon should be made if either testis is impalpable or an ectopic testis is found at the 6-week check.

Bilaterally undescended testes in the newborn always warrant investigation to rule out congenital adrenal hyperplasia (see Chapter 24). Further investigations may include:

* Ultrasound $\pm$ MRI.
* Laparoscopy.
* Endocrine investigations.

HINTS AND TIPS

Bilaterally undescended testes in the newborn may be a presentation of congenital adrenal hyperplasia and requires urgent investigation.

Management

Undescended testes carry an increased risk of malignancy, subfertility and torsion. Treatment is by orchidopexy between the age of 1 and 2 years.

Orchidectomy is indicated for a unilateral intra-abdominal testis that is not amenable to orchidopexy.

In many children, the testis may descend to its normal position in the first year of life even if it was high up in the scrotum at birth. So parents should be informed that a surgical referral will usually be made only after a year and this should not cause any harm to the child.

Inguinal hernias and hydroceles

The testis descends into the scrotum, taking with it a connecting fold of peritoneum (the processus vaginalis), which normally becomes obliterated at or around birth. Failure of the processus vaginalis to close results in an inguinal hernia or a hydrocele (Fig. 19.4).

Inguinal hernias

Inguinal hernias are more common in boys, premature babies and infants with a positive family history. A minority are bilateral. The parents notice an intermittent swelling in the groin or scrotum.

The main concern is the risk of strangulation, which is higher in young infants. Referral for prompt surgery is indicated. Danger signs requiring urgent surgical referral in the initially irreducible hernia are:

- Hardness.
- Tenderness.
- Vomiting.

Sedation, analgesia and expert manipulation allow reduction, followed by surgical repair.

Hydroceles

If the connection with the processus vaginalis is small, a hydrocele forms rather than an inguinal hernia. The swelling is painless and, being full of fluid, it transilluminates. It is possible to get above the swelling, which cannot be reduced.

Spontaneous resolution by the age of 12 months is common and treatment during infancy is not required unless the hydrocele is extremely large.

The acute scrotum

Acute pain and swelling of the scrotum is an emergency because of the possibility of testicular torsion. It occurs most frequently in the neonatal period and at puberty, but can occur at any age.

Inadequate fixation to the tunica vaginalis allows the testis to rotate and occlude its vascular supply. Doppler studies can assist in diagnosis.

Surgical exploration must not be delayed, as the testis might become non-viable. The defect is often bilateral, so the contralateral testis should also be fixed at surgery.

The differential diagnosis includes:

- Torsion of the testicular appendix (hydatid of Morgagni).
- Epididymo-orchitis.
- Idiopathic scrotal oedema.

Penile abnormalities

Penile abnormalities include:

- Hypospadias.
- Phimosis.

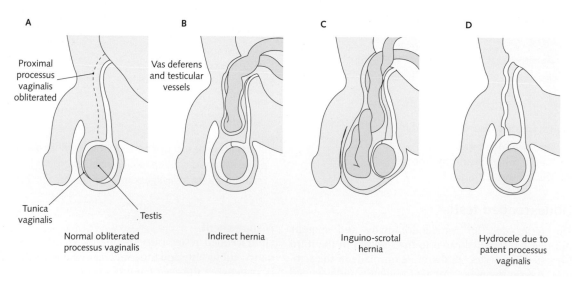

Normal obliterated processus vaginalis

Indirect hernia

Inguino-scrotal hernia

Hydrocele due to patent processus vaginalis

Fig. 19.4 (A) The normal testis. Following normal testicular descent, the processus vaginalis, an evagination of the parietal peritoneum between the internal inguinal ring and testis, disappears leaving only the tunica vaginalis around the testis. Persistence of the processus vaginalis results in an inguinal hernia (B, C), or a hydrocele (D)

Hypospadias

A spectrum of congenital abnormalities of the position of the urethral meatus occurs, ranging from mild displacement to urethral opening within the scrotum or perineum. The foreskin is incompletely closed giving a dorsal hooded appearance. Severe forms are associated with chordee (a ventral curvature of the penis), and may lead to problems with continence and fertility.

Management depends on severity; urological assessment is required.

Phimosis

Infants with hypospadias must not be circumcised: the foreskin is used for surgical correction.

Phimosis refers to adhesion of the foreskin to the glans penis after the age of 3 years. Mild degrees can be managed with periodic, gentle retraction. Paraphimosis is irreducible retraction of the foreskin beyond the glans. It leads to venous congestion and permanent damage if not reduced.

Circumcision

The foreskin is non-retractile in children and forcible attempts to retract the foreskin may result in scarring and phimosis.

Ballooning of the prepuce during urination is not uncommon and this usually resolves as the prepuce becomes more retractile.

Balanitis xerotica obliterans (lichen sclerosus) causes a thickened, scarred, white prepuce that is fixed to the glans. This, recurrent balanitis (infection of the glans) and sometimes recurrent urinary tract infection (UTI) are the only medical indications for circumcision. Most circumcisions are performed for religious reasons.

Complications of circumcision

- Haemorrhage.
- Infection.
- Damage to the glans.

The procedure should not be undertaken lightly.

Vulvovaginitis

Inflammation of the vulva and vaginal discharge is a common gynaecological complaint in pre-pubertal girls. Pre-pubertal girls have an increased risk due to lack of labial development, low oestrogen levels and more alkaline pH. Poor hygiene and tight fitting clothes are also suggested to be predisposing factors. A vulval swab might detect a yeast or streptococcal infection, which can be treated with the appropriate topical or oral therapy. It is important to think of foreign bodies if a persistent discharge is seen. Vulvovaginitis may also result from sexual abuse.

URINARY TRACT INFECTION

Infection of the urinary tract is common in children. About 3–5% of girls and 1–2% of boys will have a symptomatic UTI during childhood; boys outnumber girls until 3 months of age. UTI often presents as a non-specific illness and should be considered in all children with an unexplained fever. A history of poor flow, renal abnormalities, previous UTI and constipation should be sought.

In children, most infections are caused by *Escherichia coli* originating from the bowel flora. Other pathogens include *Proteus* (especially in boys), *Klebsiella*, *Pseudomonas* and *Enterococcus* species. The most common factor predisposing to UTI is urinary stasis. Important causes of urinary stasis include:

- Vesicoureteric reflux (VUR).
- Obstructive uropathy, e.g. ureterocoele, urethral valves.
- Neuropathic bladder, e.g. spina bifida.
- Habitual infrequent voiding and constipation.

UTIs occur:
- Predominantly in boys up to age 3 months.
- Equally in boys and girls from 3 to 12 months.
- Increasingly in girls rather than boys after age 1 year.
- UTI presents with non-specific features in infants.
- UTI must be suspected in any febrile infant with no obvious clinical source.

Clinical features

The clinical features vary markedly with age:

- In neonates and very young infants: jaundice might occur and septicaemia can develop, rapidly leading to shock.
- In infants: symptoms are non-specific; vomiting, diarrhoea, irritability, failure to thrive.
- Between 1 and 5 years of age: fever, malaise, abdominal discomfort, urinary frequency and nocturnal enuresis are the presenting features.

Fig. 19.5   Collecting a urine sample

Method	Indication
Clean catch	Method of choice for obtaining sample
Bag or pad sample	If clean catch not obtainable
Suprapubic aspirate (with ultrasound guidance)	If an urgent sample required and non-invasive technique not practical
Catheter	Only fresh samples valid for infection

- Over 5 years of age: the classic presenting features of cystitis (frequency, dysuria, fever and enuresis) or pyelonephritis (fever and loin pain) occur. Asymptomatic bacteriuria is common in school-age girls. This does not need treatment.

Diagnosis

Confirmation of diagnosis requires culture of a pure growth of a single pathogen of at least 10^4 colony-forming units per litre of urine. However, obtaining an uncontaminated urine sample from infants and children is not easy (Fig. 19.5). Specimens should be refrigerated without delay to prevent bacterial multiplication.

In children less than 3 years old urgent microscopy should be used to diagnose UTI. In over 3 s a urine dipstick can be used although false negatives occur if the urine has been in the bladder for less than an hour or the organism does not convert nitrate (e.g. enterococci).

> **HINTS AND TIPS**
>
> A urine sample should be cultured from:
> - An infant with a fever and no obvious clinical source.
> - Any child with recurrent or prolonged fever.
> - Any child with unexplained abdominal pain.
> - Any child with dysuria or frequency, enuresis or haematuria.

Treatment of the acute infection

Prompt treatment with antibiotics is indicated to prevent serious illness and reduce the risk of renal scarring. A culture should be taken before treatment, and in some instances an urgent urine microscopy will be available to confirm diagnosis pre-treatment. However, antibiotics should not be delayed in an unwell child. Treatment can be modified when culture results are available and stopped if negative. Antibiotic prophylaxis post-UTI is no longer routinely recommended.

Choice and length of treatment depends on the age of the child and whether signs or symptoms of an upper urinary tract infection (pyelonephritis) are present:

- Children <3 months: signs are non-specific, management is by parenteral antibiotics, e.g. for sepsis, and a full septic screen is often needed.
- Children >3 months with signs of pyelonephritis: IV antibiotics as needed for 2–4 days, oral antibiotics for 7–10 days.
- Children >3 months with lower UTI: oral antibiotics for 3 days.

Further investigation

Further investigation depends on:
- The age of the child.
- Whether episodes are recurrent (2 or more episodes with upper urinary tract signs, 1 upper UTI plus 1 or more lower UTI, or >3 lower UTIs).
- Presence of any atypical features (non *E. coli* UTI, failure to respond to treatment in 48 hours, sepsis, abnormal renal function).

Investigations aim to identify renal abnormalities (ultrasound scan), and reflux (with micturating cystourethrogram (MCUG)) or renal function/scarring (with static radioisotope scan (DMSA)) where appropriate.

The recommended imaging schedules (NICE guidelines 2007) are shown in Figs 19.6–19.8.

Simple advice should be given concerning measures, which can reduce recurrence risk, i.e.:
- High fluid intake.
- Regular unhurried voiding.
- Good perineal hygiene.

Fig. 19.6   Imaging schedule for infants younger than 6 months

Test	Responds well to treatment within 48 hours	Atypical UTI	Recurrent UTI
Ultrasound during acute infection	No	Yes	Yes
Ultrasound within 6 weeks	Yes (if abnormal consider MCUG)	No	No
DMSA 4–6 months following acute infection	No	Yes	Yes
MCUG	No	Yes	Yes

Fig. 19.7	Imaging schedule for children 6 months – 3 years		
Test	**Responds well to treatment within 48 hours**	**Atypical UTI**	**Recurrent UTI**
Ultrasound during acute infection	No	Yes	No
Ultrasound within 6 weeks	No	No	Yes
DMSA 4–6 months following acute infection	No	Yes	Yes
MCUG	No	No	No

Fig. 19.8	Imaging schedule for children older than 3 years		
Test	**Responds well to treatment within 48 hours**	**Atypical UTI**	**Recurrent UTI**
Ultrasound during acute infection	No	Yes	No
Ultrasound within 6 weeks	No	No	Yes
DMSA 4–6 months following acute infection	No	No	Yes
MCUG	No	No	No

- Mesangiocapillary glomerulonephritis.
- Haemolytic uraemic syndrome.

Clinical features

The presenting history will be of discoloured 'smoky' urine. Physical examination reveals signs of fluid overload such as oedema and raised blood pressure. Other features may be present depending on the underlying cause.

Diagnosis

The urine is positive for blood and protein, and microscopy might reveal red cells and casts. Renal function should be evaluated by measuring plasma urea, electrolytes and creatinine. Abdominal imaging may be required to exclude other causes of haematuria.

Investigations to determine the underlying aetiology include: throat swab, anti-DNAase B, complement C3 levels and biopsy if severe.

Management

Management centres around:

- Control of fluid and electrolyte balance by monitoring intake and output.
- Use of diuretics and antihypertensives as required.
- Treatment of underlying cause as appropriate.

The prognosis of post-streptococcal nephritis is good. However, rarely, a rapidly progressive glomerulonephritis with renal failure occurs, especially in nephritis from other causes. There is no evidence that treatment of the preceding infection prevents renal complications.

ACUTE NEPHRITIS

Acute nephritis is a clinical presentation of a group of conditions caused by inflammatory changes in the glomeruli. It is characterized by:

- Fluid retention (oedema, facial puffiness).
- Hypertension.
- Haematuria.
- Proteinuria.

In children the majority of cases are postinfectious and follow a throat or skin infection with group A β-haemolytic streptococci. Less common causes include:

- Henoch–Schönlein purpura.
- IgA nephropathy.
- Systemic lupus erythematosus (SLE).

NEPHROTIC SYNDROME

Nephrotic syndrome is characterized by proteinuria, oedema, a hypoalbuminaemia and hypertriglyceridaemia (Fig. 19.9).

The majority of childhood nephrotic syndrome is minimal change disease and is classified into steroid sensitive (90%) or steroid resistant (10%).

Clinical features

The usual presenting feature is oedema, which manifests as facial puffiness (especially around the eyes), swelling of the feet and legs and, in severe cases, gross scrotal oedema, ascites and pleural effusions.

Fig. 19.9 Comparison of acute glomerulonephritis and nephrotic syndrome

Feature	Acute glomerulonephritis	Nephrotic syndrome
Aetiology	Most often post-streptococcal	Usually idiopathic
Gross haematuria	Very common	Unusual
Hypertension	Common	Less common
Oedema	Less prominent	Prominent, generalized oedema
Urinalysis	Red cell casts, proteinuria +	Proteinuria +++
Serum C3 and C4	Usually decreased	Usually normal
Anti-DNase B/ASOT	May be positive	Negative
Treatment	Supportive	Steroids

Diagnosis

Diagnosis is confirmed by documentation of proteinuria and hypoalbuminaemia. Baseline investigations should be carried out including urea and electrolytes (U&Es), urine microscopy, C3, C4, anti-DNAse B and hepatitis serology.

The following features should prompt consideration of renal biopsy to identify rarer causes such as focal segmental glomerulosclerosis or membranoproliferative glomerulonephritis, which are usually steroid resistant:

- Age: <1 year or > 12 years.
- Macroscopic haematuria.
- Low C3.
- Failure to respond to steroid therapy.
- Hypertension.
- Renal failure.

Management

If the clinical features are consistent with classic steroid-sensitive nephrotic syndrome, treatment is begun with 4 weeks of oral steroids (prednisolone, $60 \text{ mg/m}^2/\text{day}$) with a gradually reducing regimen. Steroid resistance is defined as no remission (i.e. continued proteinuria) after 4 weeks and is associated with chronic renal failure.

Fluid balance must be closely monitored with daily weighing and salt restriction.

Several serious complications may occur including:

- Hypovolaemia (manifested by a high PCV, hypotension and peripheral vasoconstriction, treated with albumin infusion).
- Thrombosis.
- Secondary infection.
- Hyperlipidaemia; this is not usually problematic in children.

Penicillin prophylaxis is given in the acute phase to prevent secondary infection and pneumococcal vaccination is recommended.

Relapses occur in up to 70% of children; these are treated with steroids, but if frequent, additional immunosuppressants such as ciclosporin, cyclophosphamide or levamisole may be needed.

HAEMOLYTIC URAEMIC SYNDROME

This is the most common cause of paediatric acute renal failure and is associated with diarrhoea from Shiga-toxin producing *E. coli* O157:H7. This toxin results in red blood cell fragmentation (glomerular microangiopathic haemolytic anaemia) and thrombocytopenia. The kidney vasculature becomes thrombosed and infarcted.

Management is supportive and most (90%) children recover full renal function. Antibiotics are contraindicated as they induce expression and release of Shiga toxin.

Further reading

Eddy, A.A., Symons, J.M., 2003. Nephrotic syndrome in childhood. Lancet 362, 629–639.

National Institute for Health and Clinical Excellence (NICE), October 2010. Nocturnal enuresis: the management of bedwetting in children and young people (CG111). http://www.nice.org.uk/guidance/CG111.

National Institute for Health and Clinical Excellence (NICE), August 2007. Urinary tract infection: diagnosis, treatment and long-term management of urinary tract infection in children (CG54). http://www.nice.org.uk/CG054.

Neurological disorders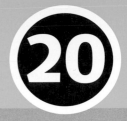

At the end of this chapter, you should be able to:
- Understand the common developmental malformations of the central nervous system
- Recognize the clinical features of raised intracranial pressure
- Know the clinical features and management of the common infections of the central nervous system
- Understand the pathogenesis, clinical presentation and management of cerebral palsy
- Understand the classification and common types of childhood epilepsy
- Identify common neurocutaneous syndromes
- Understand common neuromuscular disorders in children

The developing nervous system is susceptible to damage by a host of diverse pathological processes: inherited and acquired. Malformations, infections, trauma, genetic diseases and tumours all affect the nervous system. Several important conditions affecting the nervous system are considered elsewhere:

- Hypoxic–ischaemic encephalopathy (see Chapter 28).
- Head injury (see Chapter 29).
- Coma (see Chapter 29).
- Brain tumours (see Chapter 23).
- Neural tube defects (see Chapter 12).

MALFORMATIONS OF THE CENTRAL NERVOUS SYSTEM

If severe, these cause fetal loss or early death. They encompass such important conditions as:

- Hydrocephalus.
- Craniosynostosis.
- Neural tube defects.

Hydrocephalus

Hydrocephalus is enlargement of the cerebral ventricles due to excessive accumulation of cerebrospinal fluid (CSF). This condition is the most frequent cause of an enlarged, rapidly expanding head in newborn infants.

HINTS AND TIPS

Suspect hydrocephalus in an infant with a rapidly enlarging head circumference.

The causes include congenital malformations as well as acquired pathological mechanisms (Fig. 20.1). Hydrocephalus may be caused by:

- Intraventricular obstruction.
- Extraventricular obstruction.

Clinical features

The presenting clinical features vary with age. Dilated ventricles can be detected on antenatal ultrasound. In infants:

- The head circumference is disproportionately large and its rate of growth is excessive.
- The pressure on the anterior fontanelle is increased, sutures become separated and scalp veins are prominent. If untreated, the eyes deviate downward (setting-sun sign).

In older children, the clinical features are those of raised intracranial pressure and listed below:

HINTS AND TIPS

Signs of increased intracranial pressure:
- Altered sensorium.
- Headache.
- Vomiting (especially in the morning).
- Decerebrate/decorticate posturing.
- Abnormalities of pupillary size and reaction.
- Papilloedema.

Diagnosis

Diagnosis is confirmed by imaging. If the anterior fontanelle is still open, ultrasound is used to assess

Fig. 20.1 Causes of hydrocephalus

Intraventricular obstruction
Congenital malformation:
• Aqueduct stenosis
• Dandy–Walker syndrome
Intraventricular haemorrhage
Ventriculitis
Brain tumour
Extraventricular obstruction
Subarachnoid haemorrhage
Tuberculous meningitis
Arnold–Chiari malformation

Fig. 20.2 Meningitis: common pathogens

Bacterial
Neisseria meningitidis
Streptococcus pneumoniae
Haemophilus influenzae type B
During the neonatal period:
• Group B streptococci
• *E. coli*
• *Listeria monocytogenes*
Viral
Mumps
Enteroviruses
Epstein–Barr virus

ventricular dilatation. A computed tomography scan (CT) or magnetic resonance imaging (MRI) will establish the diagnosis and cause, and is useful for monitoring treatment and detecting complications.

Treatment

The mainstay of treatment is insertion of a ventriculo-peritoneal shunt. Complications of shunts include obstruction and infection.

Craniosynostosis

This is premature fusion of the cranial sutures. Most affected infants present soon after birth with an abnormal skull; the shape of this depends on which sutures have fused. The sagittal suture is most commonly involved, causing a long, narrow skull.

Generalized craniosynostosis is a cause of microcephaly.

In the presence of increased intracranial pressure, a craniectomy is performed.

Neural tube defects

These used to be the most common congenital defects of the CNS and are considered in detail in Chapter 12.

INFECTIONS OF THE CENTRAL NERVOUS SYSTEM

Meningitis

Acute meningitis is caused by a range of bacteria and viruses varying with age (Fig. 20.2), or more rarely by tuberculosis, fungal infections or malignant infiltration. The serious and potentially lethal nature of bacterial meningitis renders it most important. Although more common, viral meningitis is a less serious and self-limiting disease.

HINTS AND TIPS

Early signs of meningitis in infants are non-specific. Immediate treatment with parenteral antibiotics is indicated for suspected meningitis.

Bacterial meningitis

The peak incidence is in under 5-year-olds with 80% of all cases in children under 16 years. Meningococcal meningitis accounts for over half of cases and in the UK group B is the most common variety. Pneumococcal meningitis, although uncommon, affects younger children and is associated with higher fatality and neurological sequelae. Since the introduction of Hib and Men C vaccination, meningitis due to *H. influenzae* type B and meningococcus C has become rare.

The pathogens are carried in the nasal passages and invade the meninges via the bloodstream. Early symptoms and signs are non-specific, making diagnosis difficult, especially in infants.

Clinical features

There might be irritability, poor feeding, vomiting, fever and drowsiness. More specific signs develop later, including:

• A bulging fontanelle.
• Neck stiffness and photophobia in the older child.
• Seizures: beware the child diagnosed with benign febrile convulsions.

Meningococcal septicaemia may present with a characteristic non-blanching purpuric rash in conjunction with meningitis.

Diagnosis

Lumbar puncture (LP) and examination of the CSF is diagnostic. A high index of suspicion is necessary in young children in whom signs and symptoms are non-specific.

Blood cultures should be taken and LP performed as soon as possible if there are no contraindications. Treatment must not be delayed for lumbar puncture. Contraindications to LP include signs of raised intracranial pressure (depressed conscious state, papilloedema or focal neurological signs), coagulopathy and septic shock. A CT scan does not exclude raised intracranial pressure.

Rapid diagnostic tests are available for specific pathogens (see Chapter 3).

Treatment

Broad-spectrum intravenous antibiotic treatment is initiated using a third-generation cephalosporin, e.g. ceftriaxone (or cefotaxime and amoxicillin in children under 3 months). A febrile child with a purpuric rash in the community (i.e. suspected meningococcal sepsis) should be treated immediately with benzylpenicillin (IM or IV) and transferred urgently to hospital. Meningococcal septicaemia can kill within hours and early antibiotic treatment significantly reduces mortality rates.

Dexamethasone is used in children over 3 months to moderate the inflammatory response. This has been shown to reduce the incidence of some neurological sequelae, e.g. hearing loss.

Complications

Acute complications of meningitis include:

- Cerebral oedema.
- Seizures.
- Syndrome of inappropriate antidiuretic hormone secretion (SIADH).

Neurological sequelae include sensorineural deafness: all children should have their hearing tested following meningitis.

Rifampicin, ciprofloxacin or ceftriaxone should be given to all household contacts following infection with meningococcus to eradicate nasopharyngeal carriage. All bacterial meningitis should be reported to the health protection agency.

Encephalitis

In encephalitis there is inflammation of the brain substance. Acute encephalitis is usually viral. The most common causes in the UK are:

- Herpes simplex virus 1 and 2.
- Enteroviruses.
- Varicella.

The common viral exanthems (measles, rubella, mumps and varicella) can all cause encephalitis by direct viral invasion of the brain or can be complicated by an immune-mediated postinfectious encephalomyelitis.

Clinical features

The clinical features include early non-specific symptoms such as fever, headache and vomiting, followed by the abrupt development of an encephalopathic illness characterized by altered consciousness and personality and seizures.

Diagnosis and management

High-dose aciclovir should be given in all cases to cover herpes simplex until results of investigations are available.

Diagnosis is difficult acutely, but EEG and MRI might show characteristic temporal lobe abnormalities. Isolation of the causative organism may be possible from CSF or blood.

Supportive management for severe encephalitis requires:

- Admission to an intensive care unit.
- Seizure control and monitoring for raised intracranial pressure.

Postinfectious syndromes

These can affect the brain or peripheral nervous system:

- Postinfectious encephalomyelitis: delayed brain swelling caused by an immune-mediated inflammatory reaction to viral infection. It may follow any of the common viral exanthems.
- Varicella zoster typically causes an acute cerebellitis.

Acute postinfectious polyneuropathy (Guillain–Barré syndrome)

This demyelinating polyneuropathy follows 2–3 weeks after a viral infection with, for example, cytomegalovirus or Epstein–Barr virus, or infection with *Mycoplasma pneumoniae* or *Campylobacter jejuni*.

Clinical features

Guillain–Barré syndrome usually begins with fleeting sensory symptoms in the toes and fingers and progresses to a symmetrical, ascending paralysis with early loss of tendon reflexes. Autonomic involvement might occur, with dysrhythmias, and bulbar involvement can cause respiratory failure. The disease can progress over several weeks. The CSF protein is characteristically markedly raised without an increase in white cell count.

Management

Supportive care including assisted ventilation might be required. Respiratory function must be monitored closely. Specific therapy includes immunoglobulin infusion and plasma exchange. There might be residual neurological problems but in children a full recovery is expected.

CEREBRAL PALSY

Cerebral palsy (CP) is a group of conditions affecting motor function and posture due to a non-progressive lesion of the developing brain. It is useful to remember that:

- Although the lesion is non-progressive, the clinical manifestations evolve as the nervous system develops.
- Children with cerebral palsy often have problems in addition to disorders of movement and posture, reflecting more widespread damage to the brain.

The cause is unknown in many patients but identified risk factors can be categorized into antenatal, intrapartum and postnatal (Fig. 20.3). It is important to be aware that perinatal asphyxia is an uncommon cause (3–21%) of CP.

Clinical features

There might be a history of risk factors and motor delay. CP can present with:

- Delayed motor milestones.
- Abnormal tone and posturing in infancy.
- Feeding difficulties due to lack of oromotor coordination.
- Speech and language delay.

Diagnosis

The diagnosis is clinical with more than one abnormality including:

- Tone: hypertonia or hypotonia.
- Power, e.g. delay in motor milestones.

- Reflexes, e.g. brisk tendon reflexes or abnormal absence (or persistence) of primitive reflexes.
- Abnormal movements, e.g. athetosis or chorea.
- Abnormal posture or gait.

Neuroimaging, e.g. MRI, may be indicated but is not diagnostic. Other investigations may be needed, e.g. to exclude metabolic causes.

Classification

Cerebral palsy is classified according to the anatomical distribution of the lesion and the main functional abnormalities; 10% of cases are mixed.

Spastic cerebral palsy (70%)

Damage to the pyramidal pathways causes increased limb tone (spasticity), brisk deep-tendon reflexes and extensor plantar responses. Hypotonia might precede spasticity. The distribution of affected limbs allows further classification:

- Hemiparesis.
- Diplegia: all four limbs are affected, but legs more than arms.
- Quadriplegia: all four limbs are affected, arms worse than legs. There is often truncal involvement, seizures and intellectual impairment. This is the most severe form.

Ataxic cerebral palsy (10%)

Caused by damage to the cerebellum or its pathways. Features include early hypotonia with poor balance, uncoordinated movements and delayed motor development.

Dyskinetic cerebral palsy (10%)

Caused by damage to the basal ganglia or extrapyramidal pathways (e.g. in kernicterus). The clinical presentation is often with hypotonia and delayed motor development. Abnormal involuntary movements, which include chorea (abrupt, jerky movements), athetosis (slow writhing continuous movements) or dystonia (sustained abnormal postures) might appear later.

Management

Management of CP requires a multidisciplinary approach. Prognosis in early infancy can be uncertain. Motor function may be worsened by hypertonia, which is treated by physiotherapy, muscle relaxants (e.g. baclofen), botulinum toxin injections to specific muscle groups or surgical intervention. Orthopaedic intervention is often beneficial (braces, surgery, special shoes). Attention must be paid to associated problems such as sensory deficits, learning difficulties and epilepsy

---

Fig. 20.3 Causes of cerebral palsy

Antenatal (80%)
Cerebral dysgenesis
Congenital infections:
- Rubella
- Cytomegalovirus
- Toxoplasmosis

Intrapartum (10%)
Birth asphyxia

Postnatal (10%)
Preterm birth:
- Hypoxic–ischaemic encephalopathy
- Intraventricular haemorrhage
Hyperbilirubinaemia
Hypoglycaemia
Head injury
Intracranial infection:
- Meningitis
- Encephalitis

Fig. 20.4 Problems associated with cerebral palsy

Learning difficulties
Hearing and visual problems
Seizures
Gastro-oesophageal reflux
Feeding problems and failure to thrive
Recurrent pneumonia
Constipation
Speech and language problems

(25–50% of all children experience seizures) which are often difficult to control (Fig. 20.4).

EPILEPSY

Epilepsy is common, affecting 5 per 1000 school-age children. It is useful to distinguish between an 'epileptic seizure', which is a transient event, and epilepsy, which is a disease or syndrome:

- An epileptic seizure is an episode of abnormal and excessive neuronal activity in the brain that is apparent either to the subject or an observer.
- Epilepsy is a chronic disorder characterized by recurrent, unprovoked epileptic seizures.

Several important features of these definitions require emphasis. With epileptic seizures:

- The abnormal neuronal activity during an epileptic seizure can be manifested as a motor, sensory, autonomic, cognitive or psychic disturbance.
- An electrophysiological disturbance unaccompanied by any clinical change is *not* classified as an epileptic seizure.
- Many paroxysmal disturbances ('funny turns') mimic epileptic seizures (see Chapter 8).

A diagnosis of epilepsy is made in a patient in whom epileptic seizures recur spontaneously. However, it is important to recognize that an 'epileptic seizure' can be provoked in individuals who do *not* have epilepsy (for example with fever, hypoglycaemia and hypoxia).

Classification and terminology

The International League Against Epilepsy has devised a classification system for epileptic seizures and for epilepsies and epilepsy syndromes. In any patient, an attempt should be made to:

- Identify the types of seizure occurring.
- Diagnose the epilepsy or epilepsy syndrome present.

Terms such as grand mal and petit mal are outdated and should be avoided.

Fig. 20.5 Classification of epileptic seizures

Generalized
- Absence seizures
- Myoclonic seizures
- Clonic seizures
- Tonic seizures
- Tonic-clonic seizures
- Atonic seizures

Partial
 Simple (consciousness not impaired)
- With motor symptoms (Jacksonian)
- With somatosensory or special sensory symptoms
- With autonomic symptoms
- With psychic symptoms
 Complex (with impairment of consciousness)
- Beginning as simple partial seizure
- With only impairment of consciousness
- With automatisms
 Partial seizure with secondary generalization

Classification of epileptic seizures

The initial division is into (Fig. 20.5):

- Generalized seizures.
- Partial seizures (may become secondarily generalized):
- Simple
- Complex.

Classification of epilepsies and epilepsy syndromes

Some forms of epilepsy may be classified into syndromes which have a typical prognosis and respond to specific anticonvulsants.

The initial division is by seizure type (Fig. 20.6):

- Generalized epilepsies and syndromes.
- Localization: related epilepsies and syndromes.

An additional category is provided for those in which seizure type is uncertain or both focal and generalized seizures occur.

Further subdivision is according to aetiology:

- Idiopathic (or primary).
- Symptomatic: in which the cause is known or suspected.

Aetiology

Epilepsy can result from a very diverse group of pathological processes but it is important to realize that in at least 50% of children no cause will be identified, even after extensive evaluation. A specific cause (Fig. 20.7) is more likely to be identifiable in patients with partial or intractable epilepsy.

Fig. 20.6 Classification of epilepsy

Generalized epilepsies and epilepsy syndromes
Idiopathic generalized epilepsy (IGE), defined syndromes include:
- Benign familial neonatal convulsions
- Childhood absence epilepsy (CAE)
- Juvenile absence epilepsy (JAE)
- Juvenile myoclonic epilepsy (JME)

Symptomatic generalized epilepsy, defined syndromes include:
- Infantile spasms (West syndrome)
- Lennox–Gastaut syndrome
- Cerebral malformations
- Progressive myoclonic epilepsies including:
    Inborn errors of metabolism
    Neurodegenerative diseases

Localization-related epilepsies and epilepsy syndromes
Idiopathic partial epilepsy, defined syndromes include:
- Benign childhood epilepsy with centrotemporal spikes (benign rolandic epilepsy)

Symptomatic partial epilepsy, defined syndromes include:
- Epilepsy caused by focal lesions of the brain associated with:
    Cortical dysgenesis
    CNS infection
    Head injury
    AV malformations
    Brain tumours

Diagnosis

A careful history is the mainstay of diagnosis. A detailed description is required of the events before, during and after a suspected seizure (a video recording is a useful adjunct). The first aim is to distinguish true epileptic seizures from the many paroxysmal disturbances (see Chapter 8) that can mimic them:

- Breath-holding attacks.
- Reflex anoxic seizures.

Fig. 20.7 Causes of epilepsy

Cortical dysgenesis
Cerebral malformations
Genetic diseases:
- Neurocutaneous syndromes
- Down syndrome
- Fragile X syndrome
- Neurodegenerative disorders
- Inborn errors of metabolism
Cerebral tumours
Cerebral damage due to:
- Head trauma
- Hypoxia–ischaemia, including HIE
- Intracranial infection (meningitis, encephalitis)

- Vasovagal syncope (simple faints).
- Cardiac dysrhythmias.

Enquiry should be made concerning possible predisposing events (head injury, intracranial infection) and any family history of epilepsy.

Physical examination is frequently normal. Careful attention should be paid to the skin to identify the stigmata of neurocutaneous syndromes (including Wood's light examination) and to the fundi because retinal changes can provide a clue to aetiology.

Investigations

EEG

This may aid diagnosis, or identify a particular epilepsy syndrome, underlying anatomical lesion, or neurodegenerative disorder. However, a single interictal EEG will be normal in up to 50% of children with epilepsy, and non-specific or even so-called 'epileptiform' abnormalities can be found in 2–3% of normal asymptomatic children. A routine interictal EEG does not therefore prove or disprove a diagnosis of epilepsy. Additional information can be obtained from ambulatory EEG monitoring, video telemetry or recordings during sleep or after sleep deprivation.

Neuroimaging

Not all children with epilepsy require imaging. Indications for neuroimaging include:

- Focal onset seizures.
- Seizures not responsive to first line treatment.
- A focal neurological deficit.
- Children less than 2 years old with nonfebrile convulsions.

MRI is the investigation of choice as it offers greater sensitivity in the detection of small lesions, e.g. in temporal lobe or subtle cortical dysgeneses.

Other investigations

Additional specific investigations, might be appropriate if there is clinical suspicion of an underlying neurometabolic disorder, including:

- Plasma and urine amino acids.
- Biopsy of skin or muscle.
- Measurement of white blood cell enzymes.
- DNA analysis.

Some important epilepsy syndromes

Infantile spasms (West syndrome)

This is an uncommon variety of epilepsy with peak onset between 4 and 6 months of age. Myoclonic seizures

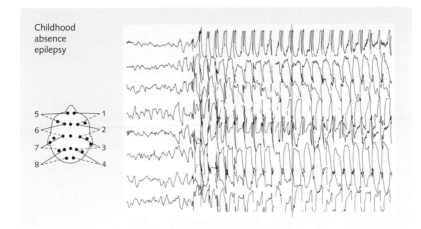

Childhood absence epilepsy

5—1
6—2
7—3
8—4

Fig. 20.8 EEG in a typical absence seizure. There is 3/s spike and wave discharge, which is bilaterally synchronous

occur, often as 'salaam attacks' – violent flexor spasms of head, trunk and limbs followed by extension of the arms. They are often multiple and can be misdiagnosed as colic. The EEG shows hypsarrhythmia, a chaotic pattern of large-amplitude slow waves with spikes and sharp waves. Seventy per cent of the patients have the symptomatic form, and important causes include tuberous sclerosis and perinatal hypoxic–ischaemic encephalopathy. The prognosis is poor but can be improved by early treatment. Treatment is with adrenocorticotrophic hormone (ACTH) or vigabatrin.

Childhood absence epilepsy

This relatively common variety of epilepsy has a peak onset at 6–7 years. The absence seizures comprise transient unawareness (blank spells), without loss of body tone. They typically last for 5–15 seconds but can be very frequent, with up to several hundred daily. Episodes can be induced by hyperventilation. The ictal EEG is characteristic with generalized, bilaterally synchronous three-per-second spike-wave discharges (Fig. 20.8). The prognosis is good with spontaneous remission in adolescence in the majority of children. Sodium valproate or ethosuximide are the first-line drugs, although medication is not required for infrequent absences.

Management of epilepsy

Effective management of a child with epilepsy involves far more than the prescription of anti-epilepsy drugs (AEDs). Both the child and parents need to be educated about the condition, the prognosis and the nature of the particular epilepsy or epilepsy syndrome.

HINTS AND TIPS

Children with epilepsy should be encouraged to participate in and enjoy a full social life. Certain activities, however, do require special precautions:
- Swimming: a competent adult swimmer supervises.
- Domestic bathing: patients should be supervised in the bath; older children should be advised not to lock the door.
- Cycling: a helmet must be worn and traffic avoided.

It is important to consider the psychological and educational implications. Overprotection by the parents should be sympathetically discouraged. Behavioural and emotional difficulties can occur in the teenage years, with loss of self-esteem, anxiety or depression. The diagnosis should be discussed with school staff. Learning difficulties are present in a proportion of children with epilepsy, but only a minority require special schooling.

Anti-epilepsy drugs (AEDs)

Not all children with epilepsy require drug treatment. AEDs are not usually started after a first uncomplicated seizure and may not be needed for infrequent myoclonic or absence seizures. First-line treatment is:

- Sodium valproate for generalized epilepsy.
- Carbamazepine for partial epilepsy.

Monotherapy should be used wherever possible and achieves total seizure control in 70% of children. Newer anti-epileptics may be appropriate for adjunctive therapy and side-effects should be considered. Blood level monitoring is rarely needed, but may identify poor compliance.

FEBRILE CONVULSIONS

A febrile convulsion is a seizure associated with fever in a child between 6 months and 6 years of age in the absence of intracranial infection or an identifiable neurological disorder.

Febrile convulsions are the most common cause of seizures in childhood and occur in about 5% of children. There might be a familial predisposition. The seizures usually occur when body temperature rises rapidly. They are typically brief (1–2 min), generalized, tonic-clonic seizures.

The underlying infection causing the fever may be viral or bacterial (commonly otitis media, tonsillitis, pneumonia or UTI).

Clinical features

Most children are well after the seizure, but it is important to exclude meningitis as this may present with seizures and fever. This may require a lumbar puncture in children in whom the seizure is atypical or there are other indicators of CNS infection. Prognosis is very good and, despite a 30% chance of recurrence, a normal neurological outcome is expected.

Management

Management includes:

- Identification and treatment of underlying infection: this might be apparent but investigations to consider include chest X-ray (CXR), blood culture, urine microscopy and culture, and lumbar puncture.

- Despite no evidence of reduction in seizures, regular antipyretics and tepid sponging are often recommended.
- Termination of a prolonged convulsion (i.e. for longer than 5–10 min) with rectal diazepam.
- Parental education (Fig. 20.9).

HEADACHE

Headache is a common presenting symptom in children, particularly with intercurrent illness. It is important to identify potentially serious causes of headache. The causes and red flag symptoms are outlined in Chapter 8.

NEUROCUTANEOUS SYNDROMES

Neurofibromatosis type 1 (von Recklinghausen disease)

Neurofibromatosis type 1 (NF1) is an autosomal dominant disorder affecting about 1 in 4000 live births. About 50% of cases result from new mutations. The important clinical features include:

- Café-au-lait patches on the skin: at least six must be present; 50% of normal individuals have at least one.
- Lisch nodules (pigmented hamartomas on the eye): usually seen after 5 years of age.
- Neurofibromas on the peripheral nerves (may be palpable).

Fig. 20.9 Information for parents about febrile seizures	
Will it happen again?	About one third of children have recurrent febrile seizures
	Recurrence is more likely if the first seizure occurs under the age of 18 months or if there is a family history
Can I prevent further episodes?	During febrile illnesses, the child should be kept cool with antipyretics, removal of clothing and tepid sponging
What should I do if a convulsion occurs?	Place child in recovery position
	Parents of children at risk of frequent or prolonged seizures can be supplied with buccal midazolam or rectal diazepam to administer if a seizure lasts longer than 5 minutes
Is it epilepsy?	Febrile seizures are not classified as epilepsy About 3% of children with febrile seizures go on to develop afebrile recurrent seizures, i.e. epilepsy, in later childhood. Risk factors for epilepsy include: • Seizures that are focal, prolonged (>15 minutes) or recur in the same illness • First-degree relative with epilepsy • Neurological abnormality

Fig. 20.10 Differences between NF1 and NF2		
Feature	NF1	NF2
Incidence	About 1/4000	About 1/50 000
Inheritance	Autosomal dominant; chromosome 17	Autosomal dominant; chromosome 22
Café-au-lait spots	Characteristic	Uncommon
Skin neurofibromas	Common	Uncommon
Lisch nodules	Characteristic	Uncommon
Family history	About 50% are inherited	Mostly new mutations
Acoustic neuromas	Uncommon	Characteristic, often bilateral
Risk of CNS tumours	Common	Common

Neurofibromatosis type 2

Neurofibromatosis type 2 (NF2) is a distinct disease due to mutations in a different gene on chromosome 22. It is much rarer than type 1 (affecting 1 in 40 000 people) and is characterized by bilateral acoustic neuromata and other CNS tumours (Fig. 20.10).

Tuberous sclerosis

This is an autosomal dominant disorder affecting 1 in 7000 live births. Up to 75% of cases represent new mutations. It is genetically heterogeneous with one disease gene on chromosome 9 and a second gene on chromosome 16.

Classically it presents with seizures, mental retardation and facial angiofibromas (adenoma sebaceum). Examination reveals hypopigmented macules (ash leaf spots), which are better seen on examination with a Wood's light.

It is a multisystem disease affecting not only the skin and brain but also the heart, kidneys and lungs.

Sturge–Weber syndrome

This sporadic disorder is characterized by:

- Unilateral facial naevus (port-wine stain) in the distribution of the trigeminal nerve.
- Angiomas involving the leptomeningeal vessels in the brain leading to seizures.
- Haemangiomas in the spinal cord.

There are abnormal blood vessels over the surface of the brain, which might be associated with seizures, hemiplegia and learning difficulties. Ocular involvement can result in glaucoma.

Brain imaging typically shows unilateral intracranial calcification with a double contour like a railway line and cortical atrophy.

NEURODEGENERATIVE DISORDERS OF CHILDHOOD

A large number of individually rare but important inherited diseases are associated with progressive neurodegeneration in childhood. Most are autosomal recessively inherited and genetic and biochemical defects have been established at a molecular level in many cases. Acquired forms do occur, such as prion disease and subacute sclerosing panencephalitis. Loss of acquired skills is the hallmark of a neurodegenerative disorder.

Clinical features

It is important to distinguish between developmental delay and developmental regression – in delayed development, milestones are not achieved in time, but once attained, they are not lost. In regression, there is a gradual loss of milestones that have already been attained. The child may have a normal initial development, only to lose those skills later, indicating a progressive disorder of the brain.

Features of neurodegenerative diseases include:

- Regression of milestones.
- Progressive dementia.
- Epilepsy.
- Visual loss.
- Ataxia.
- Alterations in tone and reflexes (depending on the precise pattern of nervous system involvement).

Parental consanguinity increases the risk of such disorders (Fig. 20.11).

NEUROMUSCULAR DISORDERS

These are best considered according to their anatomical site (Fig. 20.12) in the lower motor pathway. Genetic, infective, inflammatory and toxic factors can cause this group of diseases.

Fig. 20.11 Inherited neurodegenerative diseases – some examples

Lysosomal storage diseases
Sphingolipidosis, e.g. Tay–Sachs disease
Mucopolysaccharidosis, e.g. Hurler syndrome (MPS1)
Peroxisomal disorders
Adrenoleucodystrophy
Trace metal metabolism
Wilson's disease
Menke's syndrome

Fig. 20.12 Neuromuscular disorders

Anterior horn cell
Spinal muscular atrophy
Poliomyelitis
Peripheral nerve
Hereditary neuropathy
Guillain–Barré syndrome
Bell's palsy
Neuromuscular junction
Myasthenia gravis
Muscle
Muscular dystrophies
Myotonia
Congenital myopathies

Clinical features

The hallmark of these disorders is weakness. They can present with:

- Hypotonia.
- Delayed motor milestones.
- Weakness, fatiguability.
- Abnormal gait.

Clinical features on examination include hypotonia, muscle weakness or wasting, abnormal gait and reduced tendon reflexes.

Diagnosis

Special investigations useful in the diagnosis of neuromuscular diseases include:

- Muscle enzymes: serum creatine kinase is elevated in Duchenne and Becker dystrophies.
- Electrophysiology: nerve conduction studies and electromyography.
- Muscle or nerve biopsy.
- DNA analysis.
- Imaging: ultrasound, CT or MRI of muscle.
- Edrophonium test: for myasthenia gravis.

Muscular dystrophies

This group of inherited disorders is characterized by progressive degeneration of muscle. The most common and important is Duchenne muscular dystrophy.

Duchenne muscular dystrophy

This X-linked recessive disease affects 1 in 4000 male infants. About one-third of cases are new mutations. The disease gene encodes dystrophin, a sarcolemmal membrane protein.

Affected boys usually develop symptoms between 2 and 4 years of age. Independent walking tends to be delayed and affected children never run normally. Patients are wheelchair bound by 12 years of age and die from congestive heart failure or respiratory failure in the third decade.

Clinical features
Associated clinical features include:

- Pseudohypertrophy of calf muscles and proximal muscle weakness.
- Positive Gower's sign (evident at 3–5 years): the hands are used to push up on the legs to achieve an upright posture, indicating weakness of the pelvic girdle muscles.
- Scoliosis and contractures.
- Dilated cardiomyopathy.
- Mild learning difficulties.

Diagnosis
Most cases are confirmed by DNA analysis. Other investigations include raised serum creatine kinase (10–20 times normal) and muscle biopsy and EMG.

Management
Treatment is supportive. Walking can be prolonged by provision of orthoses and scoliosis can be helped by a truncal brace or moulded seat. Early diagnosis is important to allow identification of female carriers and genetic counselling. Respiratory symptoms can be helped with non-invasive respiratory ventilation. Cardiomyopathy worsens with age and is often the cause of death.

Becker muscular dystrophy

This disease is milder than Duchenne muscular dystrophy but is caused by a mutation in the same gene. The average age of onset is much later (in the second decade of life) with prolonged survival.

Myotonic dystrophy

This is an autosomal dominant, trinucleotide repeat condition. It is a multiorgan disorder affecting muscle, endocrine system, cardiac function, immunity and the central nervous system.

Clinical features
- Hypotonia.
- Progressive muscle wasting.

- Typical facial features: inverted V-shaped upper lip, thin cheeks and high arched palate.
- Myotonia: a characteristic feature, usually seen beyond 5 years. This is a slow relaxation of muscle after contraction, demonstrated by asking the patient to make tight fists and then to quickly open the hands.
- Arrhythmias, endocrine abnormalities, cataracts and immunologic deficiencies can also occur.

Diagnosis
This is by DNA analysis to show the CTG repeat. Serum CK is usually normal.

Management
Treatment is supportive.

Spinal muscular atrophies

Spinal muscular atrophies (SMA) are progressive degenerative diseases of motor neurons, that may onset as early as fetal life. The more severe forms present in early infancy with severe hypotonia and weakness whereas the late onset forms present in later childhood. These disorders are characterized by hypotonia, generalized weakness and absent or weak tendon reflexes. Fasciculations seen in the tongue, deltoids or biceps are characteristic and indicate denervation of the muscle. Children with the severe early onset type rarely survive beyond 2 years while intermediate forms lead to severe motor disability. Diagnosis is by muscle biopsy and identifying the genetic marker for the SMN gene. Treatment is supportive.

Further reading

Brouwer, M.C., McIntyre, P., de Gans, J., Prasad, K., van de Beek, D., 2010. Corticosteroids for acute bacterial meningitis. Cochrane Database Syst. Rev. (9), Art. No.: CD004405. http://dx.doi.org/10.1002/14651858.CD004405.pub3. http://summaries.cochrane.org/CD004405/corticosteroids-for-bacterial-meningitis.

Health Protection Agency Meningococcus and Haemophilus Forum, March 2012. Guidance for public health management of meningococcal disease in the UK. http://www.hpa.org.uk/webc/HPAwebFile/HPAweb_C/1194947389261.

National Institute for Health and Clinical Excellence (NICE), October 2004. The epilepsies: the diagnosis and management of the epilepsies in adults and children in primary and secondary care (CG20). http://www.nice.org.uk/CG020.

National Institute for Health and Clinical Excellence (NICE), September 2010. Management of bacterial meningitis and meningococcal septicaemia in children and young people younger than 16 years in primary and secondary care (CG102). http://guidance.nice.org.uk/CG102.

National Institute for Health and Clinical Excellence (NICE), December 2010. Selective dorsal rhizotomy for spasticity in cerebral palsy (IPG373). http://guidance.nice.org.uk/IPG373.

Musculoskeletal disorders 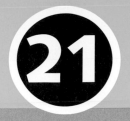 21

At the end of this chapter, you should be able to:
- Know the clinical presentation of developmental dysplasia of the hip
- Understand the common causes of hip pain and limp in children
- Recognize common infections of the bone and joints
- Know the classification, clinical features and management of juvenile idiopathic arthritis

DISORDERS OF THE HIP AND KNEE

Developmental dysplasia of the hip

This term has replaced the previous name of 'congenital dislocation' of the hip. Perinatal hip instability results in progressive malformation of the hip joint; it occurs in 1.5 in 1000 births.

Developmental dysplasia of the hip (DDH) represents a spectrum of hip instability ranging from a dislocated hip to hips with various degrees of acetabular dysplasia (in which the femoral head is in position but the acetabulum is shallow). It was previously thought to be entirely congenital, but is now known to also occur after birth in previously normal hips. There are two types:

1. Typical, which affects normal infants.
2. Teratological, which occurs in neurological and genetic conditions. Teratological DDH requires specialized management.

All babies are screened clinically but 40% will be missed and the use of national ultrasound screening remains controversial; 90% will spontaneously resolve without treatment.

Clinical features

The cause is unknown but risk factors for DDH include:

- Congenital muscular torticollis.
- Congenital foot abnormalities.
- Breech delivery.
- Family history.
- First born.
- Oligohydramnios.
- Neuromuscular disorders.
- Female sex.

Warning signs might be:
- Delayed walking.
- A painless limp.
- A waddling gait.

Asymmetrical skin creases are found in 30% of all infants and are an unreliable guide; 10% of all babies have hip clicks and this is normal.

Diagnosis

Babies are screened at birth and at the 6-week check using the Barlow and Ortolani manoeuvres. The Barlow test involves applying backward pressure to each femoral head in turn and a subluxable hip is suspected on the basis of palpable partial or complete displacement. In contrast, the Ortolani test consists of forward pressure being applied to each femoral head in turn, in an attempt to move a posteriorly dislocated femoral head back into the acetabulum. With increasing age, contractures form and these tests are then unhelpful. Typically, on examination there is limited abduction (a supine child should be able to abduct fully the flexed hip up until the age of 2 years). The femur might be shortened (Allis sign). Ultrasound scanning is diagnostic. Hip X-rays are not useful until after 4–5 months of age when the femoral head has ossified (Fig. 21.1).

Management

> **HINTS AND TIPS**
>
> Note that clinical examination will miss many hip dislocations and ultrasound of high-risk babies is indicated.

This involves:
- Fixing the hip in abduction with a Pavlik or Von Rosen harness. This is effective in children under 8 months of age.

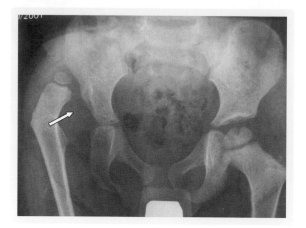

Fig. 21.1 X-ray of developmental dysplasia of the right hip in an older child. (Reproduced with permission from Crash Course: Rheumatology and Orthopaedics, 2nd edn, by Marsland, Kapoor, Coote and Haslam, Elsevier Mosby, 2008)

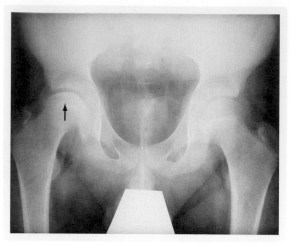

Fig. 21.2 Perthes' disease. Increased density in the right femoral head, which is reduced in height

- It is important to note that the harness must be adjusted every 2 weeks for growth and should be kept on at all times.

For children in whom the diagnosis has been delayed, open reduction and derotation femoral osteotomy needs to be performed. In these cases, accelerated degenerative changes might necessitate total hip replacement in early adult life.

Perthes' disease

This idiopathic disorder results in osteonecrosis of the femoral head prior to skeletal maturity. It results in growth disturbance associated with temporary ischaemia of the upper femoral epiphysis. This leads to a cycle of avascular necrosis with flattening and fragmentation of the femoral head. Revascularization and reossification occurs with the resumption of growth (which might not be normal); the whole cycle takes 3–4 years. Risk factors include:

- A previous family history.
- Male sex: it is five times more common in boys.

The incidence is 1 in 2000.

Clinical features

There is an insidious onset of limp between the ages of 3 and 12 years (the majority occur between 5 and 7 years). Pain, which might be intermittent, can be felt in the hip, thigh or knee. Between 10% and 20% of cases are bilateral. Abduction and rotation is limited on examination.

Diagnosis

Hip X-rays are diagnostic (Fig. 21.2). If there is doubt then serial films or MRI might be necessary.

Management

The prognosis in most children is good, especially in those under 6 years of age or if less than half of the femoral head is involved. In younger children only analgesia and mild activity restriction with bracing is needed.

In older children, and those in whom more than half of the epiphysis is involved, permanent deformity of the femoral head occurs in over 40%, resulting in earlier degenerative arthritis. In severe disease, the hip needs to be fixed in abduction allowing the femoral head to be covered and moulded by the acetabulum as it grows. Plaster, calipers or femoral or pelvic osteotomy may achieve fixation.

Transient synovitis (irritable hip)

This common self-limiting condition occurs in children between 2 and 12 years of age often following a viral infection. Typical features are:

- Sudden onset of hip pain.
- Limp.
- Refusal to bear weight on the affected side.

There is no pain at rest. Examination reveals limited passive abduction and rotation in an otherwise well and afebrile child. The critical differential diagnosis is septic arthritis, in which the child is febrile, unwell with pain at rest and refusal to move the affected joint.

Diagnosis

This is a diagnosis of exclusion and it is important to distinguish transient synovitis from septic arthritis:

- Acute-phase reactants: white blood cell count (WBC), C-reactive protein (CRP) and erythrocyte sedimentation rate (ESR).
- Blood cultures.

Hip X-ray does not enable differentiation and therefore may not be useful. If there is doubt, the joint should be aspirated for culture followed by prompt administration of intravenous antibiotics.

Management

Treatment is supportive (analgesia and avoiding strenous activity) because the condition spontaneously resolves in 2 weeks.

Slipped upper femoral epiphysis

In this relatively uncommon condition of unknown aetiology, there is progressive posterior and medial translation of the femoral head on the femoral neck through the epiphysis. Slipped upper femoral epiphysis (SUFE) occurs during the adolescent growth spurt and:

- Is most common in boys (obese and/or black).
- Is associated with delayed skeletal maturation and endocrine disorders.
- Typically presents between 10 and 15 years of age.
- Presents with limp or with hip or referred knee pain.

Thirty per cent have a family history and 20% are bilateral, although not necessarily synchronous. Diagnosis is by plain radiographs and unstable hips are an orthopaedic emergency. Complications are avascular necrosis and premature fusion of the epiphysis. Management is by pinning the femoral head or osteotomy. Non-surgical treatment is ineffective.

DISORDERS OF THE SPINE

Back pain

Back pain is uncommon before adolescence. In infants and young children it is usually associated with significant pathology such as connective tissue disorders. Referral is warranted.

In adolescence back pain may be caused by:

- Muscle spasm or soft tissue pain: this is usually a sports-related injury.
- Scheuermann's disease: this is osteochondritis (idiopathic avascular necrosis of an ossification centre) of the lower thoracic vertebrae causing localized pain, tenderness and kyphosis.
- Spondylolysis and spondylolisthesis: there is a defect in the pars interarticularis of (usually) L4 or L5 (spondylolysis). If there is anterior shift of the vertebral body – graded according to severity – there is lower back pain exacerbated by bending backwards (spondylolisthesis).
- Vertebral osteomyelitis or discitis: this presents with severe pain on weight-bearing and walking associated with local tenderness.
- Tumours: these can be benign or malignant and might cause cord or root compression.
- Idiopathic: this is a diagnosis of exclusion but pain might be exacerbated by stress and poor posture.

Scoliosis

This is lateral curvature of the spine associated with a rotational deformity and affects 4% of children. It is classified according to cause:

- Vertebral abnormalities, e.g. hemivertebra, osteogenesis imperfecta.
- Neuromuscular, e.g. polio, cerebral palsy.
- Miscellaneous, e.g. idiopathic (most common), dysmorphic syndromes.

Idiopathic scoliosis

As well as lateral curvature, there is rotation of the thoracic region, which can be demonstrated as the child bends forwards and a rib hump is noted (Fig. 21.3). More than 85% of cases occur in adolescence. It is more common in girls and often there is a family history. Pain is not a typical feature. The scoliosis is monitored clinically, radiologically and chronologically:

- Mild curves are not treated.
- Moderate curves are braced (23 hours a day until growing has stopped).
- Severe curves (>40°) require surgery that fuses the spine and therefore terminates further growth. Untreated severe curves result in later degenerative changes, pain and unwanted cosmetic appearance.

Torticollis

Acute torticollis (wry neck) is a relatively common and self-limiting condition in young children, often associated with an upper respiratory tract infection.

The most common cause of torticollis in infants is a sternomastoid tumour. A mobile non-tender nodule within the sternomastoid muscle is noticed in the first

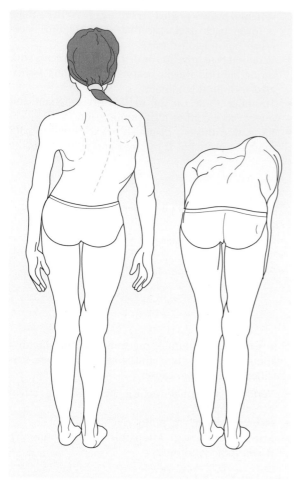

Fig. 21.3 Idiopathic adolescent scoliosis showing vertebral rotation (rib hump) when bending forward

few weeks of life. The cause is unknown. It usually resolves by 1 year and is managed conservatively by passive stretching and physiotherapy. Surgery is reserved for persistent cases.

BONE AND JOINT INFECTIONS

Osteomyelitis

Early recognition and aggressive treatment is essential for a favourable outcome in bone infections. The infection is usually haematogenous in origin or might be secondary to an infected wound. It typically starts in the metaphysis where there is relative stasis of blood. Two-thirds of cases occur in the femur and tibia. The peak incidence is bimodal, occurring in the neonatal period and in older children (9–11 years).

In all age groups, the most common pathogen is *Staphylococcus aureus*, although group B streptococci and *E. coli* occur in neonates.

Children with sickle cell disease have increased susceptibility to salmonella osteomyelitis. *M. tuberculosis* should also be considered.

> **HINTS AND TIPS**
>
> Bacterial bone and joint infections: *Staphylococcus aureus* is the most common pathogen in all age groups.

Clinical features

Infants present with fever and refusal to move the affected limb. Older children will localize the pain and are also systemically unwell. Examination reveals exquisite tenderness over the affected bone usually with warmth and erythema. Pain limits movement.

Diagnosis

The acute-phase reactants (WBC, CRP and ESR) are usually significantly elevated. Blood cultures are positive in more than half of the cases and aspiration of the bone is therefore necessary to identify the organism and its sensitivity. Bone scans are more sensitive in the early phase of the illness (24–48 hours) compared with X-rays, which tend to be normal in the first 10 days. MRI and ultrasound scans have become the chosen modalities of imaging over plain X-rays for detecting changes associated with osteomyelitis. Periosteal elevation or radiolucent necrotic areas can usually be demonstrated between 2 and 3 weeks.

Treatment

Early treatment with intravenous antibiotics is imperative until there is clinical improvement and normalizing of the acute-phase reactants. Several weeks of oral antibiotics follow. Failure to respond to medical treatment is an indication for surgical drainage.

Complications include:

- Chronic osteomyelitis.
- Septic arthritis.
- Growth disturbance and limb deformity (occurs if the infection affects the epiphyseal plate).

Septic arthritis

Purulent infection of a joint space is more common than osteomyelitis and can result in bone destruction and considerable disability. The incidence is highest in children younger than 3 years of age and is usually haematogenous in origin. Other causes include:

- Osteomyelitis.
- Infected skin lesions.
- Puncture wounds.

In infants, the hip is the most common site (the knee is the most common site in older children). *Staphylococcus aureus* is the most common pathogen in all age groups. The organisms are similar to those found in osteomyelitis and the conditions might occur together.

Clinical features

The typical presentation is a painful joint with:

- Fever.
- Irritability.
- Refusal to bear weight.

Infants often hold the limb rigid (pseudoparalysis) and cry if it is moved. There is tenderness and a variable degree of warmth and swelling on examination.

Investigation

The acute-phase reactants are usually elevated. Aspiration of the joint space might reveal organisms and the presence of white cells. The aspirate can then be cultured.

Ultrasound can identify effusions but X-rays are often initially normal or show a non-specific, widened joint space.

Management

Early and prolonged intravenous antibiotics are necessary. Surgical drainage is indicated only if the infection is recurrent or if it affects the hip.

RHEUMATIC DISORDERS

These include:

- Juvenile idiopathic arthritis (JIA).
- Dermatomyositis.
- Systemic lupus erythematosus.

Juvenile idiopathic arthritis

Juvenile idiopathic arthritis has replaced the term 'juvenile chronic arthritis'. It is diagnosed after arthritis in one or more joints for 6 weeks after excluding other causes in a child. It occurs in 1:1000 children. There are six groups and three are discussed in detail below; classification is by mode of onset over the first 6 months (Fig. 21.4). Blood investigations for antinuclear antibodies (ANA) and rheumatoid factor (RF) are helpful in classification but not diagnostic.

Systemic (previously Still's disease)

This mainly affects children under 5 years. The arthritis primarily affects the knees, wrist, ankles and tarsal bones. Other features include:

- High daily spiking fever.
- A salmon-pink rash.
- Lymphadenopathy and hepatosplenomegaly.
- Arthralgia, malaise and myalgia.
- Inflammation of pleura and serosal membranes.

There is often no arthritis at presentation. One-third will have a progressive course and the worst prognosis occurs in the younger age.

Polyarticular

Rheumatoid factor (RF) negative

This affects all ages and all joints but spares metacarpophalangeal joints (MCPs). Limitation of the motion of the neck and temporomandibular joints is seen. It has a good prognosis but disease may be prolonged.

Rheumatoid factor (RF) positive

This mainly affects females over 8 years and causes arthritis of the small joints of the hand and feet. Hip and knee joints are affected early and rheumatoid

Fig. 21.4 Classification of juvenile idiopathic arthritis

	Systemic	Polyarticular	Oligoarticular
Number of joints involved	Variable	More than four	Four or less
Joints involved	Knees Wrist Ankle and tarsal	Any joint	Knees Ankles Elbows Hips spared
Pattern	Symmetrical	Symmetrical	Asymmetrical
Rheumatoid factor	Negative	Positive or negative	Negative
Eye involvement	No	No	Yes in 30%
Clinical course	Poor in one-third	Good if rheumatoid factor negative	Good

nodules are seen over pressure points. There might be a systemic vasculitis; functional prognosis is poor.

Oligoarticular

Early onset is the most common subtype and typically occurs in young girls under 6 years with asymmetric arthritis involving knees, ankle and elbows. Antinuclear antibodies are nearly always present and one-third will develop chronic iridocyclitis (inflammation of the iris and ciliary body, which comprise the anterior uveal tract: anterior uveitis). The definition 'oligoarticular' requires that the disease affects four or fewer joints and it has a good prognosis but eye involvement is independent of the joints. There is a subclass called 'extended oligoarticular' in which more than four joints are affected after 6 months; this has a poorer prognosis.

> **HINTS AND TIPS**
>
> Ophthalmological screening with a slit lamp to detect anterior uveitis is especially important in children with oligoarticular JIA.

Diagnosis

Useful tests for the evaluation of JIA include:

- Full blood count (FBC): anaemia occurs in systemic disease.
- Acute-phase reactants: elevated.
- RF: negative in the majority.
- ANA.
- X-rays: soft tissue swelling in early stages. Bony erosion and loss of joint space later.

Management

A multidisciplinary team approach is required. This will encompass:

- Physiotherapy: to optimize joint mobility, prevent deformity and increase muscle strength.
- Medication: pain control and suppression of inflammation are provided by nonsteroidal anti-inflammatory agents (NSAIDs), e.g. ibuprofen or aspirin. Treatment depends upon current therapy, disease activity and features of poor prognosis. Oligoarticular JIA requires treatment with NSAIDs and/or glucocorticoid injection(s). Treatment can be escalated to methotrexate and subsequently a TNF-α inhibitor. For polyarticular JIA, the stepwise approach is similar to oligoarticular JIA with further escalation to a second TNF-α inhibitor. Systemic

JIA may require systemic use of glucocorticoids with escalation to interleukin-1 receptor antagonists.

GENETIC SKELETAL DYSPLASIAS

Achondroplasia

See Chapter 27.

Osteogenesis imperfecta (brittle bone disease)

Osteogenesis imperfecta is a heterogeneous group of disorders:

- Caused by mutations in type I collagen genes.
- Characterized by fragile bones and frequent fractures.

There are a total of eight types of osteogenesis imperfecta. Types 1–4 are discussed below:

- Type I (the most common form) is an autosomal dominant disorder. Affected children have recurrent fractures, blue sclerae and conductive hearing loss.
- Type II is a severe, lethal form with multiple fractures present before birth. Many affected infants are stillborn. Inheritance is usually autosomal recessive.
- Type III causes severe bone fragility but the sclerae are not blue in later life. Survival to adulthood is uncommon. This is autosomal recessive.
- Type IV is mild with a variable age of onset and only bone fragility without the other features of type I.

Management is by aggressive orthopaedic treatment of fractures to correct deformities and genetic counselling of the parents.

Further reading

Shorter, D., Hong, T., Osborn, D.A., 2011. Screening programmes for developmental dysplasia of the hip in newborn infants. Cochrane Database Syst. Rev. (9). Art. No.: CD004595 http://onlinelibrary.wiley.com/doi/10.1002/14651858.CD004595.pub2/full.

Nemeth, B., 2011. The diagnosis and management of common childhood orthopedic disorders. Curr. Probl. Pediatr. Adolesc. Health Care 41 (1), 2–28.

American College of Rheumatology, 2011. Recommendations for the treatment of juvenile idiopathic arthritis. http://www.rheumatology.org/practice/clinical/guidelines/clinician's_guide2011.pdf.

Cundy, T., 2012. Recent advances in osteogenesis imperfecta. Calcif. Tissue Int. 90 (6), 439–449.

Haematological disorders 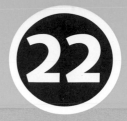 22

At the end of this chapter, you should be able to:
- Understand the normal development of the haematopoietic system
- Identify the common causes of anaemia
- Understand the clinical features and management of iron deficiency anaemia
- Understand the common types of haemolytic anaemia
- Identify the common disorders affecting haemostasis

These encompass defects in the cellular elements of the blood or in those soluble elements involved in haemostasis. Haematological malignancies are considered separately (see Chapter 23). The most common problem encountered is iron deficiency anaemia.

Normal developmental variations are important in the interpretation of changes in the blood in infancy and childhood.

HAEMATOPOIESIS

Early prenatal haematopoiesis occurs in the liver, spleen and lymph nodes. It commences in the bone marrow at about the fourth or fifth month of gestation. At birth, haematopoietic activity is present in most of the bones, especially long bones.

Cells in the peripheral blood have a relatively short lifespan. Continuous replenishment in massive amounts from the bone marrow is required to maintain adequate blood counts.

HINTS AND TIPS

Lifespan of peripheral blood cells:
- Red cells: 120 days.
- Platelets: 10 days.
- Neutrophils: 6–7 hours.

Normal developmental changes in haemoglobin

The haemoglobin (Hb) concentration and haematocrit are relatively high in the term newborn infant because of the low oxygen tension in utero. The wide range encountered, 14–20 g/dL, is accounted for by:
- Variation in umbilical cord clamping.
- The infant's position after delivery.

If cord clamping is delayed and the baby is lower than its placenta, haemoglobin and blood volume are both increased by a placental transfusion. These values subsequently decline, reaching a nadir at:
- About 7 weeks in preterm infants.
- 2–3 months for term infants.

The lower limit of normal for this 'physiological' anaemia is 9.0 g/dL. During this period, there is erythroid hypoplasia of the marrow and a change from fetal to adult haemoglobin.

HINTS AND TIPS

The haemoglobin concentration:
- Is high at birth: 14–20 g/dL.
- Falls to a nadir of 9–13 g/dL at 2–3 months in term infants.
- HbF values decline postnatally to 2% of total at 9–12 months.

ANAEMIA

Anaemia is a decrease of the haemoglobin concentration in the blood to below normal. Dietary iron deficiency is the most common cause but there are many others. Anaemia can be classified initially according to the red cell:
- Colour intensity (normochromic/hypochromic).
- Size (microcytic/normocytic/macrocytic).

Important causes based on this classification are shown in Fig. 22.1.

Fig. 22.1 Classification and causes of anaemia

Microcytic, hypochromic anaemia
  Defects of haem synthesis
  • Iron deficiency
  • Chronic inflammation
  Defects of globin synthesis
  • Thalassaemia
Normocytic, normochromic anaemia
  Haemolytic anaemias
  • Intrinsic red cell defects
      Membrane defects: spherocytosis
      Haemoglobinopathies: sickle cell disease
      Enzymopathies: G6PD deficiency
  • Extrinsic disorders
      Immune-mediated: Rh incompatibility
      Microangiopathy
      Hypersplenism
  Haemorrhage (acute or chronic)
  • Hookworm infestation
  • Meckel's diverticulum
  • Menstruation
  Hypoproduction disorders
  • Red cell aplasia, e.g. renal disease
  • Pancytopenia, e.g. marrow aplasia, leukaemia
Macrocytic anaemia
  Bone marrow megaloblastic
  • Vitamin B_{12} deficiency
  • Folic acid deficiency
  Bone marrow not megaloblastic
  • Hypothyroidism
  • Fanconi anaemia

Iron deficiency anaemia

Iron deficiency anaemia (IDA) is the commonest cause of anaemia in childhood. Unlike in adults, it usually results from inadequate dietary intake rather than loss of iron through haemorrhage.

Iron requirements

The fetus absorbs iron from the mother across the placenta:

• Term infants have adequate reserves for the first 4 months of life.
• Preterm infants have limited stores and higher demands because of their growth rate; they outstrip their reserves by 8 weeks.

Both breast milk and unmodified cow's milk are low in iron concentration (0.05–0.10 mg/100 mL). However, 50% of the iron is absorbed from breast milk, compared to just 10% from cow's milk. Most formula milks are fortified with iron and contain 10 times the concentration in breast milk (1.0 mg/100 mL); however, only 4% is absorbed.

Dietary sources of iron include red meat, fortified breakfast cereals, dark green vegetables and bread. About 10–15% of dietary iron is absorbed. Absorption is:

• Enhanced by ascorbic acid (vitamin C).
• Reduced by tannin in tea.

Iron requirements increase during adolescence, especially for girls who lose iron through menstruation.

HINTS AND TIPS

• Breast and unmodified cow's milk are low in iron.
• Iron is better absorbed from breast milk (50%) than cow's milk (10%).
• Formula milks are fortified with iron.

Causes of iron deficiency

Nutritional deficiency is common in certain at-risk groups (Fig. 22.2). Blood loss is a less common cause but might occur with:

• Menstruation.
• Hookworm infestation.
• Repeated venesection in babies.
• Meckel's diverticulum.
• Recurrent epistaxis.

Clinical features

Mild iron deficiency is asymptomatic. As it becomes more severe there might be:

• Lethargy.
• Fatigue.
• Anorexia.

On examination, the only signs might be pallor of mucous membranes.

IDA in infancy and early childhood causes developmental delay and poor growth, which is reversible by long-term oral iron treatment. Severe anaemia can cause cardiac failure.

Diagnosis

Diagnosis is confirmed by the blood count, film and iron studies.

Fig. 22.2 Dietary iron deficiency

• Prematurity
• Early introduction of unmodified cow's milk
• Delay in mixed feeding
• Poor diet (associated with low socioeconomic status, strict vegetarian diet, etc.)
• Malabsorption

While taking a history in anaemia, it is important to take a detailed dietary history. It is also important to advise parents about appropriate diet and give information regarding iron-containing foods.

Management

Primary prevention in infants can be achieved by:

- Avoidance of unmodified cow's milk.
- Iron supplementation in vulnerable infants (e.g. preterm).

Mild to moderate anaemia is treated with dietary counselling and oral iron using, for example, sodium feredetate. Therapy should be continued for 3 months after correction of anaemia to allow replenishment of iron stores.

Severe anaemia with cardiac decompensation might require transfusion. Investigation for occult gastrointestinal tract bleeding is indicated if there is a failure of response to treatment or recurrence despite an adequate intake.

Thalassaemias

The thalassaemias are a group of hereditary anaemias caused by defects of globin chain synthesis. They are classified into:

- α-Thalassaemia: reduced synthesis of α-globin chains.
- β-Thalassaemia: reduced synthesis of β-globin chains.

Mutations in the globin genes lead to a reduction or absence of the corresponding globin chains. Excess unpaired globin chains produce insoluble tetramers that precipitate causing membrane damage and either:

- Cell death within the bone marrow (ineffective erythropoiesis).

Or

- Premature removal by the spleen (resulting in haemolytic anaemia).

β-Thalassaemia

This occurs most frequently in people from the Mediterranean countries and the Middle East. There are two main types:

1. β-Thalassaemia major (homozygous).
2. β-Thalassaemia trait (heterozygous).

β-Thalassaemia major

There is usually a complete absence of β-globin chain production (genotype β^o/β^o), although some mutations allow partial synthesis (genotype β^+/β^+); haemoglobin A (HbA) cannot be synthesized.

Clinical features

Affected infants usually present after 6 months, as HbF levels decline, with severe haemolytic anaemia, jaundice, failure to thrive and hepatosplenomegaly. If untreated, bone marrow hyperplasia occurs with development of the classical facies:

- Maxillary hypertrophy.
- Skull bossing.

Diagnosis

Haemoglobin electrophoresis reveals a markedly reduced or absent HbA with increased haemoglobin F (HbF) (30–90%).

Treatment

The mainstay of treatment is regular blood transfusion, aiming to maintain the haemoglobin concentration above 10 g/dL. Unfortunately, chronic transfusion therapy is complicated by accumulation of iron in parenchymal organs including the heart, liver, pancreas, gonads and skin. Iron associated cardiomyopathy is a major cause of mortality in the second and third decades. Iron chelation is therefore vital using either oral or subcutaneous agents but does not eradicate the problem completely.

Splenectomy is useful in selected patients, and bone marrow transplantation is potentially curative. Gene therapy may also be possible in the future.

β-Thalassaemia trait

The only abnormality is a mild, hypochromic, microcytic anaemia. Most are asymptomatic. β-Thalassaemia trait can be misdiagnosed as iron deficiency anaemia. The important diagnostic feature is the raised HbA2 and about 50% have a mild elevation of HbF (1–3%) on electrophoresis.

α-Thalassaemia

This is caused by absence or reduced synthesis of α-globin genes. Most result from gene deletion. The manifestations and severity depend on the number of genes deleted (Fig. 22.3).

Genetic counselling is important in all haemoglobinopathies. Folic acid supplements are usually given but iron supplementation should be avoided.

Fig. 22.3 Clinical manifestations of α-thalassaemia variants

Variant	Number of genes deleted	Hb pattern	Clinical features
α-Thalassaemia major	Four	γ4 (Hb Bart)	Hydrops fetalis/death in utero
Haemoglobin H disease	Three	β4 (Hb H) (beyond early infancy)	Severe anaemia, persists through life
α-Thalassaemia minor	Two	Normal	Mild anaemia
Silent carrier	One	Normal	No anaemia Normal RBC indices

HAEMOLYTIC ANAEMIA

Haemolytic anaemia occurs when the lifespan of the red blood cell is shorter than the normal 120 days. Haemolytic anaemia can be caused by:

- Intrinsic red cell defects:
  - Membrane defects.
  - Haemoglobinopathies.
  - Red cell enzyme defects.
- Extrinsic defects, e.g. rhesus (Rh) incompatibility, microangiopathy and hypersplenism.

It is characterized by:

- Anaemia.
- Reticulocytosis.
- Increased erythropoiesis in the bone marrow.
- Unconjugated hyperbilirubinaemia.

Hereditary spherocytosis

This is an autosomal dominant disorder caused by abnormalities in spectrin, a major supporting component of the red blood cell membrane. About 25% of cases are sporadic due to new mutations. As the name suggests, the red cell shape is spherical and the lifespan is reduced by early destruction in the spleen.

Clinical features

The clinical features are highly variable and include:

- Mild anaemia: 9–11 g/dL.
- Jaundice.
- Splenomegaly: mild to moderate.

May be complicated by:

- Aplastic crises secondary to parvovirus B19 infection.
- Gallstones: caused by increased bilirubin excretion.

Diagnosis

Spherocytes are seen on peripheral blood film. Diagnosis is confirmed by the osmotic fragility test (spherocytes already have maximum surface area to volume and rupture more easily than biconcave red cells in hypotonic solutions), though other tests include gel electrophoresis to identify the protein defect or by molecular genetic studies.

Management

Mild disease requires no treatment other than folic acid to meet the increased demands of the marrow.

Splenectomy is indicated for more severe disease, but should be deferred until school age because of the subsequent risk of overwhelming infection. The child should receive:

- Hib, meningococcal and pneumococcal vaccines before splenectomy.
- Prophylactic penicillin for life afterwards.

Sickle cell disease

This chronic haemolytic anaemia occurs in patients homozygous for a mutation in the β-globin gene (which causes substitution of valine for glutamine in the sixth amino acid position of the β-globin chain). This causes a solubility problem in the deoxygenated state: haemoglobin S (HbS) aggregates into long polymers that distort the red cells into a sickle shape.

The heterozygous state (sickle cell trait) confers some protection against falciparum malaria; this 'heterozygote advantage' explains the high incidence of the mutation in populations originating in malarious areas such as tropical Africa, the Mediterranean, the Middle East and parts of India.

HINTS AND TIPS

Sickle cell disease:

- HbS differs from HbA by the substitution of valine for glutamine at position 6 in the β-globin chain.
- HbS forms insoluble polymers in the deoxygenated state.
- The heterozygous state confers some protection against malaria.

Sickled red cells have a reduced lifespan and are trapped in the microcirculation, causing ischaemia.

Clinical features

The synthesis of HbF during the first few months affords protection until the age of 4–6 months. Progressive anaemia with jaundice and splenomegaly then develops, and the infant might present with an episode of dactylitis or overwhelming infection. The subsequent course of the disease is punctuated by crises, of which 'vaso-occlusive' crises are by far the most common.

Vaso-occlusive crises

These episodes are often precipitated by infection, dehydration, chilling or vascular stasis. The clinical features depend on the tissue involved but episodes most commonly manifest as a 'painful' crisis, with pain in the long bones or spine. Cerebral or pulmonary infarction is less common but more serious. The latter might present as 'acute chest syndrome', which is characterized by:

- Chest pain.
- Hypoxia.
- Respiratory distress.
- Pulmonary shadowing on chest X-ray arising from a combination of infarction and infection.

In infancy, patients with sickle cell disease have a functional hyposplenism despite splenomegaly. Repeated vaso-occlusive episodes lead to infarction and fibrosis so that the spleen is no longer palpable from 5 years of age (so-called 'autosplenectomy'). These patients are, therefore, at risk of overwhelming infection with encapsulated organisms (*Haemophilus influenzae*, *Streptococcus pneumoniae*). There is an increased risk of osteomyelitis due to *Salmonella* and other organisms.

HINTS AND TIPS

The spleen in sickle cell disease:

- In infancy, there is splenomegaly.
- Recurrent infarction and 'autosplenectomy' causes the spleen to regress and become impalpable after age 5 years.
- Splenic hypofunction renders patients susceptible to infections with encapsulated organisms.

The long-term consequences of sickle cell disease include:

- Myocardial damage and heart failure.
- Aseptic necrosis of long bones.
- Leg ulcers.
- Gallstones.
- Renal papillary necrosis.

Management

Antenatal and neonatal screening is available and this allows initiation of antibiotic prophylaxis early in life. Sickle cell screening has been part of the Guthrie test since 1995. Prophylactic penicillin should be taken to prevent pneumococcal infection, there is some debate over when prophylaxis should be stopped. Daily folic acid supplements help to meet the demands of increased red cell breakdown. Pneumococcal and meningococcal vaccine should be given as well as the standard course of Hib vaccine. Hydroxyurea reduces crises in several ways, including an increase in HbF and is useful for those experiencing frequent painful crises or severe anaemia.

The treatment of a vaso-occlusive crisis includes:

- Analgesia: opioids for severe pain.
- Oxygenation.
- Maintaining good hydration with IV fluids if necessary.

Exchange transfusion, designed to reduce the proportion of sickle cells, is indicated for brain or lung infarction and priapism. Transfusion with packed red cells might be required if a sudden fall in haemoglobin occurs during an aplastic sequestration or haemolytic crisis.

Vaso-occlusive crises can result in loss of function of the limb or organ if not treated early. It is important to give adequate information to parents about its symptoms and advise them to seek medical advice early in such an event.

Serial transcranial Doppler ultrasound can identify those most at risk of stroke and allow commencement of transfusion programme or hydroxyurea. Retinopathy is also a risk and regular ophthalmology review is recommended.

Sickle cell trait

The heterozygote with sickle cell trait (HbAS) is asymptomatic unless subjected to hypoxic stress (e.g. general anaesthesia). Sickle cells are not seen on peripheral smear and diagnosis is by Hb electrophoresis. The trait is worth detecting to allow genetic counselling and precautions to be taken against hypoxaemia during flying and general anaesthesia.

Red cell enzyme deficiencies

These include glucose-6-phosphate dehydrogenase (G6PD) deficiency and the much rarer pyruvate kinase deficiency.

G6PD deficiency

This is an X-linked recessive disorder with variable clinical severity. Over 400 million people are affected worldwide, particularly in the Mediterranean, Middle Eastern, Oriental and Afro-Caribbean populations. G6PD-deficient red cells do not generate enough glutathione to protect the cell from oxidant agents. Males are more severely affected but females can manifest the phenotype.

Clinical features

G6PD deficiency is characterized by episodes of acute rather than chronic haemolysis. It can manifest with:

- Neonatal jaundice: may cause severe hyperbilirubinaemia requiring exchange transfusion.
- Haemolytic episode: induced by infection, oxidant drugs or fava beans. Intravascular haemolysis occurs with fever, malaise and the passage of dark urine (haemoglobinuria).

It is important to provide patients with information about foods and medications to avoid.

Pyruvate kinase deficiency

This is an autosomal recessive condition causing chronic haemolysis with tolerance of low haemoglobin levels. Infection (e.g. parvovirus) may precipitate severe haemolysis. Management by splenectomy is sometimes useful.

BLEEDING DISORDERS

Normal haemostasis requires a complex interaction between three factors:

- Blood vessels.
- Platelets (thrombocytes).
- Coagulation factors.

> **HINTS AND TIPS**
>
> It is unlikely that inherited bleeding disorders are present if the child has had a major haemostatic challenge, e.g. major surgery, without complications.

A bleeding diathesis can result from a deficiency or disorder of any of these elements. Clinical presentation of a generalized bleeding diathesis might include:

- Petechiae or purpura.
- Prolonged bleeding after dental extraction, surgery or trauma.
- Recurrent bleeding into muscles or joints.

Disorders of blood vessels

Injury to blood vessels provokes two responses that limit bleeding:

- Vasoconstriction.
- Activation of platelets and coagulation factors by subendothelial collagen.

Rare inherited disorders include Ehlers–Danlos syndrome associated with excessive capillary fragility and hereditary haemorrhagic telangiectasia.

Acquired disorders include vitamin C deficiency (scurvy) and Henoch–Schönlein purpura.

Henoch–Schönlein purpura

Henoch–Schönlein purpura (HSP) is a multisystem vasculitis involving the small blood vessels. It commonly follows an upper respiratory tract infection or exposure to a drug or allergen, and is immune mediated with IgA suspected to play a major role.

It is more common in boys and 75% of affected children are under 10 years old.

Clinical features

The condition affects skin, joints, gastrointestinal tract and kidneys. Clinical features are described in Fig. 22.4.

Diagnosis and management

Diagnosis is clinical. Normal platelet count and coagulation studies exclude other causes of purpura.

HSP is usually self-limiting and prognosis is excellent. Treatment is supportive with pain relief for arthralgia. Steroids may be of benefit in severe gastrointestinal disease. Most children recover within 4–6 weeks, although, rarely, chronic renal disease can develop and follow-up monitoring for hypertension and proteinuria should be arranged.

Disorders of platelets

These might be quantitative or qualitative, with the former (thrombocytopenia) being most common.

Thrombocytopenia

A decreased number of platelets (from the normal count of $150–450 \times 10^9/L$) is the most common cause of abnormal bleeding. Purpura usually occurs when the count is below $20 \times 10^9/L$. The cause might be decreased platelet production or reduced platelet survival (Fig. 22.5).

Fig. 22.4	Clinical features of Henoch–Schönlein purpura
Skin	A purpuric rash typically affects the legs and buttocks
GI tract	Colicky abdominal pain accompanied by gross or occult bleeding intussusception may occur
Joints	Pain and swelling of the large joints, e.g. knees and ankles
Kidneys	Glomerulonephritis manifested by microscopic haematuria rarely severe and progressive

---

Fig. 22.5 Causes of thrombocytopenia

Decreased production
Bone marrow failure
• Aplastic anaemia
• Leukaemia
Wiskott–Aldrich syndrome
Reduced survival
Immune-mediated thrombocytopenia
• Idiopathic thrombocytopenic purpura
  (most common)
• Secondary to viral infection, drugs
Hypersplenism
Giant haemangioma
Disseminated intravascular coagulation

Idiopathic thrombocytopenic purpura

Idiopathic thrombocytopenic purpura (ITP) is the most common cause of thrombocytopenia in childhood and refers to an immune-mediated thrombocytopenia for which an exogenous cause is not apparent. The platelets are destroyed within the reticuloendothelial system, mainly in the spleen.

Clinical features

There may be a history of recent viral illness. ITP mainly affects children between 2 and 10 years of age. Presentation is with purpura and superficial bleeding, which might be accompanied by bleeding from mucosal surfaces, e.g. epistaxis. The spleen is palpable in a minority of cases.

Diagnosis

The differential diagnosis includes:

• Acute leukaemia.
• Non-accidental injury.
• Henoch–Schönlein purpura.

A full blood count reveals thrombocytopenia but no pancytopenia. Bone marrow aspiration is unnecessary in typical ITP but should be performed where there is doubt over the diagnosis or in those who develop chronic disease. An increase in megakaryocytes (platelet precursors) is characteristic.

Treatment

In most children, the disease is acute, benign and self-limiting, and no therapy is required. However, chronic thrombocytopenia can occur in up to 20% of cases. Serious bleeding is extremely rare and platelet levels as low as $<10 \times 10^9$ are tolerated as the platelets function more efficiently. Platelet infusions are rapidly destroyed and are only useful in life-threatening emergencies. Advice regarding lifestyle (e.g. avoid contact sports) should be given.

Pharmacological intervention remains widely debated. Both immunoglobulin infusions and corticosteroids cause a rise in the platelet count; however, this has not been shown to change the risk of serious or intracranial bleeding. Current recommendations suggest treatment in:

• Life-threatening bleeding.
• Increased risk of bleeding (e.g. haemophilia).
• Prior to invasive procedures.

Teenage girls have a higher risk of chronic disease (greater than 1 year) and splenectomy might have to be used if medical therapy fails.

COAGULATION DISORDERS

Haemophilia A and B and von Willebrand disease account for the majority of inherited coagulation disorders.

Haemophilia A (factor VIII deficiency)

This is an X-linked recessive disorder due to reduced or absent factor VIII. The incidence is 1 in 5000–10 000 males. It is the result of a new mutation in one third of cases. The factor VIII molecule is a complex of two proteins:

• VIII:C: small molecular weight unit, antihaemophilic factor.
• VIII:R: large molecular weight unit, von Willebrand factor.

Clinical features

Haemophilia A results from deficiency of VIII:C. Clinical severity varies greatly and depends on the factor VIII levels (Fig. 22.6). The characteristic clinical feature is spontaneous or traumatic bleeding, which can be:

• Subcutaneous.
• Intramuscular.
• Intra-articular.

Mild haemophilia might remain undetected until excessive bleeding occurs, e.g. after dental extraction. Even severely affected boys often have few problems in the first year of life (unless circumcision is performed) but early

---

Fig. 22.6 Factor VIII levels in haemophilia A

Mild	5–25% of normal
Moderate	1–4% of normal
Severe	No detectable factor VIII activity

---

bruising and abnormal bleeding is noted from the time they begin to walk and fall over.

In later life, recurrent soft tissue, muscle and joint bleeding are the main problems. Haemarthroses cause pain and swelling of the affected joint and repeated haemorrhage might result in chronic joint disease. Life-threatening internal haemorrhage (e.g. intracranial) can follow trauma.

Diagnosis

Diagnostic evaluation reveals a prolonged activated partial thromboplastin time (APTT) with normal prothromin time (PT); factor VIII assay confirms the diagnosis.

Genetic testing is useful for other family members and prenatal diagnosis is possible.

Management

Bleeding is treated by replacement of the missing clotting factor with intravenous infusion of factor VIII concentrate. The amount required depends on the site and severity of the bleed. Prompt and adequate therapy is important to avoid chronic arthropathy; home therapy can avoid delay and minimize inconvenience.

Recombinant DNA technology is now used to produce factor VIII that is safer than the blood products previously used. Antibodies to factor VIII can develop.

Mild haemophilia can be managed with infusion of desmopressin that releases factor VIII from tissue stores.

Haemophilia B (factor IX deficiency, Christmas disease)

This is an X-linked recessive disorder caused by deficiency of factor IX. It is clinically similar to haemophilia A, but much less common. Investigation reveals a prolonged APTT and reduced factor IX activity (although presentation is heterogeneous with very variable factor IX levels). Treatment is with prothrombin complex concentrate.

von Willebrand disease

This is due to a deficiency of von Willebrand factor (VWF; VIII:R), which has two major roles:

- Carrier protein for factor VIII:C (preventing it from breakdown).
- Facilitates platelet adhesion.

Around 1% of the population is known to be affected. Inheritance is usually autosomal dominant with variable penetrance. The clinical hallmark is bleeding into the skin and mucous membranes (gums and nose).

Disseminated intravascular coagulation

Intravascular activation of the coagulation cascade may be secondary to various disease processes:

- Damage to vascular endothelium: sepsis, renal disease.
- Thromboplastic substances in the circulation, e.g. in acute leukaemia.
- Impaired clearance of activated clotting factors, e.g. in liver disease.

In disseminated intravascular coagulation (DIC) there is fibrin deposition in small blood vessels with tissue ischaemia, consumption of labile clotting factors and activation of the fibrinolytic system.

Clinical features

Clinical features are:

- A diffuse bleeding diathesis, with oozing from venepuncture sites.
- Bleeding from the lungs.
- Bleeding from the gastrointestinal tract.

Diagnosis and management

Investigations reveal:

- Prolonged prothrombin type (INR), activated partial thromboplastin time (APTT) and thrombin time (TT).
- Thrombocytopenia and microangiopathic red cell morphology.
- Hypofibrinogenaemia.
- Elevated fibrinogen degradation products.

Management is supportive with treatment of the underlying cause and replacement of platelets and clotting factors (with fresh frozen plasma).

THROMBOTIC DISORDERS IN CHILDHOOD

Recognition of thrombotic disorders in children is increasing. Although thrombosis is usually rare in children, certain genetic conditions predispose to it:

- Factor V Leiden: caused by an abnormal factor V protein that is resistant to activated protein C.

- Protein C deficiency: protein C inactivates the activated forms of factor V and VIII and stimulates fibrinolysis.
- Protein S deficiency: protein S is a cofactor to protein C.
- Antithrombin III deficiency.

HINTS AND TIPS

Thromboembolic diseases are rare in children because thrombin is inhibited more than it is in adults and is generated less readily.

Further reading

Treutiger, I., Rajantie, J., Zeller, B., et al., 2007. Does treatment of newly diagnosed idiopathic thrombocytopenic purpura reduce morbidity? Arch. Dis. Child. 92 (8), 704–707.

De-Regil, L.M., Jefferds, M.E., Sylvetsky, A.C., et al., 2011. Intermittent iron supplementation for improving nutrition and development in children under 12 years of age. Cochrane Database Syst. Rev. 2011 (12): CD009085. Review.

Bolton-Maggs, P.H.B., Stevens, R.F., Dodd, N.J., et al., 2004. General Haematology Task Force of the British Committee for Standards in Haematology. Guidelines for the diagnosis and management of hereditary spherocytosis. Br. J. Haematol. 126 (4), 455–474.

Malignant disease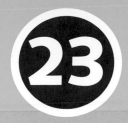

● **Objectives**

At the end of this chapter, you should be able to:
- Understand the aetiology of childhood malignancy
- Understand the types, clinical features and outline the management of childhood leukaemias
- Outline the common types of brain tumours
- Understand some of the common soft tissue tumours of childhood

CHILDHOOD CANCER

Cancer in childhood is uncommon. Only about 1:600 children aged 1–15 years will develop cancer. Despite the dramatic increases in survival rate due to new treatments, it remains an important cause of death in childhood. The spectrum of cancer in childhood is very different from that in adults (Fig. 23.1). Leukaemia accounts for over one-third of cases.

The aetiology, clinical features, investigation and management of malignant disease in childhood are considered below, before the individual diseases are described.

Aetiology

Most childhood cancers are of uncertain cause and occur sporadically in otherwise healthy children. Risk factors include:

- Genetic predisposition: genetic factors are often more evident in childhood than in adult malignancy.
- Environmental factors.
- Infections.

Malignant cells proliferate and develop abnormally because they have escaped normal control mechanisms. In younger children in particular, the malignant cells might be immature precursor cells that fail to mature into normal, differentiated functional cells.

Genetic causes of childhood cancer

During periods of rapid proliferation, a normal cell may undergo a genetic alteration that transforms it into a malignant cell. Two important mechanisms of transformation are:

- Activation of oncogenes.
- Loss of tumour suppressor genes.

Examples of childhood cancer with an identifiable genetic aetiology are shown in Fig. 23.2.

Infections

Two viruses that infect the cells of the human immune system are associated with malignancy:

- Epstein–Barr virus (EBV): EBV is present in the majority of Burkitt's lymphoma. It produces a translocation disrupting the c-myc oncogene on chromosome 8 leading to malignant change although the exact mechanism is poorly understood
- Human immunodeficiency virus (HIV): HIV/AIDS is associated with increased prevalence of malignancies (especially lymphoid).

Environmental

Carcinogens and toxins are less often a cause of childhood cancer. One important risk factor is previous treatment of malignancy in a child.

Clinical features

Cancer in childhood presents in a limited number of ways, some of which are non-specific (Fig. 23.3).

Investigations

Histological confirmation is the cornerstone of diagnosis. This is provided by biopsy (although initial biopsy is not possible at some sites, e.g. brain tumours) or bone marrow aspiration.

Imaging is a vital aid and all modalities can be useful: ultrasound, X-ray, computed tomography (CT), magnetic resonance imaging (MRI) and nuclear imaging scans. Tumour markers are useful in certain tumours, e.g. α-fetoprotein in liver tumours, urinary catecholamines in neuroblastoma.

Fig. 23.1 Relative frequencies of childhood cancer

Type	% childhood cancer
Leukaemia	35
CNS tumours	23
Lymphomas	12
Wilms' tumour	7
Neuroblastoma	7
Bone tumours	6
Other	10

Fig. 23.2 Genetic childhood cancer syndromes

Genetic cancer syndromes	Gene defect
Retinoblastoma	Chromosome 13-deletion of tumour suppressor gene
Li–Fraumeni	p53 mutation
Ataxia-telangiectasia	DNA repair defect
Down syndrome	Trisomy 21

Fig. 23.3 Childhood cancer – clinical features at presentation

Clinical feature	Type of cancer
Constitutional symptoms: fever, weight loss, night sweats	Lymphomas
A localized mass in: • Abdomen • Thorax • Soft tissue	Wilms' tumour, neuroblastoma Non-Hodgkin lymphoma Rhabdomyosarcomas
Lymph node enlargement	Lymphomas
Bone marrow failure	Acute leukaemia
Bone pain	Leukaemia, bone tumours
Signs of raised ICP	Primary CNS tumours

Management

The main therapeutic strategies available are:

- Surgery: required for biopsy, total or partial removal of solid tumours (debulking), or for removal of residual disease after chemotherapy or radiotherapy.
- Radiotherapy: has an important role in specific circumstances, e.g. brain tumours.

- Chemotherapy: has a prominent role. A number of highly effective antineoplastic agents have been developed in the last four decades. Their use is based on a number of principles (see Hints and Tips box). Most children are enrolled into clinical trials on diagnosis.

Chemotherapy may be used as:

- Primary therapy for disseminated malignancy, e.g. the leukaemias.
- To shrink bulky primary or metastatic disease before local treatment.
- Adjunctive treatment for micrometastases.

Bone marrow toxicity is the limiting factor for many therapeutic regimens. This can be circumvented by using bone marrow transplantation to 'rescue' patients after administering potentially lethal, but potentially curative, doses of chemotherapy or radiation.

Supportive care

Treatment produces many predictable and often severe side-effects in many systems. Supportive care is a vital part of treatment. Pancytopenia may occur requiring supportive treatment with blood or platelet transfusion and close monitoring/treatment of infections. Analgesia is given for pain and antiemetics are frequently needed for nausea and vomiting. Indwelling central venous catheters allow pain-free blood sampling and injections.

COMMUNICATION

Psychosocial support is very important. Diagnosis of a potentially fatal illness provokes enormous anxiety, guilt, fear and sadness. Children and their siblings need an explanation of the illness tailored to their age. Help with practical difficulties such as transport and finances might be required and support from the community nursing team is very important.

For some children, a time comes when further treatment represents postponement of inevitable death rather than prolongation of life. A decision to concentrate on palliative care is then appropriate. For survivors, long-term follow-up is required to detect and manage long-term sequelae (Fig. 23.4).

HINTS AND TIPS

Chemotherapy in childhood cancer:
- Chemotherapy is most likely to effect a cure when the malignant cell burden is small.
- Adverse effects are produced on rapidly dividing normal cells, e.g. those of the bone marrow, gastrointestinal tract and hair follicles.

Fig. 23.4 Long-term problems in survivors of childhood cancer

Secondary tumours	Leukaemia and lymphoma
Reduced fertility	From alkylating chemotherapy
Cognitive and psychosocial difficulties	Associated with methotrexate, school absence
Reduced growth and endocrine problems	From irradiated glands
Auditory	From platinum-containing drugs
Cardiac	From doxorubicin

THE LEUKAEMIAS

Leukaemias are the most common childhood malignancy (20% of all cases). They are characterized by proliferation of immature white cells. Acute leukaemias account for the majority (97%) of cases. Note that chronic myeloid leukaemia is rare and that chronic lymphocytic leukaemia is confined to adults. The malignant cells are termed 'blasts'.

The leukaemias are classified according to the white blood cell line involved:

- Acute lymphocytic (lymphoblastic) leukaemia (ALL): cells of lymphoid lineage.
- Acute myeloid leukaemia: cells of granulocytic or monocytic lineage.

Prognosis has improved significantly, mainly thanks to rigorous research programmes and high levels of trial enrolment. It continues to improve with reductions in treatment related mortality and matching of therapies to different prognostic groups.

Clinical features

In most children with acute leukaemia, there is an insidious onset of symptoms and signs arising from infiltration of the bone marrow or other organs with leukaemic blast cells. Most will have one or more of the following:

- Pallor and malaise: anaemia.
- Haemorrhagic diathesis: purpura, easy bruising, epistaxis due to thrombocytopenia.
- Hepatosplenomegaly, lymphadenopathy (50%): reticuloendothelial cell infiltration.
- Bone pain: due to expansion of marrow cavity ± periosteal involvement.
- Infection: due to neutropenia.

Investigations

Peripheral blood investigations reveal:

- Anaemia: normocytic, normochromic.

- Thrombocytopenia.
- Neutropenia: total white blood cell count (WBC) might be low, normal or high.
- Blast cells on film.

Bone marrow examination reveals replacement of normal elements by leukaemic cells.

HINTS AND TIPS

A diagnosis of leukaemia should always be confirmed by bone marrow aspiration.

Acute lymphocytic leukaemia

Acute lymphocytic leukaemia (ALL) accounts for 80% of childhood leukaemia and has a peak incidence between age 3 and 6 years. It is slightly more common in boys than girls. Lymphoblasts in these children do not successfully complete the rearrangement of immunoglobulin and T cell receptor genes necessary for full maturation. Coupled with genetic alterations, which permit them to survive and proliferate, the lymphoblasts remain 'frozen' at an early stage of development.

ALL can be classified according to cell-surface antigens (immunophenotype) into:

- Non-T, non-B cell (common) ALL: 80% are from B cell precursor lineage.
- T cell ALL: 15%.
- B cell ALL: 1%.

Clinical features

Prognosis and clinical presentation varies with subtype. T cell ALL tends to occur in older children and teenagers, with a high peripheral white cell count and mediastinal mass. The prognosis is related to tumour load and can be defined according to certain clinical and laboratory features (Fig. 23.5).

Management

Overall, 5-year survival for patients with ALL is about 85%. Children with common ALL have the best prognosis with 5-year event free survival >90%. Those with higher risk stratification have variable prognosis depending on initial response to chemotherapy.

A typical treatment regimen can be divided into five phases:

1. Induction: an intensive regimen of between three and five drugs with the aim of reducing tumour load (90% achieve remission after induction).
2. Early CNS-directed therapy/prophylaxis (may be intrathecal chemotherapy).
3. Consolidation: continued systemic therapy after remission.

Fig. 23.5 Prognostic groups in acute lymphocytic leukaemia

Factors	Good >70% cure (all factors required)	Poor <60% cure (any factor sufficient)
Age	2–9 years	<1 year
WBC	$<50 \times 10^9$ g/L	$>50 \times 10^9$ g/L
Lineage	Non-T, non-B cell	T cell or B cell
Translocation	Absence of translocation	Presence of specific translocations including Philadelphia

4. Intensification of therapy depending on risk of relapse.
5. Maintenance: chemotherapy continues for 2 years from diagnosis.

Initial preparation involves:

- Blood transfusion.
- Treatment of infection.
- Allopurinol to protect the kidneys against the effects of rapid cell lysis.

Relapses mainly occur in the bone marrow but can occur in the CNS or more rarely testes or lymph nodes. The prognosis is less good in these cases; they are treated with intensified chemotherapy and may be candidates for bone marrow transplant once remission is achieved. For those with Philadelphia translocation, monoclonal antibody therapy (imatinib) is showing some promise.

Acute myeloid leukaemia

This is classified into four subtypes depending on type of cytogenetic abnormality. Prognosis is worse than for ALL – around 85% achieve remission with chemotherapy but relapse is common and recurrence free survival ranges from 30% to 45%. Treatment approach is similar. Allogeneic bone marrow transplant has been shown to improve survival and may be offered where a suitable donor is found.

LYMPHOMAS

These can be classified into:

- Non-Hodgkin's lymphoma (NHL): more common in young children.
- Hodgkin's disease: more common in adolescents and young adults.

Non-Hodgkin's lymphoma

Non-Hodgkin's lymphomas (NHLs) are a heterogeneous group of lymphomas with different characteristics and cells of origin. NHL causes 7% of all childhood cancer and 100 cases per year are seen in the UK. They can develop in immunocompromised children with HIV infection, severe combined immunodeficiency or other severe inherited immunodeficiencies.

Clinical features

NHLs tend to be aggressive and rapidly growing, and might present with:

- Peripheral lymph node enlargement: usually B cell origin.
- Intrathoracic mass: usually T cell origin.
- Mediastinal mass or pleural effusion.
- Abdominal mass: usually advanced B cell disease.
- Gut or lymph node masses.

Subtypes of ALL and NHL might represent a continuation of the same disease.

Treatment

Chemotherapy is the mainstay of treatment but extensive surgical debulking might be required for abdominal tumours. Localized disease has a 90% survival at 5 years. Complications in the acute setting are superior vena cava syndrome and tumour lysis syndrome.

Hodgkin's disease

This is characterized histologically by the Reed–Sternberg cell. It is relatively uncommon in prepubertal children and usually presents in adolescence or young adulthood, with a slight preponderance in females.

Clinical features

The usual presentation is with painless cervical or supraclavicular lymphadenopathy. Systemic symptoms are uncommon. Metastatic disease occurs in the lungs, liver and bone marrow.

Diagnosis

Diagnosis is confirmed by histological examination of a lymph node biopsy. Classification based on histopathology identifies four subtypes of different prognosis:

1. Lymphocyte predominance: best prognosis.
2. Mixed cellularity.
3. Nodular sclerosing: most common in children and adolescents.
4. Lymphocyte depletion: least common, worst prognosis.

Treatment

The disease is staged, to determine treatment, using imaging of chest, mediastinum and abdomen. (Staging laparotomy is no longer performed in the UK.) Treatment is chemotherapy and field radiotherapy. In advanced or recurrent disease bone marrow transplant may be of benefit. The overall prognosis is good and 80–90% of patients are cured overall.

BRAIN TUMOURS

Brain tumours are the second most common form of childhood cancer and the most common solid tumour of childhood. Most are located infratentorially and present with signs and symptoms of raised intracranial pressure and cerebellar dysfunction. Metastasis is rare and diagnosis is often difficult and delayed.

> **HINTS AND TIPS**
>
> Brain tumours are the most common solid tumour of children. Two-thirds arise below the tentorium.

A classification based on histology is shown in Fig. 23.6. An example of a posterior fossa tumour with hydrocephalus is shown in Fig. 23.7.

Astrocytomas (40%)

This is a group of tumours (gliomas) that range from benign to highly malignant. They are graded I–IV by the World Health Organization (WHO) (from lowest grade, slow growing, curable by resection, to highest grade fast spreading tumours). Cerebellar astrocytomas are usually low-grade, slow-growing, cystic gliomas occurring between the ages of 6 and 9 years. Presentation might be with:

- Headache and vomiting: caused by obstructive hydrocephalus; papilloedema might be present.

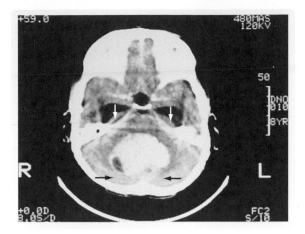

Fig. 23.7 CT of an enhancing posterior fossa tumour (black arrows) with hydrocephalus demonstrated by dilated temporal horns (white arrows)

- Cerebellar signs: ataxia, nystagmus and uncoordination.
- Diplopia, squint: sixth nerve palsy.

Supratentorial astrocytomas and gliomas are less common and present with focal neurological signs and seizures.

Brainstem gliomas (6%) present with cranial nerve palsies, ataxia and pyramidal tract signs.

Diagnosis is usually based on clinical findings and MR imaging as biopsy is hazardous. Although very low grade tumours may be curable with resection, generally prognosis is poor, with median survival less than 1 year after diagnosis despite radiotherapy.

Primitive neuroectodermal tumours (medulloblastomas) (20%)

These are the most common malignant brain tumours of childhood, with a peak incidence between the ages of 2 and 6 years, and a preponderance in boys. They usually arise in the midline and invade the fourth ventricle and cerebellar hemispheres. Unlike other CNS tumours they seed through the CNS and up to 20% have spinal metastases at diagnosis.

Presentation is usually with headache, vomiting and ataxia.

Treatment is a combined modality approach with surgical removal, CNS radiotherapy and chemotherapy all playing a part. Radiotherapy should be avoided where possible in infants and young children. Long-term complications following treatment are common. Prognosis is dependant on extent of metastasis and ranges from 20%-80% 5-year survival.

Fig. 23.6 Classification of brain tumours in childhood
Astrocytic tumours High-grade astrocytomas • Supratentorial
Low-grade astrocytomas • Cerebellar
Brainstem gliomas
Neuroepithelial tumours Primitive neuroectodermal tumours (PNET) (includes cerebellar medulloblastoma)

Craniopharyngioma (4%)

These arise from the squamous remnant of Rathke's pouch and are locally invasive. They present with:

- Visual field loss: due to compression of the optic chiasm.
- Pituitary dysfunction: growth failure, diabetes insipidus.

Most are calcified and may be visible on skull radiographs; however, MRI is the investigation of choice. Treatment is by surgical excision with radiotherapy for residual or recurrent tumour. Prognosis is good but sequelae include visual impairment and pituitary/hypothalamic dysfunction.

NEUROBLASTOMA

Neuroblastoma is a malignancy of neural crest cells that normally give rise to the paraspinal sympathetic ganglia and the adrenal medulla. It is the second most common solid tumour of childhood, occurring predominantly in infants and preschool children with a median age at diagnosis of 2 years. It is unusual in that it can regress spontaneously in very young children (stage IV-S). They can occur anywhere in the sympathetic nervous system but are most commonly found in the adrenals or abdomen.

Clinical features

The clinical features depend on the location and may include:

- Abdominal mass: a firm, non-tender abdominal mass is the most common mode of presentation.
- Systemic signs: pallor, weight loss, bone pain from disseminated disease.
- Hepatomegaly or lymph node enlargement.
- Unilateral proptosis: periorbital swelling and ecchymosis from metastasis to the eye.
- Opsoclonus-myoclonus: 'dancing-eye' syndrome caused by an immune response.
- Watery diarrhoea due to secretion of vasoactive intestinal peptide.
- Mediastinal mass on chest X-ray (CXR).

Diagnosis

Diagnosis may be suspected from characteristic clinical and radiological features (with calcium speckling of tumour). This is confirmed with:

- Biopsy demonstrating classical features on light microscopy ± immunological staining.
- Raised urinary catecholamines (vanillylmandelic acid, homovanillic acid) are useful in diagnosis and monitoring response to therapy.

- MIBG (meta-iodobenzyl guanidine), a radiolabelled tumour-specific agent, or other nuclear scan is useful to measure disease extent.

Treatment

Treatment of neuroblastoma includes:

- Surgical resection.
- Chemotherapy.
- Radiotherapy (especially for high grade tumours and complications, e.g. spinal cord compression).

Prognosis is worse for older children and those with metastatic disease. Chromosome 1p deletion and overexpression of the N-myc oncogene in tumour is associated with a poor prognosis.

WILMS' TUMOUR (NEPHROBLASTOMA)

Wilms' tumour arises from embryonal renal cells of the metanephros, there is cell proliferation without normal tubular and glomerular differentiation. It is predominantly a tumour of the first 5 years of life with a median age of presentation of 3 years of age. Sporadic and familial forms occur. Most tumours are unilateral. This is the most common childhood renal cancer, with other forms (e.g. clear cell tumours) rare.

Clinical features

The most common clinical presentation is an asymptomatic abdominal mass that does not cross the midline. Other features may include:

- Abdominal pain: due to haemorrhage into the tumour.
- Haematuria.
- Hypertension: in 25% of cases. This can be caused by compression of the renal artery or renin production by tumour cells.

Genetics and aetiology

A Wilms' tumour susceptibility gene has been recognized on chromosome 11. There is an association with a number of syndromes including Beckwith–Wiedemann syndrome (with hemihypertrophy) and WAGR syndrome. Associated abnormalities in WAGR include:

- Genitourinary tract abnormalities.
- Intellectual disability.
- Aniridia.

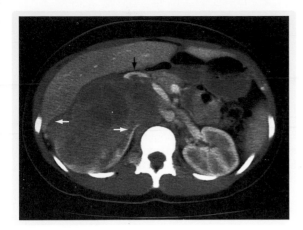

Fig. 23.8 CT scan of nephroblastoma. Wilms' tumour mass arising out of right kidney (white arrows) displacing the inferior vena cava (black arrow)

Wilms' tumour:
* Arises from embryonic renal cells.
* Usually presents as an abdominal mass in a child under 5 years old.
* Is bilateral in 5% of cases.
* Is associated with aniridia (absent iris).

Diagnosis

Diagnosis is normally made from the characteristic appearance on CT (Fig. 23.8), which shows an intrinsic renal mass with mixed solid and cystic densities, and from biopsy. A search for distant metastases, which are most common in lungs and liver, should be made.

Treatment

Treatment involves tailored chemotherapy with surgical resection of the primary tumour. Radiotherapy is used for more advanced disease. Overall, the prognosis is good, with a 90% chance of cure if there is no metastasis, although this falls to 30–40% with metastasis and unfavourable histology.

SOFT TISSUE SARCOMAS

These arise from primitive mesenchyme. The most important is rhabdomyosarcoma, but even rarer forms include fibrosarcomas and liposarcomas.

BONE TUMOURS

Primary malignant bone tumours account for 6% of childhood cancer. They are uncommon before puberty and are most common in adolescents with a preponderence in boys. The two main types are:
* Osteosarcoma: older children, most common.
* Ewing's sarcoma: younger children, less common.

Osteosarcoma

This is a malignant tumour of the bone-producing mesenchyme and is twice as common in males as females.

Clinical features

The usual presenting feature is local pain and soft tissue mass. Persistent bone pain precedes the detection of a mass. Half of all cases occur around the knee joint in the metaphysis of the distal femur or proximal tibia. Systemic symptoms are rare. Metastases are mainly to the lungs and are often asymptomatic.

Diagnosis

Bone X-ray shows destruction and a characteristic 'sunburst' appearance as the tumour breaks through the cortex and spicules of new bone are formed.

Treatment

Treatment involves surgery of primary and metastatic deposits. En bloc resection might allow amputation to be avoided. Aggressive neoadjuvant chemotherapy is important to treat micrometastatic disease. Survival has improved and is 60–80% for localized disease.

Ewing's sarcoma

This is less common than osteogenic sarcoma and is very rare in Afro-Caribbean children. It is an undifferentiated sarcoma of uncertain tissue of origin that arises primarily in bone, but occasionally in soft tissues.

It most commonly affects the long bones, especially the mid- to proximal femur, but can also affect flat bones such as the pelvis.

Clinical features and diagnosis

Pain and localized swelling are the usual presenting complaints. X-ray demonstrates a destructive lesion with periosteal elevation or a soft tissue mass (so called 'onion skin' appearance). Metastases occur to the lungs and to other bones.

Treatment

Chemotherapy is usually the initial treatment followed by radiotherapy or definitive surgical resection. Prognosis depends mainly on the extent of disease at diagnosis.

Retinoblastoma

This is a solid tumour affecting the eye and is bilateral in 40% of cases. It frequently presents with leukocoria and is a cause of an absent red reflex in the neonate. It occurs when both copies of the Rb gene (tumour suppressor) on chromosome 13 are inactivated. It may be inherited (where one copy is already inactive) or spontaneous and the determination of this pattern of inheritance played a key role in the understanding of cancer genetics. Early diagnosis and ophthalmology referral is vital to preserve visual development. Five-year survival is >90%.

LANGERHANS CELL HISTIOCYTOSIS

Formerly called histiocytosis X, this term encompasses a group of relatively rare diseases characterized by the clonal proliferation of a myeloid dendritic cell with antigenic similarities to the skin Langerhans cells. In childhood it most often presents with bony lesions, but other organs may be affected. It is not now considered a true malignancy but the potentially aggressive course and response to chemotherapy brings it within this sphere of clinical practice.

Further reading

Will, A., 2003. Recent advances in the management of leukaemia. Current Paediatrics 13, 201–216.

Ravindranath, Y., Yeager, A.M., Chang, M.N., et al., for the Pediatric Oncology Group, 1996. Autologous bone marrow transplantation versus intensive consolidation chemotherapy for acute myeloid leukemia in childhood. N. Engl. J. Med. 334, 1428–1434.

Woods, W.G., Neudorf, S., Gold, S., et al., 2001. A comparison of allogeneic bone marrow transplantation, autologous bone marrow transplantation, and aggressive chemotherapy in children with acute myeloid leukemia in remission. Blood 97 (1), 56–62

Endocrine and metabolic disorders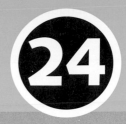

24

● Objectives

At the end of this chapter you should be able to:
- Understand the pathophysiology and management of diabetes
- Know the different types of insulin used in diabetes
- Understand the common thyroid disorders in childhood
- Recognize and know the basic principles of managing a child with congenital adrenal hyperplasia
- Have a general understanding of common inborn errors of metabolism

DISORDERS OF CARBOHYDRATE METABOLISM

Diabetes mellitus

This is a heterogeneous group of disorders, characterized by hyperglycaemia and caused by reduced or absent insulin secretion or action. Type 1 diabetes (formerly called insulin-dependent diabetes) is the most common form of childhood diabetes, although other varieties might be encountered. Type 2 diabetes is characterized by insulin resistance and its increasing incidence has been associated with childhood obesity; however, the discussion below refers to type 1. The prevalence of diabetes in children and young people is approximately 200/100 000 population.

Aetiology

There is good evidence that type 1 diabetes results from T cell-mediated autoimmune destruction of β cells in the pancreatic islets of Langerhans, perhaps triggered by environmental factors (e.g. viruses) in people with a genetic predisposition (Fig. 24.1). The incidence of the disorder is increasing in the UK.

Pathophysiology

The pathophysiological pathways are described in Fig. 24.2. Key features include:
- Insulin deficiency becomes clinically significant when 90% of the β cells are destroyed.
- Osmotic diuresis ensues when blood glucose concentration exceeds renal threshold.
- Ketoacidosis develops when insulin deficiency is severe.

Clinical features

Although type 1 diabetes can present at any age, the most common age of onset is between 7 and 15 years of age. Presenting features may include:
- Polyuria: increased frequency of urination (possibly enuresis).
- Polydipsia: increased thirst.
- Weight loss.
- Diabetic ketoacidosis.

HINTS AND TIPS

Always check for glycosuria in a child with a history of polyuria and polydipsia. Never ascribe frequency of micturition to urinary tract infection without checking for glycosuria and culturing urine. An absence of glycosuria does not exclude type 1 diabetes.

Diabetic ketoacidosis supervenes at a late stage over a short period and is characterized by abdominal pain, vomiting, features of severe dehydration and ketoacidosis (see Hints and tips box). Younger children develop more severe complications of ketoacidosis.

HINTS AND TIPS

Traps for the unwary regarding diabetic ketoacidosis include mistaking the abdominal pain for acute appendicitis and mistaking the hyperventilation for pneumonia.

Diagnosis

Diagnosis is confirmed in a symptomatic child by documenting hyperglycaemia – a random plasma glucose

Fig. 24.1 Aetiology of insulin-dependent diabetes mellitus

Genetic factors
Inherited susceptibility is demonstrated by increased incidence of IDDM in first-degree relatives: 2–5% in siblings and offspring. Concordance for identical twins is 30%. There is an 8–10 times risk for IDDM in people who are HLA-DR3, HLA-DR4, or both

Autoimmune factors
Autoimmune basis is supported by:
• Anti-islet cell antibodies
• Lymphocytic infiltration of pancreas
• Association with other autoimmune endocrine diseases, e.g. thyroiditis, Addison disease

Environmental factors
Triggers may include viruses

level >11.1 mmol/L in the absence of other acute illnesses. If there is doubt, as might occur very early in the disease process, a fasting plasma glucose >7 mmol/L or a raised glycosylated haemoglobin level will clarify the situation. Oral glucose tolerance tests are occasionally needed in children. A 2-hour plasma glucose concentration of >11.1 after ingesting 75 g of anhydrous glucose is also diagnostic.

Management

The discovery of insulin in 1922 transformed type 1 diabetes mellitus from a fatal disease into a treatable one. Initial management depends on the child's clinical condition. Long-term management of this lifelong condition rests on:

Fig. 24.2 Pathophysiology of insulin-dependent diabetes mellitus

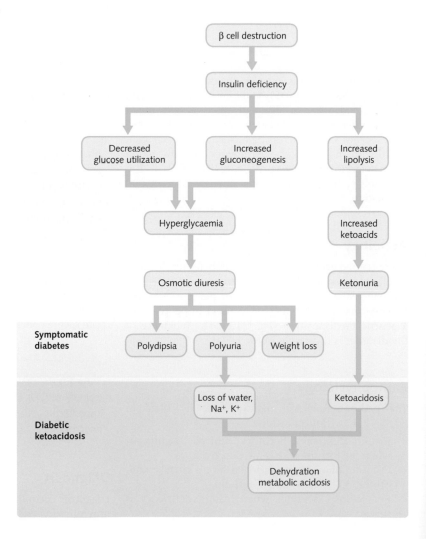

- Insulin replacement.
- Diet.
- Exercise.
- Monitoring.
- Education and psychological support.
- Management of complications: hypoglycaemia and diabetic ketoacidosis.

These are considered in turn.

Insulin replacement

The important features of insulin replacement are:

- Average requirement is 0.5–1.0 unit/kg/day. During the 'honeymoon' or remission phase, which can last for weeks or months after presentation, temporary residual islet cell function causes a reduction in insulin requirements.
- Insulin regimens (Fig. 24.3): (1) one, two or three injections daily – usually combination of short/rapid acting insulin with an intermediate acting insulin. It often comes premixed in specific ratios; (2) multiple daily injections 'basal-bolus regimen' – this involves short/rapid acting insulin injections before meals and one or more separate injections of intermediate/long acting insulin; (3) continuous subcutaneous insulin infusion using a pump.
- In the first regimen, the total daily dose is divided in a 1:2 proportion between short-acting (regular, soluble) insulin and medium-acting (isophane) insulin. Two-thirds is usually given before breakfast and one-third before the evening meal, so two injections per day are administered.
- Multiple daily injection regimens usually use ultra rapid acting insulins as they are more convenient (usually taken just before a meal, or even after the meal – the dose can be titrated according to how much the child has eaten and hence, to the blood sugar response) and results in improved glucose control.
- Injections are given subcutaneously and can be given in upper arms, outer thighs or abdomen. The site must be rotated to avoid local complications such as fat atrophy.

- During puberty, insulin requirements increase. Multiple injections may result in better glycaemic control.
- Insulin pumps have recently become widely used in type 1 diabetics and will likely become the mainstay of treatment in the future. They were invented in the 1970s, are portable and attached to the patient. The pump consists of the main pump unit and holds an insulin reservoir. The latter is attached to a long piece of tubing with a needle or cannula at the other end.

Diet and exercise

Food intake needs to match the time course of insulin absorption and be adjusted for unusual heavy exercise. Dietary management therefore encompasses:

- High fibre, complex carbohydrates: this provides sustained release of glucose and avoids rapid swings in blood glucose generated by refined carbohydrates (e.g. sweets or ice cream).
- Food intake is divided between the three main meals and intervening snacks.
- Food intake is increased before or after heavy exercise to avoid hypoglycaemia.
- Working with the dietician in carbohydrate 'counting' to plan the number of grams of carbohydrates eaten and match the insulin dose accordingly.

Monitoring

Monitoring of blood glucose concentrations is necessary to evaluate the management and control. This is performed using finger-prick samples, which are convenient and easy to take. Readings are recorded in a diary so changes to insulin regimens can be appropriately made. Twenty-four-hour profiles are more useful than single daily records. Urine testing for ketones is important if ketoacidosis is suspected; however, this is being superseded by blood ketone estimation.

The measurement of glycosylated haemoglobin (HbA1c) reflects glycaemic control over the past 6–8 weeks and allows long-term glucose control to be optimized. NICE guidelines recommend a target HbA1c level less than 7.5%, although in practice this may result in more hypoglycaemic episodes.

Fig. 24.3 Types of insulin

Type of insulin	Onset of action	Duration of action	Examples
Rapid acting	15 min	1–5 h	NovoRapid (insulin aspart), Humalog
Short acting	30–60 min	Up to 8 h	Actrapid, Humulin (soluble insulin)
Intermediate acting	1–2 h	16–35 h (peak: 4–12 h)	Insulatard, Isophane insulin (Humalin I, Hypurin)
Long acting	Steady state in 3–4 days	Constant	Levemir (insulin detemir), Lantus (insulin glargine)
Biphasic insulin	Variable	Variable	NovoMix, etc.

Education and psychological support

Children and their families require an educational programme that covers:

- A basic understanding of diabetes in lay language.
- The influence of diet and exercise on blood glucose levels.
- Practical aspects of insulin injection and blood glucose monitoring.
- Recognition and treatment of hypoglycaemia.
- Adjustments for intercurrent illness, significance of ketonuria.
- The importance of good control.

COMMUNICATION

A multidisciplinary approach is essential, involving the physician, dietician, diabetic nurse, psychologist and community nurses. Input from a dietician is a vital part of the management of diabetes. At diagnosis advice about dietary modifications should be offered and ongoing support available.

COMMUNICATION

The diagnosis of type 1 diabetes provokes strong emotional responses in the child and family, including anger, guilt, resentment and fear. Adjustment to these normal responses is facilitated by open discussion. Voluntary groups (e.g. Diabetes UK) are important sources of support.

HINTS AND TIPS

Adolescence and diabetes mellitus:
- Adolescence is often a difficult time for the diabetic.
- There might be conflict at home and with healthcare professionals.
- Problems occur with self-image, self-esteem and desire for independence.
- Poor compliance can be due to denial, apparent indifference or as a form of rebellion.
- 'Feeling well' is equated with good control and long-term risks are often ignored.
- Helpful strategies include: a united team approach, clear guidelines plus short-term goals and peer group support.

Management of complications

These can be divided into immediate complications, which include hypoglycaemia and diabetic ketoacidosis, and late complications.

Hypoglycaemia   The concentration of glucose in the blood can fall when there is a mismatch between insulin dose, time of administration, carbohydrate intake and exercise. Many young children are not aware of hypoglycaemic episodes and repeated hypoglycaemic episodes increase this lack of awareness.

Symptoms usually occur at blood glucose levels below 4 mmol/L. Initial symptoms reflect the compensatory sympathetic discharge and include feeling faint, dizzy or 'wobbly', sweating, tremulousness and hunger. More severe symptoms reflect glucose deprivation to the central nervous system and include lethargy, bizarre behaviour and – ultimately – coma or seizures. Unlike adults and older children, in young children the behavioural and neuroglycopenic symptoms predominate over autonomic symptoms.

Treatment of a 'hypo' is easily achieved at an early stage by administration of a sugary drink, glucose tablet or glucose polymer gel, which is well absorbed via the buccal mucosa, but this should be followed by a more complex form of carbohydrate. In severe hypoglycaemia, if consciousness is impaired or there is lack of cooperation, IV glucose or 1 mg of IM glucagon is administered. Eating a snack just before exercising reduces the risk of exercise-induced hypoglycaemia.

Diabetic ketoacidosis   This can occur at presentation or complicate established diabetes (e.g. if there is poor compliance or intercurrent illness). It is considered in Chapter 29.

Late complications of diabetes

Good glycaemic control reduces the incidence of long-term vascular complications of diabetes such as:

- Retinopathy.
- Nephropathy.
- Neuropathy.

Intensive control is associated with more hypoglycaemic episodes, hence may not be suitable in young children.

Hypoglycaemia

This is a common problem in the newborn (see Chapter 28) but is still seen occasionally in infants and children. It is important to diagnose because it is easy to treat and has serious consequences if unrecognized.

The various causes are best understood in relation to the normal factors determining glucose homeostasis. The major causes are listed in Fig. 24.4.

Fig. 24.4 Causes of hypoglycaemia beyond the neonatal period

Metabolic
Ketotic hypoglycaemia
Liver disease
Inborn errors of metabolism, e.g. glycogen storage disorders

Hormonal
Deficiency
- Adrenocortical insufficiency, e.g. Addison's disease, congenital adrenal hyperplasia
- Panhypopituitarism
- Growth hormone deficiency

Hyperinsulinism
- Islet cell adenoma
- Exogenous insulin-treated IDDM

---

is short and thin and becomes hypoglycaemic after a short period of starvation, for example in the early morning. Insulin levels are low and there is ketonuria. Treatment is with frequent snacks and extra glucose drinks during intercurrent illness. Spontaneous resolution occurs by the ages of 6–8 years.

HINTS AND TIPS

Regarding hypoglycaemia, at the time of blood glucose measurement, screening blood test samples should be sent for measurement of:
- Plasma insulin, growth hormone and cortisol.
- β-Hydroxybutyrate.
- Urine should be tested for ketones.
- Laboratory glucose sample.

Clinical features

Early symptoms reflect the compensatory sympathetic response and include dizziness, faintness and hunger. Signs include tachycardia, sweating and pallor. Late features are those of neuroglycopenia: altered behaviour and consciousness, headache and seizures.

Diagnosis

The precise definition of hypoglycaemia is problematic but a useful working definition is a blood glucose less than 2.6 mmol/L. This corresponds to changes in the electroencephalogram (EEG). Measurements made using a glucose-sensitive strip should always be verified by a laboratory measurement. Serum and urine should be taken during the attack for further diagnostic testing, e.g. for metabolic disorders.

Management

If the child is alert then giving a sugary drink is the first step; an unconscious child should be given 2 mL/kg IV 10% dextrose. The blood sugar should be rechecked after this dose and a further bolus given if not effective. Higher concentrations have been associated with rebound hypoglycaemia and should be avoided. Blood glucose should be monitored closely and a maintenance infusion of glucose can be given if the hypoglycaemia persists. Glucagon can be used in cases where glycogen stores are not depleted, e.g. insulin overdose.

Ketotic hypoglycaemia

The most common cause of hypoglycaemia in children 1–4 years of age, this ill-defined entity is the result of diminished tolerance of normal fasting. The typical child

THYROID DISORDERS

Thyroid hormone is critical for normal growth and neurological development in infants and children. Conditions causing hypothyroidism and hyperthyroidism occur, and the gland can also be the site of benign and malignant tumours. Worldwide, the most important condition affecting the thyroid gland is iodide deficiency, estimated to affect at least 800 million people.

Hypothyroidism

This might be present at birth (congenital hypothyroidism) or develop at any time during childhood or adolescence (acquired hypothyroidism).

Congenital hypothyroidism

This has an incidence of 1 in 4000 live births. The causes include:
- Developmental defects: thyroid agenesis or failure of migration.
- Dyshormonogenesis: inborn error of thyroid hormone synthesis (accounts for 15%, a goitre usually occurs).
- Transient congenital hypothyroidism: (e.g. ingestion of maternal goitrogens).
- Congenital pituitary lesions (rare).
- Maternal iodide deficiency: the most common cause worldwide.

Clinical features
Infants may appear clinically normal at birth. The clinical features that develop include:
- Prolonged neonatal jaundice.
- Feeding problems.

- Constipation.
- Coarse facies, large fontanelle, large tongue, hypotonia and goitre.

Diagnosis and treatment

Testing for hypothyroidism is a part of the neonatal screening in the UK and most infants are diagnosed this way. Most laboratories in the UK test for raised levels of thyroid stimulating hormone (TSH) and some laboratories in the USA measure both TSH and thyroxine (T_4). Early diagnosis and treatment with oral thyroxine can result in normal neurological function and intelligence. Acquired hypothyroidism is treated with thyroxine. Monitoring of treatment is by regular assessment of TSH and T_4.

Hyperthyroidism

Neonatal hyperthyroidism can occur in the infants of mothers with Graves' disease from the transplacental transfer of thyroid-stimulating immunoglobulins.

Juvenile hyperthyroidism

This is most commonly caused by Graves' disease, an autoimmune condition in which one type of antibody (human thyroid stimulating immunoglobulins) mimics TSH by binding and activating the TSH receptor. It usually presents during adolescence and is much more common in girls than boys.

The clinical features are similar to those seen in adults and can also include deteriorating school performance; puberty might be delayed or accelerated.

On laboratory testing, serum levels of thyroxine (T_4) and triiodothyronine (T_3) are elevated and TSH levels are depressed. Antimicrosomal antibodies are often present.

Medical therapy with carbimazole is the first line of treatment. β-Blockers can be added for relief of severe symptoms but should be discontinued when thyroid function is controlled. Subtotal thyroidectomy or radioiodine treatments are options for relapse after medical treatment. Radioiodine has not been shown to be harmful in children.

ADRENAL DISORDERS

Disorders of the adrenal cortex can result in deficiency or excess of adrenocortical hormones. The latter causes Cushing's syndrome, the most common cause of which is chronic administration of corticosteroids. Disorders of the medulla (e.g. phaeochromocytoma) are exceedingly rare.

Cortisol, the major glucocorticoid, is stimulated by pituitary adrenocorticotrophic hormone (ACTH) under a negative feedback loop. Aldosterone is the principal mineralocorticoid and is controlled by the renin–angiotensin system. The major sex steroids produced by the adrenal glands are androgens.

Adrenocortical insufficiency

Diminished production of adrenocortical hormones may arise from:

- Congenital adrenal hyperplasia (CAH): an inherited inborn error of metabolism in biosynthesis of adrenal corticosteroids.
- Primary adrenal cortical insufficiency: Addison's disease.
- Secondary adrenal insufficiency: ACTH deficiency due to pituitary disease or long-term corticosteroid therapy.

Congenital adrenal hyperplasia

Congenital adrenal hyperplasia (CAH) is a group of disorders caused by a defect in the pathway that synthesizes cortisol from cholesterol. Approximately 90% of cases are caused by a deficiency in 21-hydroxylase and 5–7% are due to 11-hydroxylase deficiency; other defects are seen but are rare. Prevalence is approximately 1 in 10 000 and the National Screening Committee are presently reviewing their policy on screening newborns for CAH, an update upon which is expected in May 2013. The condition is autosomal recessive and the gene is found on chromosome 6.

Clinical features

Clinical features are due to androgen excess and cortisol deficiency:

- Female virilization.
- Salt-wasting crises due to mineralcorticoid deficiency (this is less common with 11-hydroxylase deficiency). This leads to volume depletion, electrolyte imbalances and shock.
- Cortisol deficiency – hypoglycaemia, hypotension, shock.

It is difficult to diagnose male infants with this disorder because they have few clinical manifestations at birth. For this reason, screening programmes are currently being evaluated.

Diagnosis

Diagnosis rests on the demonstration of markedly elevated levels of 17α-hydroxyprogesterone in the serum. In the 'salt-losing' form, the characteristic electrolyte disturbance of hyponatraemia, hypochloridaemia and hyperkalaemia provides a clue to the diagnosis.

Management

Initial management of a 'salt-losing' crisis involves volume replacement with normal saline and systemic steroids. Parents are also taught to recognize early signs of illness and children should carry a steroid card to alert health professionals.

Long-term treatment involves:

- Cortisol replacement with hydrocortisone: to suppress ACTH and androgen overproduction. Growth is used as a monitor of therapy.
- Mineralocorticoid replacement: fludrocortisone if there is salt wasting.
- Surgical correction of female genital abnormalities.

HINTS AND TIPS

Congenital adrenal hyperplasia is a potentially lethal but treatable cause of vomiting and dehydration in young infants.

Primary adrenal insufficiency

Addison's disease is rare in children but can be caused by:

- Autoimmune disease.
- Haemorrhage and infarction (Waterhouse–Friderichsen syndrome).
- Tuberculosis (rare).

Physical findings include postural hypotension and increased pigmentation. Intercurrent illness or trauma can trigger an adrenal crisis (characterized by vomiting, dehydration and shock).

Secondary adrenal insufficiency

This is most commonly caused by prolonged glucocorticoid use in diseases not involving the adrenal gland, e.g. severe chronic asthma. The risk is increased by increased duration of treatment but courses less than 10 days have a low risk. Reduction of steroid doses should be slow after a prolonged course and tailored to the underlying disease. This also rarely occurs with high-dose inhaled steroids.

Fig. 24.5	Causes of Cushing's syndrome
Primary	**Adrenal tumour**
Secondary	ACTH secretion from: Pituitary tumour Ectopic ACTH production
Iatrogenic	Long-term glucocorticoid administration

HINTS AND TIPS

Steroid administration must not be stopped suddenly. If the child is sick the steroid dose should be increased. All children should carry a steroid card with them which gives clear instructions on what to do in such a situation.

Cushing's syndrome

This is a cluster of symptoms and signs caused by glucocorticoid excess, due either to endogenous overproduction of cortisol or exogenous treatment with pharmacological doses of corticosteroids. The causes are listed in Fig. 24.5.

Clinical features

The clinical features include:

- Short stature.
- Truncal obesity, 'buffalo' hump.
- Rounded 'moon' facies.
- Signs of virilization, striae.
- Hypertension.

Diagnosis

Elevated serum cortisol levels are found with absence of the normal diurnal rhythm (high midnight levels). A prolonged dexamethasone suppression test might be required to distinguish Cushing's disease (ACTH-driven bilateral adrenal hyperplasia: suppressible by dexamethasone) from Cushing's syndrome (adrenal tumour: cortisol levels not suppressed by dexamethasone). CT or MRI of the adrenal and pituitary glands might identify an adrenal tumour or pituitary adenoma. Treatment depends on the cause and might involve surgical resection and radiotherapy.

DISORDERS OF THE PITUITARY GLAND

The pituitary gland has two distinct portions: the anterior and posterior lobes. These have different embryonic origins and separate hormonal functions. Pituitary disorders in childhood are rare.

Anterior pituitary disorders

A deficiency of the anterior pituitary hormones is more common than an excess of these and might involve individual hormones or all (panhypopituitarism). Hypopituitarism in children can be caused by:

- Cranial defects, e.g. septo-optic dysplasia and agenesis of corpus callosum.
- Tumours, e.g. craniopharyngioma.
- Idiopathic hormone abnormalities.
- Trauma/surgery and radiation.

Growth restriction is a common feature, together with thyroid, adrenal and gonadal dysfunction depending on the pattern of deficiency. Isolated idiopathic growth hormone (GH) deficiency accounts for most cases of GH deficiency.

Posterior pituitary disorders

The posterior lobe (neurohypophysis) secretes arginine, vasopressin (also called antidiuretic hormone, ADH) and oxytocin.

Diabetes insipidus

This results from deficiency of ADH. It might occur as an isolated idiopathic defect or in association with anterior pituitary deficiency (e.g. due to tumours, infections or trauma).

It presents with polydipsia and polyuria. Several conditions mimic diabetes insipidus, including hypercalcaemia, chronic renal disease and psychogenic water drinking. Diagnosis is by a water deprivation test.

Syndrome of inappropriate secretion of ADH

Syndrome of inappropriate secretion of ADH (SIADH) is a common stress response and might be caused by several underlying conditions including:

- Central nervous system (CNS) disease: meningitis, brain tumours or head trauma.
- Lung disease: pneumonia.

Symptoms occur due to effects of water intoxication: these include vomiting, behavioural changes and seizures.

Diagnosis consists of:

- Hypo-osmolality with hyponatraemia.
- Normal or increased volume status.
- Normal renal, thyroid and adrenal function.
- Elevated urine sodium and osmolality.

Treatment is by treating the underlying cause and fluid restriction.

DISORDERS OF THE GONADS

These cause abnormalities of sexual differentiation (which usually present in the newborn) and disorders of puberty, which might be precocious or delayed. Disorders of sexual differentiation are covered in Chapter 12. See also Figs 24.6 and 24.7.

Disorders of puberty

During normal puberty, secondary sex characteristics are acquired and reproductive capacity is attained. Features of normal puberty in males and females are listed in Fig. 24.8. Puberty can be precocious or delayed.

Fig. 24.6   Causes of abnormal sexual differentiation

46XY males with testes and incomplete masculinization due to:
- Defects in testosterone synthesis
- Defects in androgen action, e.g. 5α-reductase deficiency
- Androgen resistance (testicular feminization syndrome)

46XX females with ovaries who are masculinized due to:
- Congenital adrenal hyperplasia
- Maternal androgen exposure

Fig. 24.7   Sex determination

An individual's sex is determined at many different levels:
- Chromosomal
- Gonadal (testis, ovary)
- Anatomical (internal and external genitalia)
- Hormonal
- Psychological
- Sex of rearing

Fig. 24.8   Features of puberty

Male genitalia	First sign is testicular growth Followed by penis enlargement Growth spurt reached 2 years later than females
Female genitalia	Initially breast development Pubic and axillary hair development follows Menses occur late

Precocious puberty

This refers to the development of secondary sexual characteristics before the age of 8 years in girls or 9 years in boys. There is an associated growth spurt. It should be differentiated from:

- Premature thelarche: isolated breast development in a very young girl. A nonprogressive, benign condition.
- Premature adrenarche: isolated early appearance of pubic hair in either sex. A benign, self-limiting condition due to early maturation of adrenal androgen secretion, although an adrenal tumour might need to be excluded.

The causes of precocious puberty are shown in Fig. 24.9. In females, it is usually due to early onset of normal puberty. In boys, it is more likely to be pathological and must be investigated.

Treatment depends on cause. Gonadotrophin-releasing hormone analogues (GnRHa) can be used to prevent puberty from progressing.

Delayed puberty

This can be defined as the absence of secondary sex characteristics at 13 years of age in girls or 14 years of age in boys. The problem is more common in boys and the majority of adolescents affected are normal. The causes are listed in Fig. 24.10.

Assessment should include pubertal staging and examination to exclude systemic disease. If indicated, helpful investigations are:

Fig. 24.9 Causes of precocious puberty

Gonadotrophin-dependent
Idiopathic, familial
CNS lesions, e.g. postirradiation, surgery, tumours, hydrocephalus

Gonadotrophin-independent
McCune–Albright syndrome (polyostotic fibrous dysplasia of bone)
Tumours of adrenals or gonads

Fig. 24.10 Causes of delayed puberty

Central causes – gonadotrophins low
Constitutional delayed puberty
Hypothalamopituitary disorders, e.g. panhypopituitarism, intracranial tumours, isolated gonadotrophin deficiency
Severe systemic disease, e.g. cystic fibrosis, severe asthma, starvation

Gonadal failure – gonadotrophins high
Chromosomal abnormalities, e.g. Klinefelter syndrome (47, XXY), Turner syndrome (45, XO)

Fig. 24.11 Categories of inborn errors of metabolism

Category	Examples
Amino acid metabolism	Phenylketonuria
Organic acid metabolism	Maple syrup urine disease
Urea cycle disorders	Ornithine transcarbamylase deficiency
Carbohydrate metabolism	Galactosaemia Glycogen storage diseases
Mucopolysaccharidosis	Hurler syndrome

- Chromosomal analysis.
- Measurement of gonadotrophin levels.

Treatment is often not required for constitutional delay, but hormone therapy (e.g. oxandrolone or low-dose testosterone) can be used to accelerate growth and induce secondary sexual characteristics in boys. Oestrogen therapy can be used in girls but care must be taken to prevent premature closure of the epiphyses.

HINTS AND TIPS

- Precocious puberty is more common in girls.
- Delayed puberty is more common in boys.

INBORN ERRORS OF METABOLISM

This term is used to describe any of the inherited disorders that result in a defect in normal biochemical pathways. Several hundred of these conditions have been described. Individually they are rare, although certain ethnic groups are at increased risk for specific diseases.

Inborn errors of metabolism are usually autosomal recessive, although some are X-linked. The main categories are listed in Fig. 24.11.

The clinical effects might be caused by accumulation of excess precursors, toxic metabolites or metabolic energy insufficiency. Clinical manifestations are non-specific and often mistaken for sepsis. Metabolic stress often precipitates symptoms, e.g. weaning, intercurrent infections and commonly during the neonatal period.

An inborn error of metabolism should be a differential diagnosis for the sick neonate. Features that may make it more likely include:

- Parental consanguinity.
- Previous neonatal or sudden infant death.

- Previous multiple miscarriages or stillbirths.
- Encephalopathic episodes.
- Severe disease in whom a diagnosis has not been forthcoming.
- Maternal HELLP (haemolysis, elevated liver enzymes, low platelet count) syndrome antenatally.

Investigations might reveal severe metabolic acidosis, hypoglycaemia or hyperammonaemia. In older children, they should be considered as a cause of:

- Progressive learning difficulties.
- Developmental delay.
- Seizures.
- Failure to thrive.
- Coarse facies.
- Hepatosplenomegaly.

Investigations that should be undertaken for an initial screen include:

- Urea and electrolytes, liver function tests, lactate and ammonia levels.
- Acid–base status and anion gap.
- Cerebrospinal fluid (CSF) lactate.
- Blood levels of glucose and amino acids.
- Urine amino acids and organic acids: ketonuria is abnormal as neonates do not readily produce ketones in the urine.

The initial treatment is generic to all disorders and includes stopping feeds and administer dextrose to stop metabolic load and further catabolism. Specific treatment for certain disorders is indicated and advice should be sought from a metabolic specialist. Correction of metabolic disturbances and ventilatory and renal support may be necessary.

Although in some conditions the prognosis is poor, the diagnosis should be made so that prenatal diagnosis can be performed in future pregnancies.

Examples of individual inborn errors of metabolism are considered briefly in turn.

Phenylketonuria

This is an autosomal recessive trait with an incidence of 1 in 10 000 live births and with a carrier rate of 1:50. In most cases, the defect lies in the enzyme phenylalanine hydroxylase, which normally converts phenylalanine to tyrosine. Hyperphenylalaninaemia occurs, with a build-up of toxic by-products, such as phenylacetic acid, which are excreted in the urine (hence phenylketonuria, PKU).

As PKU is relatively common and is treatable, newborn screening is carried out by the Guthrie test. This is carried out at several days of age because it is necessary for the infant to have been fed milk, which contains phenylalanine.

Infants with PKU are clinically normal at birth. Symptoms and signs appear later in infancy and childhood if the disorder is undetected and untreated. These include:

- Neurological manifestations: moderate to severe mental retardation, hypertonicity, tremors, behaviour disorders and seizures.
- Growth retardation.
- Hypopigmentation: fair skin, light hair (due to the block in tyrosine formation that is required for melanin production).

Treatment consists of dietary manipulation. The phenylalanine content of the diet is reduced. This should start early in infancy and is continued until at least 6 years of age. Some authorities recommend lifelong dietary restriction but the diet is unpalatable.

Females with PKU must be on dietary restriction if planning a pregnancy, because maternal hyperphenylalaninaemia is associated with spontaneous abortion, microcephaly and congenital heart disease.

Galactosaemia

This causes neonatal liver dysfunction, coagulopathy and cataracts. It has an association with *E. coli* sepsis. It is diagnosed by the presence of reducing substances in the urine and decreased or absent galactose-1-phosphate uridyltransferase in red cells. A high suspicion of this disorder should be considered in all cases of severe neonatal jaundice. Treatment is by a lactose-free diet and it is an absolute contraindication to breastfeeding.

Glycogen storage diseases

This group of conditions is caused by defects in the enzymes involved in glycogen synthesis or breakdown. There is an abnormal accumulation of glycogen in tissues. The pattern of organ involvement depends on the enzyme defect and may include liver, heart, brain, skeletal muscle or other organs. There are at least six varieties, some of which have eponyms, e.g. type 1A (von Gierke's disease; glucose-6-phosphatase deficiency). Affected children have growth failure, hypoglycaemia and hepatomegaly. Treatment is by frequent feeds throughout day and night.

Mucopolysaccharidoses

Mucopolysaccharidoses (MPS) are a group of disorders caused by defects in enzymes involved in the metabolism and storage of mucopolysaccharides. They are progressive multisystem disorders that can affect the central nervous system, eyes, heart and skeletal system. Characteristic features are:

- Developmental delay in the first year.
- Coarse facies: develop in most cases although children are normal at birth.

There are numerous types, many of which have eponymous designations, e.g. MPS I (Hurler syndrome, which is autosomal recessive). Affected children develop coarse facial features, corneal opacities, hepatosplenomegaly, kyphosis and mental retardation.

Diagnosis is made by identifying the enzyme defect and identifying the excretion in the urine of the major storage substances, the glycosaminoglycans. Treatment is by bone marrow transplant if performed early.

Further reading

National Institute for Health and Clinical Excellence (NICE), July 2004. Diagnosis and management of type 1 diabetes in children, young people and adults (CG15). (modified October 2011): http://www.nice.org.uk/CG15.

Diabetes.co.uk, http://www.diabetes.co.uk.

Gupta, N., Kabra, M., 2011. Acute management of sick infants with suspected inborn errors of metabolism. Indian J. Pediatr. 78 (7), 854–859.

Cakir, B., Teksam, M., Kosehan, D., et al., 2011. Inborn errors of metabolism presenting in childhood. J. Neuroimaging 21 (2), e117–e133.

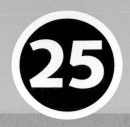
At the end of this chapter, you should be able to:
- Understand the aetiology of common childhood behavioural problems
- Understand the clinical presentations of autistic spectrum disorders
- Understand the common causes and management options for bedwetting
- Recognize the clinical features of ADHD
- Outline common behavioural problems in adolescence

Major psychoses rarely present during childhood although disturbed emotions and behavioural problems are very prevalent. The conditions encountered are, not surprisingly, age-related and range from the toddler who will not sleep to deliberate self-harm in an adolescent.

A child's personality, behaviour patterns and emotional responses are determined by an interplay between nature (genetic predisposition) and nurture (predominantly parenting). The relative importance of genes and environment remains the subject of debate and current research.

An infant's first relationship is usually with the mother and separation anxiety typically becomes evident at about 6 months to 1 year. By the second year, emotional attachments are extended to the father and other family members, and by the age of 4–5 years separation from parents can be tolerated for several hours as occurs with school attendance.

With entry into school, the importance of others – such as teachers and fellow schoolchildren – in shaping the child's psychosocial development increases.

HINTS AND TIPS

Early, strong, emotional bonding underpins normal emotional development.

Nature

There are intrinsic factors in the child that may make parenting harder, for example chronic health needs. In addition, parenting a child with autism who struggles to reciprocate affection can be especially hard.

Nurture

Families are the most powerful environmental influence on a child's emotional and behavioural development. Adequate parents will endeavour to:
- Provide love and affection.
- Provide food and shelter and protect children from physical harm.
- Exert authority to establish reasonable limits on behaviour.

Risk factors with an adverse influence are shown in Fig. 25.1.

PROBLEMS OF EARLY CHILDHOOD

Behavioural problems can relate to sleeping or eating, and tantrums are common. The rare disorder of autism might present at this time.

Sleep-related problems

Babies

An average baby sleeps for 15 hours a day in the first 2–3 months of life, sleeping for about 4 hours and waking for 3 hours at a time. After about 4 months, night-time feeds may be dropped and the baby may start to sleep through the night. The main problems encountered are infants who seem to sleep all day and awake all night. The other major problem encountered is inconsolable crying which can be due to a myriad of reasons.

Fig. 25.1 Factors associated with disturbed emotional and behavioural development

Parental factors
Parental mental health disease
Domestic violence
Drug and alcohol use
Divorce or bereavement
Intrusive overprotection or emotional rejection
Lack of or inconsistent boundary setting

Socioeconomic factors
Deprivation

Toddlers

Problems include:

- Difficulty in settling to sleep at night.
- Waking at night.
- Nightmares and night terrors.

Difficulty in getting to sleep at night

A child might not settle at night for many reasons including:

- Separation anxiety.
- Fear of darkness and silence.
- Erratic bedtime routine.

Helpful strategies include creating a predictable structure around bedtime and leaving the child alone to settle for lengthening periods.

Nightmares and night terrors

Nightmares are bad dreams that can be recalled by the child. They are common and normal unless very frequent or stereotyped in content. Reassurance is usually sufficient.

Night terrors are a form of parasomnia in which there is rapid emergence from the initial period of deep, slow-wave sleep, into a state of high arousal and confusion. The child usually cries out and is found sitting up with open eyes but disorientated and unresponsive. The child settles, with no subsequent recall of the episode. They often occur at the same time each night and waking the child briefly before the night terror is expected to occur might break the pattern.

Food refusal

Meal times can easily become a battleground. Parents often find that their toddler refuses to eat the meals provided or is a fussy eater. The child is usually well nourished with a normal rate of weight gain. Advice can be given to:

- Avoid snacking between main meals.
- Keep regular family meal times.

- Do not prolong mealtimes – if the child does not finish the meal within 20 minutes take it away but do not give any other food as a replacement.
- Try to avoid turning meals into a battleground.

Small amounts of food with gradual introduction of new foods in a relaxed, non-bargaining atmosphere is the best approach. No preschool child will voluntarily starve him- or herself, although some mothers find this difficult to believe.

Tantrums

Toddlers normally go through a period in which they are disinclined to comply with their parents' demands; this phase is sometimes referred to as 'the terrible twos'. Temper tantrums can occur in response to frustration. Parents might become demoralized in their attempts to assert control.

Management

Management strategies for 'toddler taming' include:

- Praising compliance and rewarding good behaviour.
- Avoiding threats that cannot be carried out.
- Setting reasonable limits.
- Giving clear commands.

A tantrum itself can be dealt with by ignoring it (this can be difficult, especially in a public place) or by giving the child 'time out' (removing him or her from social interaction for a short period, e.g. in a separate room).

Autism and autistic spectrum disorders

This is a pervasive developmental condition presenting in early childhood. Autism is part of a spectrum of disorders characterized by qualitative differences and impairments in reciprocal social interaction and communication combined with rigid and repetitive behaviours. It is usually evident before the age of 3 years.

Autistic spectrum disorders are present in at least 1% of children, with an excess of males to females (4:1). Autism is an organic neurodevelopmental disorder with a strong genetic component in its causation in most cases. On occasion, an identifiable cause or coexisting condition is present. No association with immunization has been found. Autistic features are found in patients with:

- Fragile X syndrome.
- Tuberous sclerosis.
- Untreated phenylketonuria.

The four main features include:

- Impaired social interaction: poor interactions with others and avoiding eye contact.

- Impaired communication: delayed speech and language development with poor comprehension.
- Restricted pattern of behaviour and interests: stereotypical patterns and lack of imaginative play and behaviour.
- Onset before 3 years of age.

In addition to these features, about two-thirds of affected children have a severe learning disability and a quarter of autistic individuals develop epileptic seizures during adolescence.

Autism is one end of a spectrum of disorders. Children can have autistic features and be socially and functionally impaired without fulfilling criteria for a diagnosis of autism. Children with Asperger's syndrome may have a normal IQ and speech but impaired social and communication skills and obsessional interests. This syndrome tends to be recognized in later childhood.

> **HINTS AND TIPS**
>
> Autism is characterized by:
> - Delayed and abnormal language.
> - Difficulty relating to others – poor social reciprocity.
> - Restricted, stereotyped interests and activities.

Management

There are no drug treatments for autism. However, specific indications do exist for symptomatic treatment of problems such as extreme anxiety or disruptive behaviour. A multidisciplinary approach is necessary with input especially from speech and language therapists and child psychologists. Special education programmes are required to meet the complex needs of the individual child. A variety of behavioural treatment programmes have been tried and it is vital that parents receive strong professional support. Only 15% of affected individuals are independent in adult life with another 15–20% functioning well with support.

Improved outcomes are seen if communicative speech is present by 5 years of age.

> **HINTS AND TIPS**
>
> Autistic spectrum disorders and the MMR vaccine:
> - Despite intense investigation, there is no evidence that links MMR and autism.
> - Autistic features often become noticeable at around the time the MMR vaccination is routinely given.
> - If parents remain concerned, the MMR vaccine can be delayed until a diagnosis is clear.

PROBLEMS OF MIDDLE CHILDHOOD

Continence disorders

Enuresis

Enuresis is the involuntary discharge of urine at an age after continence has been reached by most children (see Hints and tips box). Enuresis is usefully subcategorized as shown in Fig. 25.2.

> **HINTS AND TIPS**
>
> Urinary continence (dryness) is achieved by most girls by age 5 years and boys by age 6 years.

Nocturnal enuresis

Nocturnal enuresis, or 'bedwetting', is the involuntary voiding of urine during sleep beyond the age at which dryness at night has been achieved in a majority of children. Children under 5 years of age who regularly wet the bed can be regarded as normal. About 1 in 6 5-year-olds regularly wets the bed; this drops to 1 in 20 at age 10 years.

Nocturnal enuresis is usefully classified into:

- Primary, in which dryness has never been achieved.
- Secondary, in which it has.

The aetiology of primary nocturnal enuresis is multifactorial with genetic, emotional and cultural factors contributing. Organic causes of either are uncommon but include:

- Urinary tract infection.
- Polyuria due to diabetes mellitus or chronic renal failure.
- Neuropathic bladder.
- Faecal retention causing bladder neck dysfunction.

Fig. 25.2 Classification of enuresis

Primary or secondary?
Children with primary enuresis have never been continent for a period of at least 3 months
Secondary enuresis is incontinence after a prolonged period of bladder control

Nocturnal or diurnal?
Nocturnal enuresis occurs only at night (85% enuretic children)
Diurnal enuresis occurs during the day (5% enuretic children)
10% have a mixed type

History and examination

The history should establish the frequency (50% or more wet nights over 2 weeks is severe) and time of night that wetting occurs. The presence of any daytime urgency or wetting should be established as this suggests an underlying cause. A family history might be present and an assessment should be made of any emotional stresses either at school or at home.

Physical examination must include:

- A review of growth and measurement of blood pressure to identify unrecognized renal failure.
- Careful abdominal palpation to exclude an enlarged bladder.
- Inspection of the genitalia.

The spine and overlying skin should be inspected for any deformity, hairy patch or sinus and the neurology of the lower limbs examined thoroughly. Investigation is usually not indicated but may include urinalysis if features of diabetes or UTI are present.

Management

Nocturnal enuresis can be broadly divided into those children who sleep very deeply and so fail to recognize the signals from the bladder and those children who secrete insufficient levels of antidiuretic hormone (ADH) at night and so continue to produce large amounts of urine. The management depends of which broad category the child falls into. If it is the former a bell and pad alarm may be more successful. Desmopressin treatment is more effective for the latter. For both groups a supportive non-punitive attitude from the parents is required. Reassuring the child that it is a common problem and not shameful can help. A description of how the bladder works can also be useful. Simple measures such as cutting down fluid intake and caffeine in the evening and ensuring the bladder is completely emptied prior to bed help.

Bell and pad alarms work by waking the child at the onset of wetting. The child should be encouraged to go to the toilet to complete voiding. Gradually the child learns to wake before voiding starts. Desmopressin tablets work by increasing ADH levels in the body and so reduce the volume of urine produced.

Parents often employ techniques such as 'lifting' to reduce wet beds. This involves taking the child to the toilet while still asleep half way through the night. This should be discouraged as the child will learn that voiding while in a drowsy state is normal and may perpetuate the problem.

Encopresis (faecal soiling)

Encopresis is involuntary faecal soiling at an age beyond which continence should have been achieved (normally about 4 years). Children with encopresis fall into two main groups:

- Retentive: rectum loaded with faeces, leading to overflow incontinence (the majority).

- Non-retentive: without constipation, i.e. neurogenic sphincter disturbance or psychiatric illness.

A number of factors predispose to chronic stool retention. These include:

- Environmental problems: lack of toilet facilities, harsh toilet training.
- Idiopathic: some children's rectums only empty occasionally, perhaps due to poor coordination with anal sphincter relaxation.
- Idiopathic constipation: e.g. due to dehydration or an anal fissure leading to chronic retention.
- Organic constipation: associated with Hirschsprung's disease, drugs or hypothyroidism.

Once established, a large bolus of faeces in the rectum might be impossible for the child to expel. The loaded rectum becomes dilated and might habituate to distension, so the child is unaware of the need to empty it. Psychological factors can be both a cause and a result of encopresis. Soiling disturbs the child and can have a profound impact in school, social life and in the family.

Onset of soiling in middle childhood, without coexistent constipation, suggests a primary psychiatric cause. It might occur in the setting of a chaotic family with high levels of emotional deprivation, neglect and disturbed behaviour.

Diagnosis

Assessment must include a full bowel history, assessment of the family's psychological functioning and careful examination of the neurological system and abdomen. Abdominal palpation may reveal a faecal mass. Rectal examination in children is only performed rarely by those competent to interpret the findings.

Management

The key objective in management of encopresis due to faecal retention is to empty the rectum as soon as possible. This is done via an escalating faecal impaction regimen of oral laxatives, e.g. a macrogol (see constipation, Chapter 18). Regular defecation should then be encouraged by:

- Regular laxatives.
- Star charts.
- Sitting on the toilet after meals.
- Dietary changes: increased fibre and adequate hydration.

The distended rectum will take several weeks to shrink to normal size. It is unusual for the problem to persist into adolescence.

Attention-deficit hyperactivity disorder (ADHD)

The three hallmarks of ADHD are:

- Inattention beyond what is normal for the child's age.
- Hyperactivity.
- Impulsiveness.

Incidence and aetiology

There is some variation in diagnostic criteria between the USA (DSM-IV) and the UK (ICD-10). Current National Institute for Health and Clinical Excellence (NICE) guidelines suggest that ADHD can be diagnosed where there is hyperactivity/impulsivity and/or inattention meeting either ICD-10 or DSM-IV criteria which:

- Are present for at least 6 months.
- Persist in two or more settings (home and school).
- Impair function.

Hyperkinetic syndrome is a more severe subtype of ADHD with a prevalence of 1 in 200 (ADHD affects 2–9% of schoolchildren). Hyperkinetic syndrome is four times more common in boys than girls and is characterized by severe inattention, hyperactivity and impulsivity.

Twin studies suggest a genetic contribution to aetiology. Perinatal problems and delays in early development appear to be more common in hyperkinetic syndrome. Disturbed relationships, such as might occur with an emotionally rejecting parent or institutional upbringing, seem to exacerbate it.

HINTS AND TIPS

Hyperkinetic syndrome is a severe subtype of ADHD. It is more common in boys than girls.

Clinical features

Features of ADHD:

- Inattention: manifests as an easily distracted child who changes activity frequently and does not persist with tasks.
- Hyperactivity: an excess of movement with persistent fidgeting and restlessness that can be distinguished from normal high-spirited, energetic behaviour by the interference with normal social functioning.
- Impulsiveness: acting without reflection: affected children act impetuously and erratically.

Although these features might be present in the pre-school years, they often come to clinical attention with the increased demands of the classroom. Physical examination should include a search for:

- Developmental delay, clumsiness.
- Deficits in hearing or vision and specific learning difficulties.
- Dysmorphic features.

Most children do not have a sudden onset or an identifiable brain disorder and do not need special investigations such as electroencephalography or brain imaging. Up to 50% of children will have a co-morbid psychiatric disorder.

HINTS AND TIPS

Parents may self-diagnose children with ADHD: it is important to have a definitive diagnosis made by a specialist to enable the child to access appropriate services, particularly in the school setting.

Management

A behaviour-modifying and educational approach is the mainstay of treatment but drug treatment should be considered if these strategies fail. It is important to explain the nature of the disorder to the parents and school staff. Parent support groups might provide reassurance and help.

Behavioural therapy

About 50% of children respond to behavioural therapy comprising:

- A structured environment.
- Positive reinforcement.
- Cognitive approaches (e.g. cognitive behavioural therapy) emphasizing relaxation and self-control.

Extra help in the classroom and modification of the curriculum might be required. Group or family therapy may also be of benefit.

Drug therapy

Where behavioural therapy is ineffective, central stimulant medication can be used in conjunction. Medication is not recommended in preschool children. In school age children the mainstay is methylphenidate (Ritalin). Side-effects include slowing of growth and hypertension. A drug holiday should be given once per year. Atomoxetine may be useful where tics are present, and dexamfetamine is considered where both have failed. Immediate drug therapy may be indicated where there is severe functional impairment.

Alternative therapies

Numerous alternative therapies have been advocated. It is not generally recommended that additives/colourings should be eliminated. Diets can have a role in a minority of children and the parents' observations that a particular food aggravates hyperactivity should be heeded.

Hyperactivity itself does not usually persist as a predominant feature into adulthood. However, affected children tend to do poorly at school and low self-esteem together with antisocial traits might turn them into disadvantaged adults.

Symptoms diminish over time but approximately half will continue to have symptoms in adolescence and adulthood.

Recurrent pain syndromes

Recurrent pain without an organic cause is not uncommon in children. The usual sites are the abdomen, head or limbs.

A strict dichotomy between organic and psychological causation for recurrent pain is unhelpful and explains only a minority of cases. In most cases the pain is best explained as dysfunctional, a result of mild individual differences in physiology that render the child vulnerable to pain in response to stress.

HINTS AND TIPS

- Apley's law: the further the pain is from the umbilicus, the more likely it is to be organic.
- The more localized limb pain is, the less likely it is to be 'growing pains'.
- Measure the blood pressure and examine the fundi in a child with recurrent headaches.

Clinical features and diagnosis

The history should establish:

- Onset, frequency and duration of the pain and associated symptoms.
- Family functioning.
- Stressors, e.g. bullying at school.

Physical examination is directed towards excluding an organic cause (Fig. 25.3). Investigations have a low yield if physical examination is normal and should be kept to a minimum. Full blood count, erythrocyte sedimentation rate and urinalysis might be indicated.

Management

For dysfunctional pain, normal activity should be encouraged. Symptomatic relief should be offered

Fig. 25.3 Organic causes of recurrent pain	
Site	**Cause**
Abdominal pain	Genitourinary problems: UTI, obstructive uropathy Gastrointestinal disorders: constipation, inflammatory bowel disease, peptic ulcer
Headache	Refractive disorders Migraine Hypertension Raised intracranial pressure
Limb pain	Neoplastic disease, e.g. leukaemia, bone tumour Orthopaedic: Osgood–Schlatter disease

(e.g. mild analgesics) and the patient should be encouraged to keep a symptom diary. It is important to provide psychological support, and to emphasize to parents that this is usually not malingering.

School refusal

Repeated absence from school might be due to illness or truancy but in a few cases it is due to school refusal, i.e. an unwillingness to attend because of severe anxiety. School refusal might be associated with:

- Separation anxiety (under 11 years).
- Adverse life events (bereavement, moving).
- Stressors (bullying).

School refusers tend to be good academically but may be oppositional at home.

True school phobia is seen in older, anxious children, who typically have problems beginning school in the autumn and returning to school after weekends and holidays. Unlike school refusal, they are poor academically and have a lack of desire rather than anxiety about school.

Management

Management requires an early, graded return to school with support for the parents and treatment of any underlying emotional disorder. Two-thirds of school refusers will return to school regularly.

Selective mutism

Selective mutism is an anxiety disorder where there is an inability to speak in specific social situations despite the ability to speak normally. It is rare, affecting around 0.5% children typically aged 3–6 years. The majority of cases resolve spontaneously; however, individual or family therapy may be required. It can be exhibited in response to abuse, especially sexual abuse.

PROBLEMS OF ADOLESCENCE

This is a period during which a number of important disorders might present, including emotional disorders such as anxiety and depression, conduct disorders and disorders of eating.

Eating disorders

Eating disorders are common with a lifetime prevalence of 5–7% of women. Incidence is highest in teenage girls (around 50 per 100 000) although the presence of eating disorders in boys is being increasingly recognized. Aetiology is felt to be multifactorial with risk factors including feeding difficulties in infancy, premorbid obesity and adverse life events or family history of eating disorders. There are several forms including anorexia nervosa, bulimia nervosa and binge eating. They are all associated with abnormal body image.

Anorexia nervosa

Anorexia nervosa is the maintenance of low bodyweight due to preoccupation with weight and body image. It is characterized by:

- Weight less than 85% of expected bodyweight.
- Intense fear of gaining weight or being fat.
- Disturbed body image: feeling fat when actually emaciated.
- Denial of the danger of serious weight loss or low bodyweight.
- Amenorrhoea for at least three cycles (in postmenarchal girls).

It may present as failure to gain weight appropriately rather than loss of weight. The prevalence rate is 1% with a peak age of onset of 14 years (and girls outnumbering boys by 20 to 1). The aetiology is unknown. The patient often displays obsessive, overachieving, perfectionist and controlling personality traits.

Clinical features and diagnosis

Physical examination may reveal:

- Emaciation and muscle wasting.
- Fine lanugo hair over trunk and limbs.
- Bradycardia and poor peripheral perfusion.
- Slowly relaxing tendon reflexes.

Laboratory investigations may reveal:

- Reduced plasma proteins, vitamin B_{12} and ferritin.
- Endocrine abnormalities: elevated cortisol, reduced T_4, luteinizing hormone and follicle stimulating hormone.

Management and prognosis

The immediate aim is to make a therapeutic alliance with the patient to restore normal bodyweight. Most patients are managed on an outpatient basis, with goal setting and psychological interventions (including cognitive behavioural therapy and family therapy). Initial goal should be a gain of 500 g per week. In severe cases, failing to respond to outpatient intervention, inpatient treatment is necessary. This can be difficult because affected young people might hide food and lie about their weight. Tube feeding might be required if there is continued weight loss in hospital. Where there is severe undernutrition the patient should be monitored carefully for refeeding syndrome. Treatment will also encompass management of physical aspects of anorexia, e.g. gradual weaning off laxative and dental hygiene.

Prognosis is variable with an eventual 5% mortality rate from malnutrition, infection or suicide. Fifty per cent make a good recovery, 30% show partial improvement and 20% have a chronic relapsing course. Good prognostic factors are:

- Young age at onset.
- Supportive family.
- Insight and improved self-esteem.

Bulimia nervosa

Bulimia is a disorder characterized by abnormal body image, low self-esteem and regular binge eating with associated inappropriate behaviours to avoid weight gain, e.g. vomiting or laxative abuse. Weight may be low but individuals are often in the normal range or overweight. Clinical features include hypotension, tachycardia, dry skin, menstrual abnormalities. In addition where there is vomiting after binges there may be parotid enlargement or calluses on the fingers. Management is similar to anorexia nervosa with cognitive behavioural therapy playing a key role.

Emotional disorders

Depression

Depression as a clinical syndrome is more than just a transitory low mood or misery in response to adverse life circumstances. It is characterized by:

- Persistent feelings of sadness or unhappiness.
- Ideas of guilt, despair and lack of self-worth.
- Social withdrawal.
- Lack of motivation and energy.
- Disturbances of sleep, appetite and weight.

It is increasingly recognized in prepubertal children but is predominantly a problem of adolescence. Aetiology is multifactorial but there is a clear genetic contribution. Dysfunctional families or adverse life events might contribute.

Management

General interventions should be offered for mild depression including advice on self-help information, exercise, sleep hygiene and anxiety management. If this persists or for moderate to severe depression, treatment is therapy based (cognitive behavioural therapy, individual and family therapies). Medication should be offered in conjunction with therapy where symptoms are severe or not improving, with fluoxetine recommended as first-line.

HINTS AND TIPS

- Suicide is the third most common cause of death in adolescents and young adults.
- Most intentional overdoses are not taken with suicidal intent but an important minority are, so psychiatric evaluation is important in all cases.

Anxiety

Anxiety disorders are increasingly recognized as a problem in childhood; the National Institute for Mental Health (NIMH) estimates a prevalence of around 8%. Anxiety is often a part of normal development and recognizing where it becomes pathological can be challenging. Management is with cognitive behavioural therapy and occasionally anxiolytics.

Deliberate self-harm

The prevalence of deliberate self-harm, particularly cutting of the skin, has increased in recent years. It is more common in girls and encompasses mutilation of the skin as well as the ingestion of medications. There can be a variety of triggers and it may occur as a one-off in response to a life event or be part of a chronic pattern. Young people who seek help should be treated sympathetically and undergo a psychological evaluation for risk of suicidality. Then they should be offered psychological support.

Chronic fatigue syndrome

This refers to generalized fatigue persisting after routine tests and investigations have failed to identify an obvious underlying cause. It is classically exacerbated by mental and physical exertion and usually associated with non specific pain in muscles and joints. Headaches, sleep difficulties, depressed mood, sore throat, tender lymph nodes and abdominal pain can also occur. A full history and examination is important to characterize symptoms and basic screening tests are important to exclude other diagnoses, e.g. anaemia and hypothyroidism. Diagnosis requires persistent fatigue in combination with at least four associated symptoms.

Management and prognosis

A multidisciplinary approach is valuable. Management is usually with cognitive behavioural therapy or graded exercise programmes in addition to symptomatic control, e.g. of myalgia.

Psychosis

Psychosis is uncommon in childhood and is more likely to be organic in origin. Chronic disorders such as schizophrenia and bipolar affective disorder might present in adolescence. The prevalence of drug abuse in this age group renders drug-induced psychosis an important problem.

Further reading

National Institute for Health and Clinical Excellence (NICE), October 2010. Nocturnal enuresis: the management of bedwetting in children and young people (CG111). http://www.nice.org.uk/guidance/CG111.

National Institute for Health and Clinical Excellence (NICE), September 2008. Attention deficit hyperactivity disorder: diagnosis and management of ADHD in children, young people and adults (CG72). http://www.nice.org.uk/CG72.

National Institute for Health and Clinical Excellence (NICE), September 2005. Depression in children and young people: identification and management in primary care, community and secondary care (CG28). http://www.nice.org.uk/CG28.

National Institute for Health and Clinical Excellence (NICE), January 2004. Eating disorders: core interventions in the treatment and management of anorexia nervosa, bulimia nervosa and related eating disorders (CG9). http://www.nice.org.uk/CG009.

National Institute for Health and Clinical Excellence (NICE), August 2007. Chronic fatigue syndrome/ myalgic encephalomyelitis (CG53). http://guidance.nice.org.uk/CG53.

Volkmar, F.R., Pauls, D., 2003. Autism. Lancet 362, 133–141.

Wong, P., 2010. Selective mutism: a review of etiology, comorbidities, and treatment. Psychiatry 7 (3), 23–31.

Social and preventive paediatrics

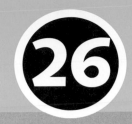

At the end of this chapter, you should be able to:
- Understand the importance of prevention in child health
- Outline the current UK immunization schedule
- Know the contraindications to routine immunization in children
- Understand the importance of neonatal screening
- Recognize the different types of child abuse
- Outline the causes and prevention of sudden unexpected death in infancy
- Understand some of the legal issues pertaining to paediatrics

This includes all aspects of promoting health and preventing illness such as child health surveillance, immunization, health education and accident prevention. In addition, community paediatric services are closely involved with the problems of child abuse, adoption and foster care, and children with special needs. Important legislation concerning children and health in the UK exists, in particular the Children Act and the Education Act.

PREVENTION IN CHILD HEALTH

There remains a high level of morbidity from preventable conditions including:

- Infectious diseases.
- Congenital disorders.
- Accidents.
- Malnutrition.
- Obesity.

Strategies for prevention include:

- Immunization.
- Screening.
- Child health surveillance.
- Health promotion and education.

Immunization

Immunization has conferred more benefit on the world's children than any other medical advance or intervention. It has allowed the prevention of many major diseases such as diphtheria and polio, which killed or disabled millions of children, and the complete eradication of smallpox. In recent times, the highly successful introduction of immunization against *Haemophilus*

influenzae type b (Hib) has dramatically reduced the incidence of invasive infections such as Hib meningitis and epiglottitis.

Immunization is effective against major bacterial diseases, such as diphtheria and tuberculosis (TB), and viral diseases, such as measles, mumps, rubella and hepatitis. Bacille Calmette–Guérin (BCG) vaccination against TB is effective in some parts of the world. However, a vaccine has yet to be developed against the important parasitic disease, malaria.

Immunity: active and passive

Immunity can be induced either actively (long term) or provided by passive transfer (short term) against a variety of bacterial and viral agents. Active immunity is induced by using:

- A live, attenuated form of the pathogen, e.g. measles, mumps, rubella vaccine (MMR) or BCG vaccine for TB.
- An inactivated organism, e.g. inactivated poliomyelitis vaccine (IPV), pertussis.
- A component of the organism, e.g. Hib, pneumococcal vaccine, hepatitis B and meningitis C.
- An inactivated toxin (toxoid), e.g. tetanus vaccine, diphtheria vaccine.

In many individuals, live, attenuated viral vaccines promote a full, long-lasting antibody response after one dose. Several doses of an inactivated version or toxoid are usually required.

Passive immunity is conferred by the injection of human immunoglobulin. There are two main types:

- Human normal immunoglobulin (HNIG).
- Specific immunoglobulins for tetanus, hepatitis B, rabies and varicella zoster (VZIG).

Routes of administration are:

- By mouth: oral polio vaccine (superseded by IPV in the UK).
- Intradermal: BCG.
- Subcutaneous or intramuscular injection: all other vaccines.

In infants, the upper outer quadrant of the buttock or the anterolateral aspect of the thigh are the recommended sites for the injection of vaccines.

Immunization schedule

In the UK, the schedule for primary immunization has been changed recently to include pneumococcal vaccine and human papilloma virus vaccination for girls. This schedule provides earlier and more effective protection against haemophilus, pneumococcal and pertussis infections, which are more dangerous to the very young.

The new schedule is shown in Fig. 26.1.

> **HINTS AND TIPS**
>
> The timing of childhood immunization is critical: too early and the immune response might be inadequate, too late and the child could acquire the disease before being protected.

Indications and contraindications to immunization

Every child should be protected against infectious diseases and a refusal to immunize should only be accepted if the risks are understood by the parents.

Special risk groups can be identified for whom the risk of complications from infectious disease is high and who should be immunized as a priority. These include children with:

- Chronic lung and congenital heart disease.
- Down syndrome.
- HIV infection.
- Low birth weight.
- Asplenic or hyposplenism.

General contraindications

These include:

- Acute illness with fever >38°C: postpone until recovery has occurred.
- A definite history of a severe local or general reaction to a preceding dose.

Live vaccines: special risk groups Live vaccines pose a risk for certain individuals whose immunity is impaired. These include children:

- Being treated with chemotherapy or radiotherapy for malignant disease.

Fig. 26.1 UK immunization schedule

Age	Vaccine	Comments
2 months	Diphtheria, tetanus, pertussis, polio and *Haemophilus influenzae* type b (DTaP/IPV/Hib); (pneumococcal vaccine) PCV	Two injections
3 months	DTaP/IPV/Hib; meningitis C (Men C)	Two injections
4 months	DTaP/Hib/IPV; Men C; PCV	Three injections
12–13 months	Hib/Men C/PCV and measles mumps and rubella (MMR)	Three injections
3 years 4 months to 5 years	dTaP/IPV or DTaP/IPV and MMR	Two injections
13–18 years	Td/IPV	One injection
Girls aged 12–13 years	Human papillomavirus vaccine (HPV)	Three injections at 0, 1–2 months and 6 months

- On immunosuppressive treatment after organ or bone marrow transplant.
- On high-dose systemic steroids.
- With impaired cell-mediated immunity, e.g. severe combined immunodeficiency syndrome.
- Who are HIV positive; they can receive all routine vaccines except BCG. Infants born to mothers with HIV should have two negative HIV PCR tests prior to BCG immunization.

> **HINTS AND TIPS**
>
> - MMR is not associated with autism.
> - Premature infants should start the immunization schedule according to chronological age (i.e. 2 months from birth).
> - The flu vaccine should be offered to children with chronic disease (e.g. asthma, coeliac disease, sickle cell disease).

Specific contraindications

Particular vaccines are contraindicated in certain circumstances:

- Measles vaccination is contraindicated if there is a previous anaphylactic reaction to neomycin. MMR is usually safe for those with egg allergies. However, if previous anaphylaxis has occurred to egg then consider giving the MMR under hospital supervision.

- Pertussis: it is debatable whether this vaccine has ever caused brain damage and the current acellular pertussis vaccine is safer than the previous cellular vaccine. There are no specific contraindications (in particular, a family or personal history of epilepsy is not a contraindication). In an evolving neurological disorder immunization may be delayed until it has stabilized.

'False' contraindications

The following are *not* contraindications to immunization:

- Family history of adverse reaction to immunization.
- Prematurity (infants <28 weeks should have first immunization in hospital).
- Stable neurological conditions, e.g. cerebral palsy.
- Asthma, eczema, hay fever.
- Over the age recommended in standard schedule.
- Minor afebrile illness.
- Child's mother being pregnant.

Adverse reactions associated with specific vaccines are shown in Fig. 26.2.

Screening

An effective and worthwhile screening programme should satisfy certain criteria:

- The condition screened for should be an important health problem.
- There should be a sensitive and specific test.
- Treatment should improve the condition.

Fig. 26.2 Adverse reactions associated with specific vaccines

Vaccine	Minor reaction	Major reaction
Diphtheria/ tetanus	Local	Neurological (very rare)
Pertussis	Fever, crying	Convulsions (1:300000) Encephalopathy (very rare)
Polio	–	Vaccine-associated polio (1 in 2 million)
MMR	Fever, rash, arthropathy	Encephalopathy (very rare) Thrombocytopenia
BCG	Local abscess	Adenitis

- It should be cost-effective.
- The screening method should be acceptable to child and parents.

Screening can be targeted at a 'high-risk' population or carried out opportunistically when a patient presents for some other reason at the relevant age.

Child health promotion

A programme of health surveillance is undertaken to identify important conditions that have a better outcome if diagnosed and treated early (e.g. congenital dislocation of the hip and deafness). This programme includes:

- Neonatal examination.
- 6–8 week check.
- 12 month review
- 30 month review
- School entry.

Neonatal examination

Full physical examination with particular emphasis on:

- Eyes (presence of red reflex).
- Heart (detection of murmurs or absent femoral pulses).
- Hips (congenital dislocation).
- Testicles (undescended testes).

Hearing is tested by otoacoustic emission and brainstem auditory evoked potentials in all babies in the first few days. Guthrie test: Usually between days 5 and 8, a heel prick blood sample is taken to screen for:

- Phenylketonuria.
- Cystic fibrosis.
- Congenital hypothyroidism.
- MCADD (medium chain acyl CoA dehydrogenase deficiency).
- Sickle cell disease.

6–8 week check

Physical examination as per the neonatal examination. In addition:

- Growth: weight, length and head circumference.
- Development: alert, makes eye contact, smiles, head control.
- Vision and hearing (explore parental concerns).

Assessment should also be made of the family's adjustment to the new infant, quality of parent–child interactions and signs of maternal depression.

12 month review

- General health.
- Assess growth and development.

- Health promotion to include accident prevention, dietary and dental advice.
- Parenting advice (boundary setting, encourage reading to child).

30 month review

This is done by the health visitor but in some areas it is no longer performed.

- General health and growth.
- Assess development: with emphasis on social and communication skills.
- Parenting advice on toilet training, temperament and behaviour, early years education.

School entry

- Growth: height and weight.
- Hearing and vision tests.
- Review immunization status.
- Assess if any additional help will be required at school.

CHILD ABUSE

The National Society for the Prevention of Cruelty to Children (NSPCC) estimates that approximately 1 in 4 adults reports being maltreated during childhood. Two children per week die in the UK due to child abuse. Child abuse can be considered under four main categories but they often overlap (Fig. 26.3).

Diagnosis

Certain families and children are at particular risk. The three most recognized risk factors are domestic violence, mental health issues and abuse of drugs and alcohol. However, other factors such as poor parenting role models, social deprivation and isolation are often implicated. Young children under the age of 3 years and babies born prematurely or with health needs are at particular risk.

Suspicions of abuse may arise from a healthcare professional such as the GP or health visitor, from the school or from a concerned neighbour or relative. Diagnosis is difficult and stressful for all concerned.

Fig. 26.3 Types of abuse

Physical (non-accidental injury)
Sexual
Emotional
Neglect

Types of abuse

Physical abuse or non-accidental injury (NAI)

Certain features in the history of a physical injury should raise the suspicion that it might be non-accidental (Fig. 26.4). Any injury can be accidental or inflicted but certain injuries are more likely to be due to abuse, e.g. burns or bites. Fractures in a non-ambulant child are concerning. Rib fractures require considerable force and so in the absence of major trauma (e.g. road traffic accident) raise suspicions. Multiple bruises of differing ages and in unusual locations are worrying. Accidental bruises usually occur over bony prominences and if they are found in other areas suggest non-accidental injury. Violent shaking of a baby might tear the vessels that cross the subdural space leading to subdural haemorrhage. This is associated with irritability, retinal haemorrhages and signs of raised intracranial pressure.

Neglect

Neglect is failing to provide the basic needs of a child. It can manifest as faltering growth, developmental delay, poor hygiene or not prioritizing the child's health needs (e.g. missed appointments).

Emotional abuse

This includes rejection of a child, persistent criticism, belittling or threats. It can also occur when a parent fails to appreciate the developmental age of a child, for example reversal of the parent–child role. Fabricated and factitious illness can also be considered emotional abuse. Occasionally this can progress to induced illness which is also a form of physical abuse.

Sexual abuse

Child sexual abuse (CSA) can involve either sex at any age, but is more common in girls. It has been defined as the involvement of dependent, immature children or adolescents in sexual activities that they do not fully

Fig. 26.4 Features of non-accidental injury

History
Delay in seeking medical help
Differing or changing history from witnesses
Mechanism inconsistent with injury or developmental stage of child
Previous concerns about non-accidental injury
Parents' level of concern inappropriate

Examination
Signs of neglect
Unusual affect of child, e.g. withdrawn or overly affectionate with strangers
Multiple injuries of differing ages
Injuries suggestive of an implement, e.g. belt marks

understand and are unable to give informed consent to. A normal physical examination does not exclude abuse. The majority (80%) of abuse is conducted by someone known to the child. Exposing children to sexual images is also considered abuse.

Management

Diligent note keeping is vital as the records may be required for legal proceedings. Body map diagrams should be used to record findings and photographs taken with consent. If child abuse is suspected in the UK, the local Child and Families Social Work Team must be informed.

The first priority is to treat any injury or illness. Following this a decision should be taken on ensuring a place of safety for the child. If the parents are the suspected perpetrators accommodation by a foster carer may be required. If possible this is done with parental consent but if not legal enforcement may be required. Senior staff should be involved from the beginning because experience is required in handling what is always a very difficult situation.

Investigations are often indicated to exclude any organic cause for the signs and symptoms (e.g. a bleeding diathesis in bruising). Further investigations may be directed at detecting occult injuries, for example a skeletal survey to look for old fractures and imaging of the brain and ophthalmology review if a shaking injury is suspected. Forensic samples must be taken in suspected sexual abuse and this examination should be conducted by a specialist in this field.

In most cases, further management will involve evaluation of the family by social workers and the convening of a Child Protection Conference involving all the professionals involved in the child's life. A decision will be made on whether to make the child subject to a child protection plan, whether court proceedings are required and whether the child can be returned safely to the family. The child protection plan will define the kind of intervention and level of supervision required.

SUDDEN INFANT DEATH SYNDROME

Sudden infant death syndrome (SIDS) is defined as the sudden death of an infant under 1 year of age, which remains unexplained after the performance of a complete post-mortem examination and examination of the scene of death. In the UK approximately 300 infants die suddenly each year; however, this has fallen by 70% with the implementation of risk reduction.

Risk factors are numerous but include:

- Sleeping prone ('back to sleep' campaign).
- Smoking in the household.
- Overheating at home.
- Co-sleeping especially on a sofa or chair under the influence of drugs and alcohol.
- Pre-term birth.

All paediatric units should have a protocol on dealing with SIDS. The police will often be involved and information should be collected jointly to prevent the parents having to repeat information at such a stressful time. The family will need support and counselling and there are numerous agencies that provide ongoing help and support.

CHILDREN AND THE LAW

The principal legislation concerning children and health in the UK is contained in:

- The Children Act (England and Wales 1989, Scotland 1995).
- The Education Act (1993).
- The UN Convention on the Rights of the Child (1989).

The Children Act

This integrates the law relating to private individuals with the responsibilities of public authorities towards children. It aims to strike a balance between family independence and child protection. The essential components include:

- Parental responsibilities are defined. Responsibilities replace rights. Parents have the prime responsibility for their children and this is retained in all circumstances except adoption.
- The welfare of the child is paramount. The wishes and feelings of the child must be respected and courts should ensure that any orders made positively benefit the child or children concerned.
- Professionals are encouraged to work in partnership with parents.
- Defines responsibilities for 'children in need'. Local authorities are required to provide supportive services to assist parents in bringing up their children.
- The court must consider the child's race, religion, culture and language.
- A child should remain with his or her family whenever possible.
- Describes court orders in relation to custody and access, and child protection. The latter includes: Emergency Protection Order, Child Assessment Order, Care and Supervision Order, Police Protection Order.

Foster care

The purpose of foster care is to provide a safe, temporary placement for a child who is at physical, emotional or social risk. Common reasons for foster placement include:

- Child abuse.
- Death or ill health of parents.
- Babies awaiting adoption.

Foster care does not provide legal rights and these remain with the natural parents, local authority or courts. Attempts are made to place children with other family members where possible.

Adoption

The annual number of adoptions in the UK has fallen in recent years, thought to be due to wider use of contraception and abortion and also to the greater social acceptance of single parenthood.

Most children requiring adoption are in local authority care with foster parents or in a children's home. Unfortunately many are older, disabled or have suffered abuse or neglect and are less likely to be adopted.

Adoption is a legal procedure encompassing several important features:

- It is arranged by registered agencies.
- Adopters must be aged over 21 years.
- An adoption cannot be reversed except in exceptional circumstances.
- An adopted child loses all legal ties with his or her birth parents and the adoptive parents assume parental responsibility.
- The original parents have no right of access, although contact for older children is often maintained.
- The natural parents must give informed consent, unless they cannot be found or are judged unlikely to ever be able to look after the child adequately.
- The child lives with the adoptive parents for 3 months before the order is finalized.
- At age 18, an adopted child is entitled to his or her original birth certificate.

Consent to medical care

A person older than 18 years can legally give his or her own consent and this cannot be overridden. Between 16 and 18 years consent can be given by the young person but refusal of life-saving treatment is not permitted.

Below 16 years consent can be obtained from:

- A person who holds parental responsibility.
- The child if the doctor considers that the child is of sufficient understanding to make an informed decision (Gillick or Fraser competent principle).

However, it is good practice to inform the parents if the child/young person agrees.

> **HINTS AND TIPS**
>
> - If a child is deemed competent, the parents cannot override consent.
> - Immediate life-saving treatment does not require consent.

If the parent(s) of a child younger than 16 years refuse a life-saving treatment, a court can give consent.

Parental responsibility (PR) is held by:

- The mother.
- The father if:
  - Married to the mother at the time of birth
  - Named on the birth certificate (applies since 1 December 2003)
  - Registered or court order of PR.
- Under a legal order (emergency protection order, interim care order, residence order).
- Legal guardian or step-parent with a PR order.

Confidentiality

A person aged 16 years and over has full rights to confidentiality. However, the duty of confidentiality owed to a patient under 16 years of age is as great as that owed to any other person. Information can be disclosed to parents only if it is in the interests of the child.

THE CHILD WITH A DISABILITY

Many children have complex and long-lasting neurodevelopmental disabilities that require early identification and support in the community. It is useful to define some of the terms used:

- Impairment: any loss or abnormality of physiological or anatomical structure.
- Disability: any restriction or loss of ability in performing an activity (in a way considered normal for a particular age) that is caused by an impairment.
- Handicap: a disadvantage for an individual arising from a disability that prevents the achievement of desired goals.

For example, an intraventricular haemorrhage with periventricular leucomalacia (impairment of motor tracts) might cause a hemiparesis (the disability), resulting in difficulty playing the piano (handicap). The use of the term 'handicap' with its connotation of dependency has fallen out of favour.

Presentation of children with disabilities

The commonest disabilities encountered:

- Cerebral palsy.
- Social and communication disorders (e.g. autism).
- Behavioural problems (e.g. ADHD).
- Genetic conditions (e.g. Down syndrome, Prader–Willi syndrome, etc.).
- Global developmental delay (often idiopathic).
- Hearing or visual impairment.
- Learning difficulties.

Examples of how different problems tend to present at different ages are shown in Fig. 26.5.

Telling parents about a disability

Diagnosis of a disability might be sudden and unexpected, or the culmination of protracted concern and investigation. In any event, the news is likely to provoke reactions of grief accompanied by anger, guilt, despair or denial. The initial interview requires sensitive handling.

HINTS AND TIPS

Breaking news to parents about a disability:
- They should be told as soon as possible.
- They should be told together, not separately.
- Tell them in a quiet place with a colleague, e.g. a nurse.
- Adopt an honest and direct approach.
- Arrange a period of privacy for the parents after the initial interview.
- Arrange a second meeting to allow questions after the news has been assimilated.

Fig. 26.5 Presentation of disabilities by age

Age	Disability
Neonatal period	Chromosomal abnormality or syndrome, e.g. Down syndrome Hypoxic–ischaemic encephalopathy
Infancy	Cerebral palsy
Severe visual or hearing impairment
Preschool	Speech and language delay
Abnormal gait
Global developmental delay
Loss of skills from neurodegenerative disorder
School age	Learning difficulties – specific or general

Assessment

It is necessary to assess what a child is able to do and what the main difficulties are in several areas:

- Hearing, language and communication.
- Vision and coordination.
- Physical health and mobility.
- Behaviour and emotions.
- Social interactions and self-care, including continence.
- Learning disabilities.

Medical problems commonly encountered in children with disabilities are shown in Fig. 26.6.

Management: the multidisciplinary team

Management of a severe or complex disability requires a multidisciplinary clinical team, working with social services, local education authorities and voluntary agencies. The balance changes with age:

- Pre-school children: community-led child development team, voluntary agencies.
- School-age children: education authorities, community health services.
- School leavers/young adults: social services, community disability teams.

Members of the child development team will usually include:

- Paediatricians.
- Physiotherapists.
- Occupational therapists.
- Speech and language therapists.
- Dieticians.
- Psychologists.
- Social workers.
- Nurses and health visitors.

Fig. 26.6 Medical problems in children with neurodisability

System	Problem
Nervous system	Vision and hearing impairment
Epilepsy
Behavioural disorders, e.g. sleep disturbance, head banging
Skeleton	Postural deformities, e.g. scoliosis, contractures
Dislocation of hips
Gastrointestinal tract	Feeding difficulties
Faltering growth
Gastro-oesophageal reflux
Constipation or faecal incontinence
Respiratory system	Recurrent pneumonia

Statementing

Education authorities have a duty to identify children with special needs and provide appropriate resources. A detailed assessment is undertaken with reports from the educational psychologist, members of the multidisciplinary team and the parents. The resulting 'statement' sets out the child's educational and non-educational needs and the provision of services required to meet those needs. Regular reviews of the statement are also undertaken.

Further reading

Department of Health, 2006. Immunization against infectious disease. HMSO, London.http://www.dh.gov.uk/en/Publicationsandstatistics/Publications/PublicationsPolicyAndGuidance/DH_079917.

Foundation for the Study into Infant Deaths, http://fsid.org.uk.

National Institute for Health and Clinical Excellence (NICE), July 2009. When to suspect child maltreatment. http://guidance.nice.org.uk/CG/Wave12/11.

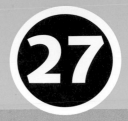
Objectives

At the end of this chapter, you should be able to:
- Know the common patterns of inheritance of genetic disorders
- Know more about common genetic disorders
- Know the principles of genetic counselling

The human genome comprises 46 chromosomes, which include 22 pairs of autosomes and 1 pair of sex chromosomes. With the mapping of the human genome, our understanding of genetics has increased exponentially and continues to develop at a rapid rate. Many genetic disorders are common during childhood and infancy; those that are associated with a poor prognosis and a short lifespan are not seen during adulthood. As our understanding of genetics has advanced, many new diagnostic technologies have become clinically relevant and therapies for genetic diseases are emerging.

Clinical manifestations are highly variable but it is worth remembering that many dysmorphic syndromes have a genetic basis.

HINTS AND TIPS

Dysmorphism and syndromes:
- Dysmorphism is an abnormality in form or structural development, often manifested in the facial appearance and often due to an underlying genetic disorder.
- A syndrome is a recognizable pattern of structural and functional abnormalities or malformations known or presumed to be the result of a single cause. Dysmorphism is often a feature.
- Syndromes might be of unknown cause, due to teratogens (e.g. fetal alcohol syndrome), chromosomal anomalies (e.g. Turner syndrome) or single gene disorders (e.g. Marfan syndrome).

BASIC GENETICS

Some useful definitions are shown in Fig. 27.1. The key symbols used in drawing a family tree are shown in Fig. 27.2.

SINGLE GENE DISORDERS

Disorders of single nuclear genes are recognizable because of their Mendelian pattern of inheritance, which can be:

- Autosomal dominant.
- Autosomal recessive.
- X-linked.

More than 13 000 single gene disorders have been identified so far. Examples of important single gene disorders are shown in Fig. 27.3.

AUTOSOMAL DOMINANT DISORDERS

An affected person has just one copy of the abnormal gene. The disease manifests in the heterozygote. Each offspring has a 50% chance of inheriting the abnormal gene and thus, being affected. A typical pedigree of an autosomal dominant (AD) disorder is shown in Fig. 27.4. The features of an AD pedigree are:

- Several generations with affected individuals.
- Equal numbers of males and females are affected.
- Male-to-male transmission occurs.

Several complicating factors can occur. These include:

- Variable expression: the pattern and severity of disease varies in affected individuals within the same family.
- Non-penetrance: some individuals with the disease allele have no clinical signs or symptoms.
- Sporadic cases: a new mutation in the ovum or spermatocyte of a parent will give rise to a 'sporadic' case with no family history of the disease. The recurrence risk for new offspring from those parents is then very low.

Fig. 27.1 Basic genetics: some definitions

Term	Definition
Karyotype	A display of the set of chromosomes extracted from a eukaryotic somatic cell arrested at metaphase
Genome	The totality of the DNA contained within the diploid chromosome set of a eukaryotic species and within extranuclear structures such as the mitochondrial genome
Gene	A sequence of DNA occupying its own place (locus) on a chromosome and containing the information necessary for biosynthesis of a gene product such as a protein or ribosomal RNA molecule
Allele	Any one of the variations of a gene or polymorphic DNA marker found in the members of a species. Numerous alleles may exist, but any individual usually possesses at most two alleles of the gene or polymorphic marker
Genotype	The pair of alleles of a variable gene possessed by an individual, or the pairs of alleles of any number of variable genes possessed by an individual
Phenotype	The entire physical, biochemical, and physiological make-up of an individual as determined by genotype and environment

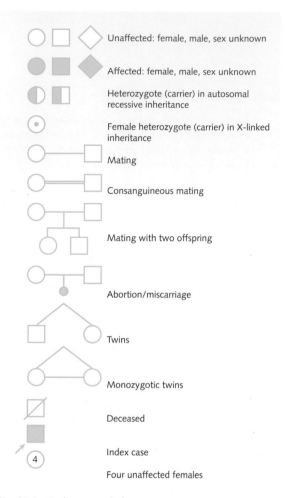

Fig. 27.2 Pedigree symbols

New mutations are common in some AD disorders. For example, over 80% of individuals with achondroplasia have unaffected parents.

Achondroplasia

This autosomal dominant disorder is characterized by short limbs, large head and abnormalities in neurology. The gene is found on the short arm of chromosome 4 and is a fibroblast growth receptor gene (FGFR3 gene). It affects 1 in 2500 births; typical clinical features are shown in Fig. 27.5.

AUTOSOMAL RECESSIVE DISORDERS

An affected individual has two copies of the abnormal gene inherited from each parent and is said to be homozygous for the disease alleles. Heterozygous carriers (with only one abnormal copy) are often unaffected, but may display a mild phenotype in some conditions. Many recessive disorders are caused by mutations in the genes coding for enzymes. As half of the normal enzyme activity is usually sufficient, a person with only one mutant allele will not normally be affected.

Fig. 27.3 Single gene disorders: examples

Autosomal dominant

Myotonic dystrophy
Marfan syndrome
Neurofibromatosis type 1
Tuberous sclerosis
Achondroplasia
Autosomal recessive
Cystic fibrosis
Thalassaemia
Sickle cell disease
Congenital adrenal hyperplasia
Inborn errors of metabolism (majority), e.g. phenylketonuria
X-linked recessive
Haemophilia A and B
Duchenne muscular dystrophy
Fragile X syndrome
Glucose-6-phosphate dehydrogenase (G6PD) deficiency
Colour blindness (red–green)

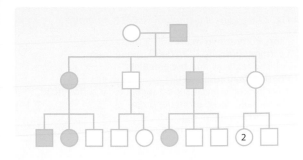

Fig. 27.4 Typical pedigree with autosomal dominant inheritance

Fig. 27.5	Major clinical features of achondroplasia
Limbs	Shortened limbs: proximal > distal Bow legs
Neurological	Hydrocephalus Motor developmental delay Normal intelligence
Spine	Short stature Thoracolumbar kyphosis Lumbar lordosis
Ear	Recurrent otitis media

A typical pedigree of an autosomal recessive disorder is shown in Fig. 27.6.

- Autosomal dominant disorders are often caused by mutations in a gene encoding a structural protein.
- Autosomal recessive disorders are often caused by mutations in a gene encoding a functional protein, such as an enzyme.

The risk of each child being affected when both parents are carriers is 25%. Males and females are equally likely to be affected. There is usually no positive family history other than affected individuals within the sibship.

Parental consanguinity increases the risk of a recessive disease occurring in the offspring. Everyone probably carries at least one recessive disease gene allele. A couple who are first cousins are more likely to have inherited the same abnormal recessive disease gene allele from their common ancestor.

Certain recessive disorders show a founder effect. Affected individuals have inherited a founder mutation that occurred on an ancestral chromosome many generations ago. Carrier rates may be high within inbred populations (e.g. Tay–Sachs disease in Ashkenazi Jews).

Important autosomal recessive diseases are described elsewhere, including cystic fibrosis (Chapter 17), thalassaemia, sickle-cell disease (Chapter 22), congenital adrenal hyperplasia (Chapter 24) and inborn errors of metabolism (Chapter 24).

X-LINKED DISORDERS

Several hundred disease genes are found on the X chromosome and give rise to the characteristic pattern of X-linked inheritance. Most X-linked disorders are recessive. Female carriers have an abnormal allele on one X chromosome but are protected by their second, normal allele. The male is hemizygous for the gene because he has only a single X chromosome. The abnormal allele is not balanced by a normal allele and he manifests the disease.

A typical pedigree for X-linked recessive inheritance is shown in Fig. 27.7.

The characteristic features are:

- Males only are affected.
- Females are carriers and are usually healthy.
- Females might show mild signs of the disease depending on the pattern of X-chromosome

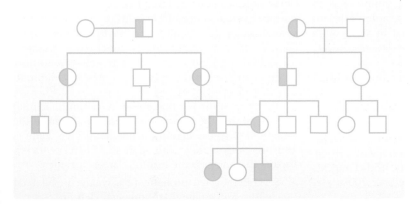

Fig. 27.6 Pedigree of an autosomal recessive disorder

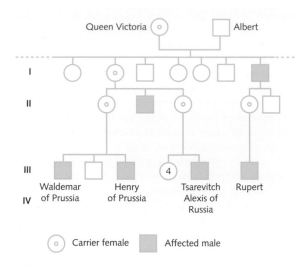

Fig. 27.7 Typical pedigree for X-linked recessive inheritance. Haemophilia in a royal family

---

Fig. 27.8 Clinical features of fragile X syndrome

More common in males
Learning difficulty (IQ 20–80, mean 50)
Autistic features and hyperactivity
Physical features:
• Dysmorphic facial appearance, i.e. large forehead, long face, large prominent ears
• Macrocephaly
• Macro-orchidism – more common after puberty

• The number of repeats becomes amplified when the gene is inherited from a mother but not usually when inherited from a father.
• One-third of female carriers have mild learning difficulties.
• 'Normal transmitting males' occur, who pass the disorder on to their grandchildren through their daughters.

Cytogenetic analysis or direct DNA analysis confirms the diagnosis.

Ornithine transcarbamylase deficiency

This is an X-linked recessive disorder caused by mutations in the gene for the urea-cycle enzyme that causes hyperammonaemia. Males are most severely affected and usually present with an overwhelming and sometimes fatal illness a few days after birth when protein-containing feeds are given.

Up to 30% of female carriers manifest symptoms, depending on the pattern of lyonization in hepatic cells (the enzyme is expressed in the liver). They might present with learning difficulties or headache and vomiting after high-protein meals.

MULTIFACTORIAL DISORDERS

These conditions are believed to be caused by a combination of genetic susceptibility, due to the interaction of several genes (polygenic) and environmental (nongenetic) factors. Multifactorial inheritance accounts for several common birth defects as well as a number of other important diseases with onset in childhood or adult life (Fig. 27.9).

A feature of the familial clustering of multifactorial diseases is that the recurrence risk is low, often in the range 3–5% (most significant for first-degree relatives and decreases rapidly with more distant relatedness). Factors that increase the risk to relatives include:

• Severely affected proband (e.g. greater in bilateral cleft lip and palate than unilateral cleft lip).

---

inactivation (note that in any cell only one X chromosome is transcriptionally active – the Lyon Law).
• Male infants of female carriers have a 50% chance of being affected; female infants have a 50% chance of being a carrier.
• Daughters of affected males are all carriers.
• Sons of affected males are never affected because a father passes his Y chromosome to his son (i.e. there is no male-to-male transmission).

New mutations are common, so there might be no family history. Several important X-linked recessive diseases, including haemophilia (Chapter 22) and Duchenne muscular dystrophy (Chapter 20), are discussed elsewhere. Additional examples are fragile X syndrome and ornithine transcarbamylase deficiency.

Fragile X syndrome

This is an example of a trinucleotide repeat disorder. After Down syndrome, this is the most common cause of severe learning impairment (mental retardation) with an incidence of 1 in 3600 men and 1 in 4000–6000 women. The disorder is due to expansion of a triplet repeat (CGG) in the FRAXA gene FMR1.

The clinical features of fragile X syndrome are listed in Fig. 27.8.

A number of unusual features are accounted for in part by the triplet repeat amplification:

• The number of repeats determines status: normal individuals have fewer than 50 triplet repeats, carriers with a 'pre-mutation' have 50–200 triplet repeats and affected men or women have over 200 triplet repeats.

Fig. 27.9 Conditions with multifactorial inheritance

Congenital malformations
Neural tube defects
Orofacial clefts (lip and palate)
Pyloric stenosis
Talipes
Common diseases
Asthma
Insulin-dependent diabetes mellitus (IDDM)
Epilepsy
Hypertension
Atherosclerosis
Psychiatric disorders, e.g. autism

- Multiple affected family members.
- The affected proband is of the less often affected sex (if there is a difference in the M:F ratio of affected individuals).

In many multifactorial disorders, the environmental factors remain obscure.

CHROMOSOMAL DISORDERS

An alteration in the amount or nature of the chromosomal material is seen in 5 in 1000 live births and is usually associated with multiple congenital anomalies and learning difficulties. A high proportion (40%) of all spontaneous abortions are caused by chromosome abnormalities.

Most chromosome defects arise de novo. They are classified as abnormalities of number or structure, and might involve either the autosomes or the sex chromosomes. Examples of important chromosomal disorders are shown in Fig. 27.10.

Fig. 27.10 Chromosomal disorders

Type	Class	Name	Defect
Numerical	Autosomal	Down syndrome Edwards syndrome Patau syndrome	Trisomy 21 Trisomy 18 Trisomy 13
	Sex chromosomes	Klinefelter syndrome Turner syndrome	47, XXY 45, XO
Structural	Deletions	Prader–Willi syndrome Cri-du-chat syndrome Wilms tumour with aniridia	15q deletion 5p deletion 11p deletion

---

Fig. 27.11 Indications for chromosome analysis

- Phenotype consistent with known chromosomal disorder
- Multiple congenital abnormalities
- Dysmorphic features
- Spontaneously aborted or stillborn fetuses
- Leukaemia, some solid tumours
- Complex genital anomaly

The indications for chromosome analysis are shown in Fig. 27.11. Chromosome studies are carried out on dividing cells. Most commonly, T cells from peripheral blood are used after stimulation of mitosis with phytohaemagglutinin.

Chromosomal abnormalities

Three autosomal trisomies are found in live born infants; others are not compatible with life and are found only in spontaneously aborted fetuses. These are:

- Down syndrome: trisomy 21 (1:700 live births).
- Edward syndrome: trisomy 18 (1:8000 live births).
- Patau syndrome: trisomy 13 (1:15 000 live births).

Trisomy refers to the fact that three, rather than the normal two copies of a specific chromosome are present in the cells of an individual. Trisomies occur because of a meiotic error called non-dysjunction in the gamete of mother or father.

Down syndrome

Trisomy 21 is the most common autosomal trisomy compatible with life. The extra chromosomal material can result from non-dysjunction, translocation or mosaicism.

Non-dysjunction
Ninety-five per cent of children with Down syndrome have trisomy 21 due to non-dysjunction. The pair of chromosomes 21 fails to separate at meiosis, so one gamete has two copies of chromosome 21. Fertilization of this gamete gives rise to a zygote with trisomy 21.

Ninety per cent of non-dysjunctions are maternally derived and the risk rises with maternal age, increasing steeply in mothers over 35 years (Fig. 27.12).

Fig. 27.12 Risk of Down syndrome (for live births) by maternal age at delivery

Maternal age (years)	Risk
All ages	1:700
20	1:1500
30	1:900
35	1:380
40	1:85
44	1: 35

However, because a higher proportion of pregnancies occur in younger women, most children with trisomy 21 are born to women under 35 years of age. The recurrence risk for parents of children with trisomy 21 increases to 1–2% (unless the age-related risk is higher).

Translocation

Four per cent of Down syndrome children have 46 chromosomes with a translocation of the third chromosome 21 to another chromosome (most commonly 14). Three-quarters of cases are de novo and, in one-quarter, one of the parents has a balanced translocation involving one chromosome 21. If the mother is the translocation carrier, the recurrence risk might be as high as 15%; if the father is the carrier, the risk is 2.5%.

Mosaicism

In 1% of cases the non-dysjunction occurs during mitosis after formation of the zygote so that some cells are normal and some show trisomy 21. The phenotype might be milder in mosaicism.

Clinical features

Down syndrome is often suspected at birth because of the characteristic facial appearance but the diagnosis can be difficult on clinical features alone. A senior paediatrician should confirm clinical suspicion. Rapid chromosomal analysis is performed via FISH (fluorescence in situ hybridization) but may not exclude mosaicism. A complete karyotype is performed to confirm the initial result. The phenotypic features are listed in Fig. 27.13.

Fig. 27.13 Clinical features of Down syndrome	
Dysmorphic facial features	Round face
	Epicanthic folds, flat nasal bridge
	Protruding tongue
	Small ears
	Brushfield spots on iris
Other dysmorphic features	Single palmar creases
	Flat occiput
	Incurved little fingers
	Gap between first and second toes (sandal toe gap)
	Small stature
Structural defects	Cardiac defects in 50%
	Duodenal atresia
Neurological features	Hypotonia
	Developmental delay
	Mean IQ = 50
Late medical complications	Increased risk of leukaemia
	Respiratory infections
	Hypothyroidism
	Alzheimer's disease
	Atlantoaxial instability

Management and prognosis

Parents need information about the implications of the diagnosis and the assistance available from professionals and self-help groups. Feelings of disappointment, anger and guilt are common. Genetic counselling for recurrence risks will be required. A cardiology review and echocardiogram should be arranged shortly after birth because of the association with cardiac defects. Life expectancy in Down syndrome has increased and issues relating to employment and living situations in adulthood will need to be addressed. Screening for diseases associated with Down syndrome should be performed throughout life (e.g. hypothyroidism, coeliac disease).

COMMUNICATION

Treatment of trisomy 21 involves a multidisciplinary approach. In addition to the healthcare agencies there are many voluntary organizations, e.g. the Down's Syndrome Association, offering help and support to affected families.

Edwards syndrome (trisomy 18)

The characteristic phenotype for Edwards syndrome is microcephaly and micrognathia with associated cleft lip/palate, ocular abnormalities (including palpebral fissures, hypertelorism and ptosis); hands are often clenched with overlapping fingers, and talipes and absent radii may also feature. Systemic abnormalities include congenital cardiac malformations, renal disease, exomphalos, atresia and developmental delay. Most die in infancy.

Patau syndrome

Patau syndrome is caused by trisomy 13. It is characterized by polydactyly, low set ears, talipes, cutis aplasia and cleft palate. There are problems with the CNS (low IQ, microcephaly and holoprosencephaly), microphthalmia and other eye problems, abnormal genitalia and renal malformation and it is associated with cardiac malformation. A small proportion survive to adulthood – those with mosaicism have better prognosis but most die in early childhood.

Sex chromosome disorders

Turner syndrome

In this condition, there are 44 autosomes and only one normal X chromosome. It affects 1 in 2500 live born females. Various underlying chromosomal defects are seen:

- In 55% of girls, the karyotype is 45, XO.
- In 25%, there is a deletion of the short arm of one X chromosome, or a so-called isochromosome with duplication of one arm and loss of the other.

- In 15%, there is mosaicism due to postzygotic mitotic non-dysjunction (45, XO/46, XY).

The incidence does not increase with maternal age and the recurrence risk is the same as the general population risk.

Clinical features and diagnosis

The clinical features are shown in Fig. 27.14. Diagnosis may be made:

- Prenatally by ultrasound scan.
- At birth by presence of puffy hands and feet (lymphoedema) or a cardiac abnormality.
- During childhood because of short stature.
- In adolescence because of primary amenorrhoea and lack of pubertal development.

Diagnosis is confirmed by a blood karyotype.

Management

Therapy with growth hormone improves final height. Ovarian hormones are not produced due to the gonadal dysgenesis (streak ovaries). Oestrogen therapy is given at the appropriate age (11 years) to produce maturation of secondary sexual characteristics including breast development. Towards the end of puberty, progestogen is added to maintain uterine health and allow monthly withdrawal bleeds (periods). Although pregnancy can occur naturally, most patients are infertile. Pregnancy can be achieved with in vitro fertilization. Treatment may also be necessary for other abnormalities, e.g. surgical correction of coarctation of the aorta.

Klinefelter syndrome

Klinefelter syndrome is characterized by one or more extra X chromosomes, most commonly 47 XXY karyotype. The phenotype is of:

- Tall stature with long legs.
- Small testes.
- Gynaecomastia.
- Learning difficulties.

Treatment with testosterone may be needed to stimulate development of secondary sexual characteristics.

Structural chromosomal abnormalities

These arise from chromosome breakage and include deletions, duplications, inversions and unbalanced translocations. Deletions are the most common. Most arise de novo but they can also arise from inheritance of an unbalanced translocation. Examples of conditions associated with chromosomal deletions include:

- Cri-du-chat syndrome: caused by deletion of short arm of chromosome 5 (5p-). Affected children have profound mental retardation and a cat-like cry.
- Prader–Willi syndrome: caused by deletions of the paternal copy of 15q11-13.
- Angelman syndrome: caused by deletions of the maternal copy of 15q11-13.

MITOCHONDRIAL INHERITANCE

Mitochondrial disorders are inherited maternally. Examples include:

- Mitochondrial encephalopathy, lactic acidosis, stroke-like episodes (MELAS).
- Mitochondrially inherited diabetes mellitus.

Fig. 27.14 Clinical features of Turner syndrome

Dysmorphic features

Lymphoedema of hands and feet (at birth)
Neck webbing
Widely spaced nipples
Wide carrying angle (cubitus valgus)
Short stature
Structural and functional abnormalities
Gonadal dysgenesis
Congenital heart disease, particularly coarctation of the aorta
Renal anomalies
Specific learning difficulties – visuo-spatial

The mitochondria contain genetic material as a 16.5-kilobase circular chromosome. They have no introns and a mixture of normal and abnormal mitochondria (heteroplasmy) can exist within tissues. It is worth noting the similarities between mitochondrial and prokaryotic genetics.

POLYMERASE CHAIN REACTION

This is a technique of obtaining a large amount of DNA copied from a small initial sample. It has applications in detection of specific DNA sequences or differences in genes. Its main clinical use is in detection of mutations and rapid diagnosis of bacterial or viral infection. It has a very high sensitivity and is being increasingly used in clinical practice.

HINTS AND TIPS

Information base in genetic counselling:
• Magnitude of risk.
• Severity of disorder.
• Availability of treatment.
• Parental cultural and ethical values.
  Options in antenatal genetic counselling:
• Not to have offspring.
• To ignore the risk.

• Antenatal diagnosis and termination of pregnancy.
• Pre-implantation diagnosis.
• Artificial insemination by donor or ovum donation.

GENETIC COUNSELLING

This is usually carried out as a specialist service by trained medical staff. The main aim is to provide information about hereditary disorders so that parents will have greater autonomy and choice in reproductive decisions.

HINTS AND TIPS

The basic elements of counselling include:
• Establishing a diagnosis: this might involve physical examination of proband and family members and special investigations including DNA, cytogenetic and biochemical analysis.
• Estimation of risk: the risk for future offspring is determined by the mode of inheritance of the disease.
• Communication: information must be conveyed in an unbiased and non-directive way and all the possible options should be discussed.

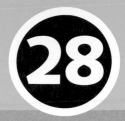
At the end of this chapter, you should be able to:
- Define some of the terms used in perinatal statistics
- Understand the influence of maternal health on the infant
- Understand the physiology of a normal newborn
- Understand common problems of the preterm infant
- Understand some of the problems seen in term infants
- Understand the common infections of the newborn

Fetal and neonatal life are best regarded as a continuum. Many factors from before conception to delivery influence the health of the newborn infant.

Introduction: perinatal statistics and definitions

Terms used in perinatal statistics are defined in Fig. 28.1.

Nearly half of all neonatal deaths occur in the first 24 hours. The perinatal mortality rate in developed countries has fallen steadily over the last 20 years and seems to be approaching an irreducible lower limit set by deaths from lethal malformations. However, disadvantaged people continue to have the highest rates of perinatal deaths and congenital malformations.

MATERNAL AND FETAL HEALTH

Mother and fetus are a single physiological unit and any serious maternal disease or condition can affect the fetus. Action to optimize the chances of a healthy baby can begin even before conception. The chance of a good outcome can be enhanced by:

- Avoiding smoking, excess alcohol and medication.
- Avoiding infections: rubella immunization before pregnancy, avoiding exposure to toxoplasmosis (via cat's litter) and listeriosis (unpasteurized dairy products).
- Folic acid supplements reduce the risk of neural tube defects.
- Optimizing treatment of maternal conditions such as obesity, hypertension and diabetes mellitus.
- Genetic counselling for couples at risk of inherited diseases.

FETAL ASSESSMENT AND ANTENATAL DIAGNOSIS

Methods for assessing the growth, maturation and well-being of the fetus are available. They include:

- Ultrasound: for assessing age and growth.
- Doppler blood flow studies.
- Fetal echocardiography: to assess congenital cardiac defects.
- Fetal MRI: more detailed assessment of abnormalities seen on ultrasound.

Antenatal diagnosis is now available for many disorders using the methods shown in Fig. 28.2. In addition to invasive fetal investigation it is possible to detect free fetal nucleic acids in the maternal blood stream from the fifth week of pregnancy. At present this is used to detect known paternal alleles not found in the maternal genome but has potential for much wider application.

Antenatal diagnosis can allow the option of termination to be offered in certain disorders, therapy to be given, or neonatal management to be planned in advance. Medical treatment can be given to the fetus via the mother or directly (e.g. fetal blood transfusion for anaemia in severe rhesus isoimmunization).

MATERNAL CONDITIONS AFFECTING THE FETUS

Organogenesis occurs during the embryonic period (weeks 2–9) with many organs structurally complete by the end of the second trimester. Therefore, conditions and medications occurring in the first and second trimesters lead to organ dysfunction or structural abnormality.

Fig. 28.1 Definitions for perinatal statistics	
Term	**Definition**
Still birth	A fetus born after 24 weeks of gestation who shows no signs of life after delivery
Low birthweight	A baby weighing 2500 g or less at birth
Neonatal period	First month of life
Perinatal mortality rate	Still births and deaths within the first 6 days per 1000 live and still births (i.e. total births)
Neonatal mortality rate	Deaths of live born infants during the first 28 days of age per 1000 live births

The fetus can be affected by:

- Maternal diseases: diabetes mellitus, thyrotoxicosis and autoimmune disorders (e.g. systemic lupus erythematosus, myasthenia gravis and thrombocytopenia).
- Maternal drugs, e.g. medications, alcohol and narcotics.
- Maternal infections: congenital infections.

Maternal diseases

Diabetes mellitus

Diabetes mellitus can cause both neonatal and fetal problems.

Potential fetal problems include:

- Congenital malformations: there is a three-fold increase (especially cardiac malformations).

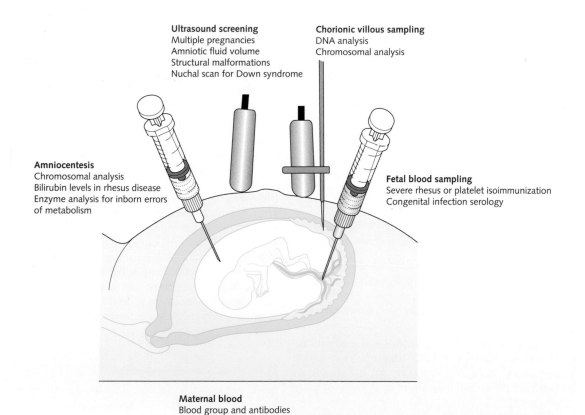

Ultrasound screening
Multiple pregnancies
Amniotic fluid volume
Structural malformations
Nuchal scan for Down syndrome

Chorionic villous sampling
DNA analysis
Chromosomal analysis

Amniocentesis
Chromosomal analysis
Bilirubin levels in rhesus disease
Enzyme analysis for inborn errors of metabolism

Fetal blood sampling
Severe rhesus or platelet isoimmunization
Congenital infection serology

Maternal blood
Blood group and antibodies
Hepatitis B, HIV
Maternal serum α–fetoprotein for neural tube defects
Test for Down syndrome risk estimation

Fig. 28.2 Antenatal diagnosis: various methods and the disorders they are used to diagnose

- Macrosomia: the fetal insulin response to hyperglycaemia promotes excessive growth, which predisposes to difficulties during delivery.

Potential neonatal problems include:

- Hypoglycaemia: transient early hypoglycaemia occurs due to fetal hyperinsulinism; early feeding can usually prevent this.
- Respiratory distress syndrome (RDS).
- Polycythaemia (haematocrit >0.65).

Maternal drugs affecting the fetus

Drugs taken by the mother might cause congenital malformations (Fig. 28.3), adverse effects by their pharmacological action on the fetus or placenta, or transient problems at birth.

HINTS AND TIPS

Maternal drugs and the fetus:
- Teratogenic drugs taken during organogenesis can cause spontaneous abortions or congenital malformations.

Fig. 28.3 Maternal medication that can harm the fetus

Drug	Adverse effects
Cytotoxic agents	Congenital malformations
Phenytoin	Fetal hydantoin syndrome (growth retardation, microcephaly, hypoplastic nails)
Sodium valproate	Neural tube defects
Carbamazepine	Growth retardation, craniofacial abnormalities
Warfarin	Interferes with cartilage formation, risk of cerebral haemorrhage, and microcephaly
Progestogens (androgenic)	Masculinization of fetus
Diethylstilboestrol	Adenocarcinoma of vagina
Thalidomide	Limb shortening (phocomelia)
Drug abuse	
Alcohol	Fetal alcohol syndrome (characteristic facies, septal defects, mental retardation)
Opiates (heroin/methadone)	Growth retardation, prematurity, drug withdrawal in neonate (tremors, hyperirritability, seizures)
Cocaine	Spontaneous abortion, prematurity, cerebral infarction

- Drugs given during labour can have adverse effects, e.g. analgesics and anaesthesia (suppression of spontaneous breathing at birth), sedatives (sedation, hypotension).
- IV fluids: excess hypotonic fluids can cause hyponatraemia.

Maternal infections and the fetus

A number of infections acquired by the mother could affect the fetus or newborn (Fig. 28.4). Transmission can occur in utero, during labour or postpartum (Fig. 28.5).

Rubella

For rubella, see Chapter 13.

Varicella zoster

More than 85% of women of childbearing age have evidence of past infection with chickenpox, so a minority of pregnant women are at risk.

Infection in the first trimester does not usually cause fetal damage but about 2% develop 'congenital varicella syndrome' characterized by:

- Cicatricial skin lesions (scars).
- Malformed digits and limbs.
- Cataracts, chorioretinitis.
- CNS damage.

Fig. 28.4 Maternal infections transmitted to the fetus in utero

Toxoplasmosis
Rubella
Cytomegalovirus
Varicella zoster
HIV
Treponema pallidum (syphilis)
Listeria monocytogenes

Fig. 28.5 Infections acquired during delivery

Group B haemolytic streptococci
E. coli
HIV
Hepatitis B
Herpes simplex
Gonococci
Chlamydia trachomatis
Echoviruses

The principal problem is infection acquired late in pregnancy, particularly within 5 days before and 2 days after delivery. The fetus receives a high viral load but little in the way of maternal antibodies. Severe infection can ensue with a mortality of up to 5%.

Exposed susceptible women can be treated with varicella zoster immune globulin (VZIG) and aciclovir. Infants exposed in the high-risk period should also be treated with VZIG. Intravenous aciclovir should be used if lesions develop in the newborn infant.

Cytomegalovirus

For cytomegalovirus, see Chapter 13.

Human immunodeficiency virus (HIV)

Vertical transmission from mother to infant can occur in utero, during birth or postnatally by breastfeeding. The exact risk of infection by each of these routes is uncertain but overall vertical transmission rate is now less than 1% (see Chapter 13).

Pregnant women are routinely screened for HIV. Prevention of transmission centres around reducing maternal viral load, appropriate method of delivery (women with a low viral load may be suitable for vaginal delivery. Postnatal treatment of the neonate is tailored depending on maternal control and any drug-resistance. Usually zidovudine is given for the first 6 weeks. Mothers are advised not to breast feed to reduce the risk of postpartum transmission.

Toxoplasmosis

Infection with the protozoan parasite *Toxoplasma gondii* occurs from the ingestion of raw or undercooked meat, or from oocytes excreted in the faeces of infected cats. Most infections are asymptomatic. Serological epidemiological studies show that in some countries (e.g. France and Austria), 80% of women of childbearing age are immune, whereas in the UK only 20% have antibodies.

Transmission is unlikely where the mother has seroconverted prior to pregnancy. The risk of fetal infection following acute infection depends on the gestational age – transmission is more likely where seroconversion occurs later in pregnancy; however, more serious disease occurs where the transmission is in the first trimester. About 10% of infected infants have clinical manifestations at birth, which can include:

- Hydrocephalus.
- Intracranial calcification.
- Chorioretinitis.
- Neurological damage.

Infants with asymptomatic infection may still develop chorioretinitis in later life.

NORMAL NEONATAL ANATOMY AND PHYSIOLOGY

There are characteristic features of newborn anatomy and physiology that are important and these are considered in turn.

Size and growth

The average term infant in the UK weighs about 3500 g. Boys weigh approximately 250 g more than girls. Infants of 2500 g or less are classified as 'low birthweight'. This important category is considered separately.

During the first 3–5 days, up to 10% of birthweight is lost. This is regained by 7–10 days. In the first month, average weight gain per week is 200 g.

Skin

The newborn skin is immature, with a thin epithelial layer and incompletely developed sweat and sebaceous glands. Combined with the high surface area to body mass ratio, this renders the baby prone to heat and water losses.

Numerous benign skin lesions occur (see Chapter 15). The skin is covered with a greasy protective layer, the vernix caseosa.

Head

The average occipitofrontal head circumference is 35 cm. Significant moulding of the head might occur during birth. Two soft spots or fontanelles are present. The anterior fontanelle closes between 9 and 18 months of age and the posterior closes by 6–8 weeks.

Respiratory system

Changes occur at birth that allow the newborn to convert from dependence on the placenta to breathing air for the exchange of respiratory gases:

- In utero, the airways and lungs are filled with fluid that contains surfactant in the later stages of pregnancy. Oligohydramnios can lead to pulmonary hypoplasia.
- The lung fluid is removed by the squeezing of the thorax during vaginal delivery and by reduced secretion and increased absorption mediated by fetal catecholamines during labour and after birth.
- Surfactant lines the air–fluid interface of the alveoli and reduces the surface tension thereby facilitating lung expansion. This is associated with a fall in pulmonary vascular resistance.

Newborn infants breathe mainly with the diaphragm. The rate is variable and normally ranges between 30 and 50 breaths/min. Brief (up to several seconds) self-limiting apnoeic spells might occur during sleep. Small babies are obligate nose-breathers.

Cardiovascular system

Major changes in the lungs and circulation allow adaptation to extrauterine life.

In the fetal circulation, the right-sided (pulmonary) pressure exceeds the left-sided (systemic) pressure. Blood flows from right to left through the foramen ovale and ductus arteriosus (Fig. 28.6). At birth, these relationships reverse:

- Left-sided (systemic) pressure rises with clamping of umbilical vessels.

- Right-sided (pulmonary) pressure falls as the lungs expand and the rising PO_2 triggers a prostaglandin-mediated vasodilatation.
- The foramen ovale and ductus arteriosus close functionally shortly after birth. The ductus closes due to muscular contraction in response to rising oxygen tension.
- Certain forms of congenital heart disease are 'duct-dependant', i.e. flow through the duct is necessary for oxygen delivery and closure of the duct precipitates sudden deterioration (see Chapter 16).

Gastrointestinal system

Most infants over 35 weeks' gestation have developed the coordination necessary to 'latch on' and feed from breast or bottle. At term, the secretory and absorbing

Fig. 28.6 Fetal circulation

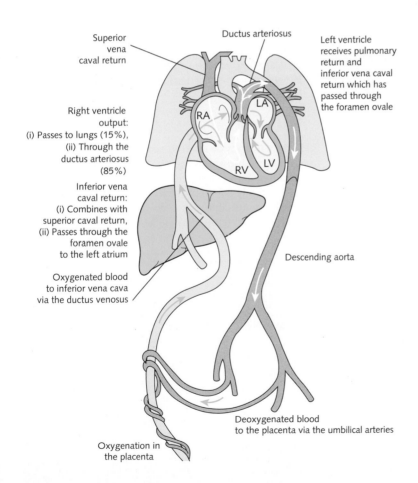

Superior vena caval return

Ductus arteriosus

Left ventricle receives pulmonary return and inferior vena caval return which has passed through the foramen ovale

Right ventricle output:
(i) Passes to lungs (15%),
(ii) Through the ductus arteriosus (85%)

Inferior vena caval return:
(i) Combines with superior caval return,
(ii) Passes through the foramen ovale to the left atrium

Oxygenated blood to inferior vena cava via the ductus venosus

RA
LA
RV
LV

Descending aorta

Deoxygenated blood to the placenta via the umbilical arteries

Oxygenation in the placenta

surfaces are well developed, as are digestive enzymes, with the exception of pancreatic amylase.

Meconium is usually passed within 6 hours and delay beyond 24 hours is considered abnormal.

With normal feeding meconium is replaced by yellow stool by day 3 or 4. Immaturity of the liver enzymes responsible for conjugation of bilirubin is responsible for the 'physiological jaundice' which can occur from the second day of life.

Genitourinary system

Urine production occurs during the second half of gestation and accounts for much of the amniotic fluid. The infant might micturate during delivery (unnoticed) and should void within the first 24 hours of life. Renal concentrating ability is diminished in neonates.

Haematopoietic and immune system

The newborn's red cells contain fetal haemoglobin (HbF) which has a higher affinity for oxygen than adult haemoglobin. The haemoglobin concentration of cord blood ranges from 15 to 20 g/dL (mean 17 g/dL). A large volume of blood is present in the placenta and late clamping causes this blood to enter the baby. This can lead to polycythaemia. In the preterm baby it is advantageous.

The neonatal immune system also is incomplete compared to older children and adults:

- Impaired neutrophil reserves.
- Diminished phagocytosis and intracellular killing capacity.
- Decreased complement components.
- Low IgG_2, leading to infections with encapsulated organisms.

The presence of maternal antibody in babies born greater than 30 weeks' gestational age provides some protection against infection.

Central nervous system

The central nervous system (CNS) is relatively immature at birth. Myelination is incomplete and continues during the first 2 years of life.

A limited behavioural response repertoire is sufficient for survival, comprising a sleep and wake cycle, sucking and swallowing, and crying:

- Newborn infants sleep for a total of 16–20 hours each day.
- The touch of a nipple on the baby's face initiates the sequence of rooting, latching on and the complex coordination of lip, tongue, palate and pharynx required for sucking and swallowing.
- Crying (without tears) is the main means of communication.

BIRTH

The short journey down the birth canal from the intrauterine environment to the external world is potentially hazardous. Various risk factors can be identified during labour, the most important of which is prematurity. The problems of the preterm infant are dealt with separately. Here we consider:

- Normal care and resuscitation of the term newborn.
- Problems of hypoxic insult around birth, and birth injuries.

Assessment and care at a normal birth

The infant is usually delivered after a short period of oxygen deprivation and begins to breathe within a few seconds. The Apgar score is a useful quantitative assessment of the infant's condition (Fig. 28.7) and is commonly determined at 1, 5 and 10 minutes after birth. The Apgar score is influenced by several factors including intrapartum asphyxia, maternal sedation or analgesia, the gestational age and any cardiac, pulmonary or neurological disease in the infant. Most babies will establish respirations spontaneously after delivery or if apnoeic respond to airway opening manoeuvres. However, a few will need more extensive resuscitation (see Fig. 28.8).

Perinatal asphyxia

Perinatal asphyxia refers to a condition in which the fetus is acutely deprived of oxygen. The majority of insults occur antenatally (70%) with only a small proportion (5%) arising solely due to intrapartum events. A cause may be clearly identifiable, e.g. placental abruption, maternal cardiac arrest, fetomaternal haemorrhage, etc.; however,

Fig. 28.7 Apgar score evaluation of the newborn			
Criteria	*Score*		
	0	**1**	**2**
Heart rate	Absent	<100 beats/min	>100 beats/min
Respiratory effort	Absent/ weak	Irregular/ gasping	Regular
Muscle tone	Limp	Some flexion	Active movements
Reflex response to stimulation	None	Weak	Cries
Colour	Blue or pale	Extremities blue	Pink

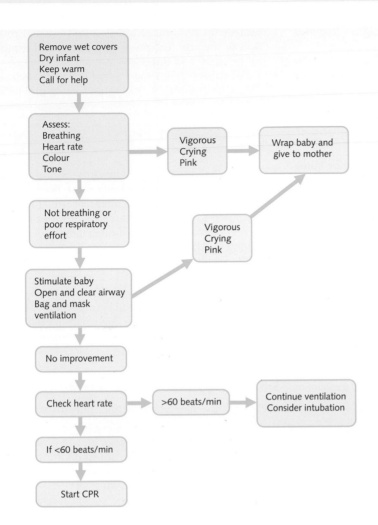

Fig. 28.8   Neonatal resuscitation

more often the aetiology is unclear. Risk factors include pre-eclampsia, abnormal placenta, sepsis and intrauterine growth restriction (IUGR). The incidence has fallen to 1.5–6 per 1000 live births.

The insult produces fetal hypoxia, hypercapnia and acidosis which manifest during labour as:

- Abnormalities in fetal heart rate: fetal bradycardia (rate under 120 beats/min), fetal tachycardia (rate over 160 beats/min) or an abnormal pattern of deceleration during or after uterine contractions.
- Acidosis: significant acidosis (pH < 7.20) on fetal scalp blood sampling.
- Meconium staining of the liquor.

These signs are an indication for prompt delivery of the fetus. Hypoxic insults affect all organ systems (the brain is relatively protected due to autoregulatory mechanisms, therefore by the time neurological symptoms are manifested other organ systems may have suffered significant damage Fig. 28.9.

The postnatal symptoms and signs are classified as mild, moderate or severe.

Fig. 28.9   Complications of perinatal asphyxia (severe)

Organ	Complication
Brain	Hypoxic–ischaemic encephalopathy
Heart	Hypoxic cardiomyopathy, hypotension
Lungs	Persistent pulmonary hypotension
Guts	Ileus and necrotizing enterocolitis
Kidneys	Acute tubular necrosis
Blood	Disseminated intravascular coagulation

Hypoxic–ischaemic encephalopathy

This describes the neurological manifestations of perinatal hypoxic injury. It may be classified using the Sarnat criteria as:

- Mild: initial lethargy followed by a period of hyperalertness with irritability, tone is normal and there are no seizures. There may be impaired feeding for 1–2 days. There are no focal signs. Prognosis is good.

- Moderate: there is hypotonia with reduced movements and decreased conscious level. Seizures are often seen. Variable prognosis.
- Severe: coma with absence of spontaneous movement, absent reflexes. Seizures are usually seen and may be frequent. Multiorgan failure is often present. Morbidity and mortality are high.

Neuronal injury occurs in two phases: the acute injury caused by hypoxia at time of the event and the reperfusion injury which occurs between 6 and 72 hours post-insult. Supportive care is therefore vital in minimizing damage and reducing morbidity. Total body cooling has been shown to reduce neurodisability in moderate to severe hypoxic–ischaemic encephalopathy (HIE) (TOBY trial). This involves inducing hypothermia for 72 hours followed by gradual rewarming to protect the brain from reperfusion damage. It does not reduce mortality rates but improves outcomes in survivors. Neurological function and seizures can be monitored using an amplitude-integrated EEG (the cerebral function monitor (CFM)) and provides some indication of prognosis.

In addition to cooling close supportive management is needed including:

- Respiratory support.
- Anticonvulsants for seizures.
- Fluid restriction.
- Circulatory support with inotropes if necessary.

MRI and EEG can assist in predicting the outcome. Cystic lesions or cerebral atrophy may appear in the ensuing weeks.

BIRTH INJURY

Physical injury during labour and delivery is now relatively uncommon, partly because the availability of caesarean section obviates the need for heroic attempts at vaginal delivery. Predisposing factors include:

- Breech presentation.
- Cephalopelvic disproportion.
- Macrosomia.
- Assisted delivery: manual or instrumental (forceps or ventouse extraction). Injuries can occur to soft tissues, nerves or bones.

Common injuries include:

- Bruising.
- Cephalohaematoma: (haematoma of the scalp, limited by suture lines, usually benign) especially following ventouse delivery.
- Brachial plexus injury: e.g. Erb's palsy, especially following shoulder dystocia. The hand is held in the waiter's tip position (adduction and internal rotation of the arm, extension of forearm, and flexion of the wrists and finger).
- Facial palsies: following forceps delivery, often resolves spontaneously, may cause feeding problems.

DISEASES OF THE NEWBORN

Much neonatal care is directed towards the problems of low-birthweight infants, especially those born prematurely, many of whom require intensive care. It is therefore useful to consider the disorders of low-birthweight and term infants separately, although there is, of course, significant overlap.

Size and gestational age

Newborn infants might be small because they have been born preterm or because they are small in relation to their gestational age (small for dates). Some useful definitions are shown in Fig. 28.10.

Small for gestational age infants

These infants have intrauterine growth restriction (IUGR), which can be caused by:

- An intrinsic fetal problem: poor growth is symmetrical, with head circumference proportionally reduced, e.g. chromosomal disorders, small normal fetus and congenital infections.
- Placental insufficiency: poor growth is asymmetrical, with brain growth relatively spared (an adaptive response), e.g. maternal pre-eclampsia, hypertension, renal disease, sickle cell disease and multiple pregnancy.

The fetus with IUGR is at risk from hypoxia and death and is closely monitored using cardiotocography and Doppler ultrasound to profile blood flow velocity in the uterine and umbilical arteries.

Fig. 28.10 Definitions for size and gestational age	
Term	**Definition**
Preterm	Gestation <37 completed weeks
Post-term	Gestation >42 completed weeks
Low birthweight	<2500 g
Very low birthweight	<1500 g
Extremely low birthweight	<1000 g
Small for gestational age	Birthweight <10th centile for gestational age
Large for gestational age	Birthweight >90th centile for gestational age

Postnatal problems encountered by the fetus with IUGR include:

- Hypothermia.
- Hypoglycaemia from low fat and glycogen stores.
- Increased risk of periventricular leucomalacia (see intracranial lesions).
- Polycythaemia (haematocrit >0.65).

Large for gestational age infants

The most common cause of macrosomia is maternal diabetes mellitus. Potential associated problems include birth asphyxia from a difficult delivery and birth trauma, especially from shoulder dystocia.

The preterm infant

About 3 in every 100 babies are born prematurely (before 37 weeks' gestation) and are classified as 'preterm'. Most weigh less than 2500 g and are therefore 'low-birthweight' babies. These infants provide much of the work in neonatal units and account for 60% of neonatal deaths.

The major problems encountered by preterm infants are determined by the immaturity of their organ systems, particularly the lungs (Fig. 28.11). The limits of

Fig. 28.11	Major problems in preterm infants
Temperature	Hypothermia
Respiratory	Respiratory distress syndrome Pneumothorax Chronic lung disease Pneumonia Pulmonary hypertension
Cardiac	Patent ductus arteriosus Hypotension
Gastrointestinal	Feed intolerance Vomiting and gastro-oesophageal reflux Jaundice Necrotizing enterocolitis
Infection	Group B streptococci Staphylococcus epidermidis Gram-negative cocci Fungi, e.g. Candida species
Nervous	Intraventricular haemorrhage Retinopathy of prematurity Developmental delay Cerebral palsy
Bone	Osteopenia of prematurity
Fluids and electrolytes	High transepidermal water loss Hypoglycaemia
Haematology	Anaemia

viability are currently in the region of 23–24 weeks' gestation.

Characteristics of the preterm infant

There is physiological immaturing of major organ functions:

- Temperature control: heat production is low (no brown fat, limited muscle activity). Heat loss is high (high surface area to volume, lack of fat insulation).
- Blood and circulation: hypotension, easy bruising and bleeding.
- Respiratory system: narrow nasal airways, soft thoracic cage, poor cough reflex, unstable respiratory drive with irregular breathing and apnoea. Alveolar collapse due to surfactant deficiency.
- Gastrointestinal tract: uncoordinated suck or swallow (before 32–34 weeks). Regurgitation common. Increased severity and incidence of 'physiological' jaundice.
- Renal function: tendency to lose sodium but unable to excrete fluid load. Oedema and hyponatraemia might occur.
- Immune system: active and passive immunity are both limited.

General care of the preterm infant

Some basic principles apply to the care of all preterm infants. These are considered separately from the specific problems that arise in different systems.

Predelivery care

Prevention of preterm labour is not possible at present. Various techniques have been attempted with limited success including bed rest, progesterone supplementation and cervical sutures for women with a history of premature labour or cervical shortening, and tocolytic drugs, e.g. atosiban or ritodrine. Once labour has started it can be delayed for a short time (hours to days) by using tocolytic drugs. This might give time for corticosteroids to be administered.

> **COMMUNICATION**
>
> Parents should be given the opportunity to speak to a paediatrician prior to the delivery of a premature infant and, if possible, visit the neonatal unit. At this time, they should be made aware of the possible complications of preterm delivery and the chances of survival and disability. It is also important to tell them what happens soon after delivery and briefly about the resuscitation. They should also be prepared for a long stay in the neonatal intensive care.

Stabilization at birth

Delivery should ideally take place in a location with full paediatric backup, including a neonatal intensive care unit. At birth the baby should be handled gently, dried and placed under a source of radiant heat.

Many preterm infants of 28 weeks' gestation or less will not achieve adequate spontaneous ventilation and will require intubation or nasal continuous positive airways pressure (CPAP). Surfactant administration is considered in infants <28 weeks at this stage.

COMMUNICATION

Parents often want to know the chances of survival of an extremely premature infant. The EPICURE 2 study showed that babies born at less than 23 weeks have a 1% chance of survival. By 24 weeks over a third survive and around 20% with no disability. By 28 most babies survive and do not have major disability although minor learning difficulties can occur.

Body temperature

Preterm infants rapidly lose heat. Strategies for maintaining body temperature include:

- Ambient temperature and humidity: incubators provide a controlled microenvironment.
- Insulation with clothing, including a hat to prevent excessive heat loss from the relatively large head.
- Radiant heat: used predominantly in the resuscitation area, but it causes excessive fluid loss over prolonged periods, extremely premature infants should be placed in a plastic bag for resuscitation to minimize fluid loss.

HINTS AND TIPS

Body temperature in the preterm infant:
- Heat loss is excessive due to high surface area to volume ratio, poor insulation and transepidermal water loss.
- Heat generation is limited by reduced muscular activity, lack of brown fat and inability to shiver.

Avoiding infection

Meticulous attention to hand-washing before and after handling is the most important safeguard against transmitting infection. Good skin care will reduce the incidence of *Staphylococcus epidermidis* infection.

Nutrition and fluids

Infants of 34 weeks' gestation or more are usually able to take oral feeds of milk from breast or bottle. Although preterm infants can digest and absorb enteral feeds, their sucking and swallowing reflexes might be ineffective and some or all of the feeds must be delivered through a small-bore nasogastric or orogastric tube. The approach to giving nutrition and fluids therefore depends on the size and maturity of the individual baby.

The majority of small preterm infants (under 150 g) require their fluid and calorie requirements intravenously during the first few days. Feeds should be introduced gradually particularly in low birthweight and growth restricted infants.

If enteral feeds by mouth or nasogastric tube are not tolerated, more prolonged maintenance of nutrition is achieved by total parenteral nutrition. A mixture of amino acids, dextrose, lipids and electrolytes is given intravenously via a long line, the lumen of which is placed centrally in the vena cava.

Which milk for preterm infants? Breast milk is better tolerated than artificial feeds, and has many additional benefits including protection against necrotizing enterocolitis (NEC). Breast milk fortifier and electrolytes can be added to breast milk and preterm formulas may be used if breast milk is not available.

Supplements Preterm infants need supplements of phosphate ($\pm$ vitamin D) to ensure adequate bone mineralization. A multivitamin preparation is usually given once full enteral feeding is established and continued until age 5, with an iron supplement from 4 weeks of age until weaned.

DISORDERS OF THE PRETERM INFANT

Respiratory disorders

Surfactant deficiency (hyaline membrane disease, respiratory distress syndrome)

This syndrome is caused by a deficiency of surfactant associated with immaturity of the type II pneumocytes. Surfactant is a lipoprotein that lowers surface tension in the alveoli and prevents collapse of the alveoli during expiration. At post-mortem, an exudate of proteinaceous hyaline material is seen in the alveoli and terminal bronchioles (hence, the alternative term 'hyaline membrane disease' for this disorder).

Surfactant deficiency occurs in the majority of infants <30 weeks' gestation and significant numbers of preterms >30 weeks. It is uncommon in term infants but may occur in infants of diabetic mothers. It tends to be worse in boys and hypoxia, acidosis, hypothermia, meconium and pulmonary haemorrhage exacerbate surfactant deficiency.

Clinical features

Respiratory distress is the major feature. This might be present from birth or could develop within the first 4 hours. The signs include:

- Tachypnoea.
- Cyanosis.
- Subcostal and intercostal recession.
- Expiratory grunting.

The disease displays a spectrum of severity from mild to severe and life threatening. A chest X-ray (CXR) will show a diffuse granular or 'ground glass' appearance of the lungs and an air bronchogram outlining the larger airways.

Management

Glucocorticoids given antenatally for 48 hours stimulate fetal surfactant production but many preterm births occur without this period of warning. Effective stabilization at birth of infants at risk reduces the severity of the disease. The mainstays of management include:

- Artificial surfactant therapy (e.g. Curosurf).
- Oxygen.
- Assisted ventilation.

Exogenous surfactant therapy given after birth reduces mortality and morbidity and many babies can be rapidly weaned off ventilatory support after treatment.

An increased concentration of inspired oxygen is required and in more severe disease this needs to be supplemented with continuous positive airways pressure via the nasal airways or mechanical ventilation. Ventilation is guided by monitoring of the arterial blood gas tensions (PaO_2 and $PaCO_2$). High frequency oscillatory ventilation can be used when conventional ventilation fails. Complications of RDS are shown in Fig. 28.12.

Surfactant deficiency itself resolves spontaneously in 3–7 days as endogenous surfactant is produced. Extremely preterm, very low-birthweight infants have immature lungs in addition to surfactant deficient and may require ventilator support for longer.

Fig. 28.12 Complications of respiratory distress syndrome	
Pulmonary	Pneumothorax
	Interstitial emphysema
	Secondary infection
	Chronic lung disease
Non-pulmonary	Intraventricular haemorrhage
	Patent ductus arteriosus

- Mechanical ventilation can cause acute lung injury.
- Over-ventilation (especially large volumes) is harmful and contributes to chronic lung disease.
- Oxygen should be used with care and a lower oxygen saturation limit set to minimize retinopathy of prematurity (ROP) and other adverse effects of hyperoxia.

Apnoeic attacks

Many small, preterm infants display 'periodic respiration' with some spells of very shallow breathing or complete cessation of breathing for up to 20 seconds. This reflects immaturity of the respiratory centre.

Apnoeic is defined as cessation of respirations for at least 20 seconds (10 seconds if associated with bradycardia). Predisposing factors include:

- Respiratory distress syndrome (RDS).
- Hypoxia.
- Sepsis – especially meningitis.
- Cranial pathology, especially haemorrhage.

The differential diagnosis includes seizures, which can mimic apnoeic attacks.

Apnoea alarms set to respond at an appropriate interval are useful for alerting staff to the need for action. Breathing will usually start again with physical stimulation. Caffeine is used in premature infants to prevent apnoeic episodes (and seems to improve neurodevelopmental outcome). Ventilatory support might be needed if severe.

Cardiovascular problems

Patent ductus arteriosus

A patent ductus arteriosus (PDA) is a common problem in preterm infants and is often associated with RDS. Failure of closure occurs because of gestational immaturity and hypoxia.

As the pulmonary vascular resistance falls, blood is shunted across the ductus from left to right. The clinical features are a widened pulse pressure with prominent peripheral pulses, tachycardia and a systolic murmur. This shunt often causes difficulty in weaning ventilated infants. Diagnosis is by echocardiography.

Management

Spontaneous closure may occur but treatment is used if the duct is causing significant problems (difficulty weaning ventilation, signs of heart failure, growth failure). Supportive management with fluid restriction and adequate oxygenation might be sufficient, but a prostaglandin inhibitor, such as ibuprofen, or indometacin may be effective, especially with early intervention. Surgical closure is occasionally required, especially in ventilator dependent infants.

Intracranial lesions

Preterm infants are at risk of:

- Intracranial haemorrhage: into the germinal matrix or ventricles.
- Ischaemia: of the periventricular white matter.

Risk factors for both include pneumothorax, asphyxia, hypovolaemia, hypotension and hypoxia in association with RDS. Hydrocephalus is a late complication of intracranial haemorrhage. Serial cranial ultrasounds are used to diagnose bleeds or ischaemia.

Gastrointestinal problems

Necrotizing enterocolitis

Necrotizing enterocolitis (NEC) is a necrosis of the intestine involving usually the distal ileum or proximal colon. The aetiology is uncertain but established predisposing factors include:

- Preterm birth.
- Intrauterine growth restriction (IUGR).
- Polycythaemia.
- PDA.
- Asphyxia.
- Early rapid enteral feeding with formula milk: early feeding with breast milk is protective.

Clinical features include abdominal distension, vomiting and bloody stools. Abdominal X-rays might show dilated, thick walled, static bowel loops, free air or intramural gas (a pathognomonic finding). Bowel perforation may occur in 20–30%. Mortality is high (up to 30%).

Fig. 28.13 Respiratory distress in term infants

Pulmonary
Transient tachypnoea of the newborn
Pneumonia
Pneumothorax
Meconium aspiration
Persistent fetal circulation
Milk aspiration
Diaphragmatic hernia
Non-pulmonary
Congenital heart disease
Severe anaemia
Metabolic acidosis

Management

This comprises:

- Large bore nasogastric tube (free drainage) and parenteral nutrition.
- Antibiotics: penicillin, gentamicin and metronidazole.
- In severe cases, surgical resection of the necrosed segment might be required.

Long-term sequelae and prognosis

Although the majority of preterm infants survive intact without sequelae, a number of significant problems can persist, especially in the very low-birthweight group. These include:

- Retinopathy of prematurity (retrolental fibroplasia).
- Chronic lung disease of prematurity (bronchopulmonary dysplasia).
- Neurodevelopmental problems.

Retinopathy of prematurity

This is a disorder occurring in premature infants whose retinas are incompletely vascularized at birth. There is abnormal vascular proliferation in response to insults including hyperoxia (but also hypotension and hypoxia). This may progress to fibrosis, retinal detachment and blindness.

All infants weighing less than 1500 g, or <32 weeks' gestational age or requiring significant respiratory or cardiovascular support should have their eyes screened 6–8 weeks after birth by indirect ophthalmoscopy until 36 weeks' corrected gestational age. Most cases resolve spontaneously but laser therapy might be indicated for severe disease.

Chronic lung disease of prematurity

Chronic lung disease (CLD) of prematurity or bronchopulmonary dysplasia is defined as requiring supplemental oxygen beyond 36 weeks' corrected gestation or 28 days of age, whichever is later. It occurs in newborns who, for any reason, require prolonged assisted ventilation with high pressures and high concentrations of oxygen. It is particularly common in very low-birthweight infants and positive pressure ventilation causing volutrauma, oxygen toxicity and inflammation (possibly secondary to infection) are all believed to contribute. The CXR shows widespread opacities with patchy translucent areas.

Management

- Respiratory support: assisted ventilation or continuous positive airways pressure and supplemental O_2 as needed, with efforts to minimize further damage.

- Dexamethasone is effective in weaning from ventilatory support but increases the risk of neurodevelopmental impairment, so is used only in severe cases.
- Strict attention to nutrition.
- Prophylaxis against respiratory syncytial virus (RSV).

Bronchiolitis, particularly due to RSV, is a major risk to infants with CLD; in recent years a monoclonal antibody (palivizumab) has been developed as prophylaxis and is recommended for vulnerable infants.

Complete recovery of lung function may occur as the child grows; however, a significant proportion of children will continue to have decreased lung function and increased incidence of asthma and respiratory infections.

Neurodevelopmental problems

The prospects for normal survival in preterm infants are good, especially for those weighing more than 1500 g at birth. However, very low-birthweight infants and those with a gestation period of under 28 weeks are at risk of a range of neurodevelopmental problems including:

- Cerebral palsy.
- Cognitive delay.
- Visual impairment.
- Hearing loss.
- Seizures.
- Behavioural problems.
- Educational difficulties.

A 24 week infant has around a 60% chance of survival, and only a 30% chance of survival without moderate to profound neurodisability. This improves with babies born later but all should have regular monitoring of developmental progression. Low-birthweight infants also show educational disadvantages into adulthood.

DISORDERS OF THE TERM INFANT

Respiratory disorders

Respiratory distress in term infants is characterized by:

- Tachypnoea.
- Cyanosis.
- Nasal flaring and recession.
- Expiratory grunting.

The causes are considered in Chapter 12 and are listed again in Fig. 28.13.

The pulmonary causes are considered in turn.

Transient tachypnoea of the newborn

This is caused by delay in reabsorption of fetal lung fluid and is more common after birth by caesarean section. There is early onset of mild to moderate respiratory distress and the CXR shows prominent pulmonary vasculature and fluid in the horizontal fissure. Treatment with increased ambient oxygen might be required. The condition usually settles spontaneously but antibiotic cover is given because infection cannot be ruled out in the early stages.

Pneumonia

Early onset, congenital pneumonia is acquired prenatally, especially when the membranes have been ruptured for more than 24 hours before the onset of labour. It is most commonly caused by the group B haemolytic streptococcus. Respiratory distress is the chief sign and the condition can mimic surfactant deficiency in preterm infants. Preterm infants with respiratory distress are therefore given antibiotics. Chlamydia should be suspected if there is concurrent purulent conjunctivitis.

Treatment

This comprises:

- Respiratory support with oxygen and ventilation if severe.
- Careful fluid balance and nutrition.
- Intravenous antibiotics.

Pneumothorax

A pneumothorax can occur spontaneously but is most commonly seen as a complication of positive pressure ventilation. Tension pneumothorax results in a sudden deterioration in the infant's condition manifested by cyanosis and hypotension. Diagnosis is confirmed by transillumination with a fibre-optic cold light source, or CXR. Urgent treatment by needle thoracostomy or insertion of a chest drain is indicated.

Chylothorax

This refers to the accumulation of lymphatic fluid in the pleural cavity and is usually iatrogenic, following surgery or birth trauma. Rarely, it may be due to a congenital abnormality of the lymphatic system or associated with various syndromes, e.g. trisomy 21. But most often, it is idiopathic and a cause is never found. It needs drainage using a percutaneous chest drain and often resolves subsequently. Dietary elimination of long chain fatty acids may hasten resolution.

Meconium aspiration

Passage of meconium into the amniotic fluid is triggered by fetal distress in term or post-term infants. The infant is at risk of inhaling meconium and developing meconium aspiration syndrome. This severe condition causes respiratory distress and cyanosis and has a high mortality rate. Suctioning of thick meconium from the trachea under direct vision after delivery is indicated if causing obstruction. However, most severe cases are probably due to antenatal aspiration in utero and cannot be prevented by suction at delivery.

Persistent pulmonary hypertension of the newborn

This condition is characterized by high pulmonary vascular resistance and is usually found in term or post-term infants. There is right-to-left shunting of blood at atrial and ductal levels with severe cyanosis. Persistent fetal circulation may be primary or secondary to birth asphyxia, meconium aspiration, respiratory distress syndrome or severe sepsis.

Raised pulmonary pressures on echocardiography are diagnostic (and excludes cyanotic congenital heart disease). A CXR shows a normal cardiac shadow and pulmonary oligaemia.

Management

Is mainly supportive and includes:

- Oxygenation.
- Assisted ventilation with sedation.
- Inhaled nitric oxide for pulmonary vasodilatation.
- Extracorporeal membrane oxygenation for severe cases.
- Sildenafil has shown promise in clinical trials as a potential treatment.

Milk aspiration

Aspiration of milk or stomach contents into the lungs may occur especially in:

- Preterm infants with RDS or neurological problems.
- Infants with chronic lung disease of prematurity.
- Infants with cleft palate.
- Infants with tracheo-oesophageal fistula.
- Reflux (see Chapter 18).

Diaphragmatic hernia

See Chapter 12. This congenital malformation:

- Occurs in 1 in 3000 live births.
- Is usually left-sided (80–85%).
- Is often diagnosed antenatally.
- Has a high mortality, despite surgery, due to coexisting pulmonary hypoplasia.

Gastrointestinal and hepatic disorders

Congenital anomalies of the gastrointestinal tract including cleft lip and palate, tracheo-oesophageal fistula,

duodenal stenosis or atresia, and exomphalos or gastroschisis are considered in Chapter 12.

Small bowel obstruction

This presents with:

- Persistent, bile-stained vomiting.
- Delayed or absent passage of meconium.
- Abdominal distension.

Important causes are listed in Fig. 28.14.

Diagnosis is made on clinical features and abdominal X-ray. Treatment depends on the cause and is often surgical. In the presence of meconium ileus it is important to exclude cystic fibrosis.

Large bowel obstruction

Hirschsprung's disease or rectal atresia can cause this.

Hirschsprung's disease

Congenital aganglionic megacolon, or Hirschsprung's disease, is a genetic disorder in which there is absence of ganglion cells from the myenteric and submyenteric plexuses of a segment of the large bowel (see Chapter 18).

Jaundice

Clinical jaundice appears in newborns when the serum bilirubin exceeds 80–120 µmol/L and is covered in Chapter 12. Identifying jaundice is vital as it may indicate underlying problems such as infection and early treatment can prevent bilirubin encephalopathy from deposition of unconjugated bilirubin in the brain.

Haematological disorders

Haemolytic diseases of the newborn are considered with jaundice.

Haemorrhagic disease of the newborn

This is caused by a relative deficiency of the vitamin-K-dependent coagulation factors II, VII, IX and X. It characteristically affects the fully breastfed infant between the third and sixth day of life, because breast milk does not contain adequate amounts of vitamin K. Mothers

Fig. 28.14 Causes of small bowel obstruction
Duodenal atresia
Midgut volvulus and malrotation
Gastroschisis and exomphalos
Meconium ileus

taking anticonvulsant drugs that interfere with vitamin K metabolism, such as phenytoin, are at increased risk.

Bleeding usually occurs from the gastrointestinal tract but can rarely be intracranial or from the umbilical stump.

A single intramuscular dose of vitamin K prevents this disease but three doses of oral vitamin K can also be given. It is important that all three doses are administered.

Neonatal abstinence syndrome

Neonatal abstinence syndrome (NAS) is a cluster of withdrawal symptoms that develop in babies of substance abusing mothers. This may be due to recreational drug abuse, e.g. heroin or in infants of mothers on a methadone programme.

Clinical features
This includes yawning, sweating, jitteriness and pyrexia. More severe symptoms include seizures or tremors, high pitched or inconsolable cry, projectile vomiting and watery diarrhoea.

Diagnosis
There is often a history of maternal drug abuse; this should be confirmed by urine toxicology in both mother and infant. Scoring charts are used to monitor infants at risk and dictate management. These babies are also at high risk of other diseases like hepatitis B, C and HIV, so the mother's serology should be checked.

Management
If withdrawal scores are high treatment is initiated with oral morphine and gradually weaned over the next few days to weeks. It is also important to evaluate the social situation and liaise with drug and alcohol services, social services and the health visitor.

Infections

The newborn infant is vulnerable to infection by bacteria, viruses and fungi. In utero, infection can take place across the placenta or by ascending the birth canal.

After birth, the skin and umbilicus are colonized by staphylococci, the gut by *Escherichia coli* and the upper respiratory tract by streptococci. Important bacterial pathogens in the neonate include:

- Group B β-haemolytic streptococci (GBS).
- *E. coli.*
- *Staphylococcus epidermidis:* a particularly important causes of line sepsis in preterm babies on intensive care.

The range of acquired infections in the newborn is shown in Fig. 28.15.

Fig. 28.15 Acquired infections in the newborn

Minor infections
Skin pustules
Paronychia
Acute mastitis
Conjunctivitis
Thrush
Major infections
Septicaemia
Meningitis
Pneumonia
Urinary tract infection
Ophthalmia neonatorum

Minor infections

Skin pustules and paronychia
These are caused by staphylococcal infection and typically occur in moist areas such as the groin and axillae. Inflammation of the skin in the area of a nail fold might evolve into a pustular lesion. Treatment with oral flucloxacillin is indicated in severe cases but most resolve spontaneously.

Acute mastitis
This is an inflamed swelling under the nipple in a febrile infant. It is usually caused by *Staphylococcus aureus* infection in an engorged neonatal breast. Flucloxacillin is the antibiotic of choice.

Conjunctivitis
A 'sticky eye' in the first day or two of life is often due to chemical irritation and clears spontaneously. Conjunctivitis with a purulent discharge might be due to:

- Staphylococci, streptococci, *E. coli.*
- Gonococci: ophthalmia neonatorum (see below) – usually between days 2 and 5 of life.
- *Chlamydia trachomatis:* usually between days 7 and 10 of life.

Gonococcal and chlamydial infections are notifiable diseases and need systemic antibiotic treatment because the risk of scarring and blindness is high. Erythromycin or a cephalosporin is used and ophthalmological review is mandatory. It is also important to treat the parents.

Thrush (moniliasis)
Infection with *Candida albicans* can affect the mouth or nappy area. Oral thrush appears as white plaques on the tongue and inside of the mouth. Nystatin suspension 1 mL (100 000 units) after feeds for 7–10 days is usually effective. Perineal thrush responds to topical nystatin.

Major infections

Septicaemia

Neonatal sepsis carries a high mortality and morbidity and can be rapid and fulminant. As signs are non-specific (Fig. 28.16), a low threshold for investigation and empirical treatment with antibiotics is needed. As this results in a high number of treated infants, to reduce unnecessary antibiotic usage antibiotics are stopped after 48 hours if cultures are negative (the incidence of false negative blood cultures is lower in neonates than adults).

The incidence of serious acute infections in the newborn period is about 3 per 1000 live births in the UK.

Initial presentation is often non-specific and outlined in Fig. 28.16.

Specific signs relating to a site of infection may then emerge. These include:

- Tense fontanelle, seizures: meningitis.
- Respiratory distress: pneumonia.

Group B streptococcal infection

About 20–30% of pregnant women are colonized with group B streptococcus, which, although asymptomatic in the woman, may cause sepsis in the neonate with high morbidity and mortality. It may present early (within the first week) or late (after the first week). Early disease is associated with a worse outcome but can be reduced with preventive measures (including antepartum treatment of mothers, careful observation and early treatment of neonates particularly at risk).

Diagnosis   If systemic infection is suspected, prompt investigation is essential. The following investigations are performed to confirm the diagnosis and identify a causative organism.

- 'Septic' screen: blood, urine and cerebrospinal fluid (CSF) cultures (including CSF gram staining) with or without CXR.
- Rapid antigen testing on blood and CSF.

Treatment   Group B streptococcal (GBS) infection is usually sensitive to penicillin and aminoglycosides (e.g. gentamicin) are added for additional synergistic effects.

Fig. 28.16   Signs suggestive of neonatal infection

Irritability or lethargy
Persistent tachycardia
Tachypnoea or grunting
Frequent apnoeas or bradycardias and desaturations
Poor response to handling
Acute onset of pallor
Temperature instability
Feeding intolerance

Meningitis

Neonatal meningitis is usually due to a different range of pathogens from that in the older infant or child. In infants, the infective organisms include:

- Group B streptococci.
- *E. coli.*
- *Listeria monocytogenes.*

Meningeal infection usually follows septicaemia. Clinical features include poor feeding, irritability and temperature instability. Fullness of the anterior fontanelle and fits are late signs.

Diagnosis   Lumbar puncture is required to confirm the diagnosis.

Treatment and outcome   High-dose intravenous antibiotics for 14–21 days are required. Penetration of drugs occurs through the inflamed meninges. Mortality has reduced from around 30–60% to 10% but morbidity remains unchanged with a high incidence of neurological impairment in survivors.

Pneumonia

This is most commonly due to the group B streptococcus. Respiratory distress is the chief presenting sign together with features of septicaemia.

Urinary tract infection

The most common pathogen is *Escherichia coli*, with other Gram-negative organisms occasionally responsible. There is a relatively high incidence of underlying congenital anomalies or vesicoureteric reflux.

Symptoms and signs are usually non-specific. Urine must be cultured in all infants with poor feeding, lethargy, vomiting, failure to thrive and jaundice.

Urine is obtained by clean catch for microscopy and culture; any bacteriuria or pyuria is considered diagnostic of urinary tract infection (UTI).

IV antibiotics are used for treatment; imaging is needed (see Chapter 19 for details).

Further reading

Wood, N.S., Marlow, N., Costeloe, K., et al., for the EPICure Study Group, 2000. Neurological and developmental disability after extremely preterm birth. N. Engl. J. Med. 343, 378–384.

Resch, B., 2011. The challenge of early diagnosis of bacterial infection in neonates. Journal of Neonatal Biology 1, e101. http://dx.doi.org/10.4172/jnb.1000e101.

Azzopardi, D., Brocklehurst, P., Edwards, D., et al., for the TOBY Study Group, 2008. The TOBY Study. Whole body hypothermia for the treatment of perinatal asphyxial encephalopathy: a randomised controlled trial. BMC Pediatr. 8, 17.

Reducing mother to child transmission of HIV infection in the United Kingdom. Update Report of an Intercollegiate Working Party. July 2006. Royal College of Paediatrics and Child Health.

NICHD Neonatal Research Network (NRN): Extremely preterm birth outcome data. http://www.nichd.nih.gov/about/org/cdbpm/pp/prog_epbo/epbo_case.cfm.

Accidents and emergencies 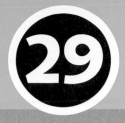 29

ACCIDENTS

Accidents in children are extremely common and are the leading cause of death between the ages of 1 and 14 years. The pattern of accidents varies with age (Fig. 29.1). Road traffic accidents account for the majority of fatal accidents (Fig. 29.2). Child abuse needs to be considered in any child presenting with injury.

Trauma

Physical trauma causing multiple serious injuries is an important cause of death. Early, appropriate management of the multiply injured child is vital to reduce mortality and long-term morbidity. Injuries to the head are the most important class of local injury.

Major trauma

Initial assessment and management is described in Fig. 29.3. Events during the first 'golden hour' determine the outcome. Once the initial steps of immediate resuscitation have been carried out, a careful secondary survey of the complete child must be undertaken to detect and treat all injuries (Fig. 29.4).

Head injury

Minor head injuries in children are very common and most children recover without ill effect. A small minority, about 1 in 800 of those admitted, develops serious complications such as intracranial haemorrhage. Causes of head injury include:
- Road traffic accidents (RTAs): the most common cause of severe and fatal head injuries.
- Falls from trees, windows, bicycles, etc.
- Child abuse: especially 'shaking' injuries in infants.

Damage to the brain might be primary or secondary (Fig. 29.5).

The history should establish:
- The mechanism of injury.
- Was consciousness lost?
- Subsequent symptoms: vomiting, drowsiness, seizures, bleeding from nose or ears.
- Anterograde amnesia >5 minutes.

Clinical features

Clinical examination should look for the following signs:
- Head: external injury including haematoma, laceration, depressed fracture. In babies, the anterior fontanelle tension provides a useful indicator of intracranial pressure. Look for blood or cerebrospinal fluid leak from the ears or nose.
- Central nervous system: assess Glasgow Coma Scale/AVPU scale, fundi and pupillary reflexes. Examine for focal neurological signs.
- General: full examination to exclude other injuries.

Diagnosis

Investigations include:
- Cranial computed tomography (CT): (see Fig. 29.6: NICE Guideline CG56 2007). If the CT scan is normal but the infant or child remains unwell or symptomatic, then discharge should be delayed with a low threshold for admission and observation.
- Skull X-ray: not routinely indicated, useful only if non-accidental injury is suspected.

Minor and moderate injuries

These are the majority. Admit to hospital for observation if:
- History of seizure or loss of consciousness.
- Declining level of consciousness.

Fig. 29.1 Accidents in childhood

Toddlers are prone to:
Falls
Scalds
Drowning
Accidental ingestion
Choking

School-age children are prone to:
Falls while climbing
Road traffic accidents

Fig. 29.2 Causes of death in childhood

	Causes of fatal accidents
Age range	**Leading cause of death (highest at top)**
4–52 weeks	Congenital abnormalities Sudden unexpected death in infancy Infection
1–4 years	Trauma Congenital abnormalities Cancer Infection
5–14 years	Trauma Cancer Congenital abnormality Infection

- Severe headache or persistent vomiting.
- Skull fracture.
- Suspected non-accidental injury.
- Child has a bleeding tendency.
- Supervision at home is inadequate.

If the child is well enough to be discharged, the parents should be given written instructions to bring the child back if there is severe headache, recurrent vomiting or a declining level of consciousness.

If admitted, neurological observations should be made at intervals dictated by the child's clinical state and existing guidelines. In all cases of head injury particular attention should be paid to analgesic control and titrated according to the child's response.

HINTS AND TIPS

Non-accidental injury should be suspected if:
- The mechanism of injury or history is incompatible with the infant or child's stage of development.
- The injury does not fit with the mechanism offered.
- Inappropriate care or concern by the parent/carer or delay in presentation.

Severe injuries

These usually occur in the context of multiple major trauma requiring intensive care.

Additional measures in severe head injury are directed towards the management of complications such as raised intracranial pressure, intracranial bleeding, seizures and risk of infection.

Urgent referral to a neurosurgeon is indicated if there is any evidence of an expanding haematoma, such as:

- Declining level of consciousness.
- Focal neurological signs.
- Depressed skull fracture.
- Signs of rising intracranial pressure: bradycardia, rise in systolic blood pressure and irregular respirations.

Burns and scalds

Scalds from contact with hot liquids are the most common form of thermal trauma in childhood (most of the fatalities are from house fires but those are due to gas and smoke inhalation rather than burns). Burns and scalds can be non-accidental. Toddlers are most at risk of accidental scalds.

Assessment

The extent, depth and distribution of the injury should be estimated (Figs 29.7 and 29.8 and see Hints and tips box).

HINTS AND TIPS

- Electrical burns are usually full thickness.
- Most scalds are deep, partial thickness.

Diagnosis

Investigations should include:

- Full blood count: packed cell volume may be increased with significant hypovolaemia.
- Urea and electrolytes.
- Group and save (if burns are greater than 15–20).
- Serum albumin.

HINTS AND TIPS

Location of the burn is important, as well as extent:
- Face – potential airway involvement, scarring.
- Hands – contractures and functional loss.
- Genitalia – difficult to nurse, risk of infection.

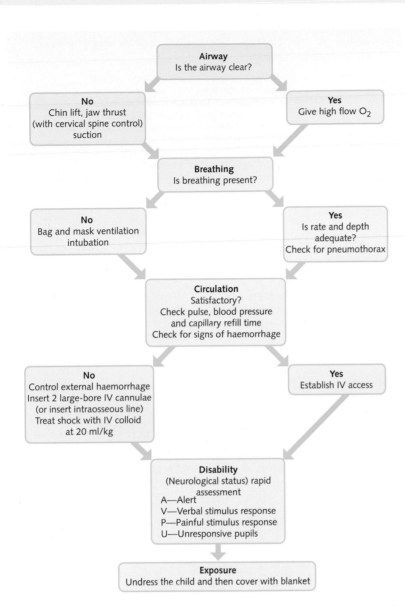

Fig. 29.3 Major trauma. Initial assessment and management – A, B, C, D and E

Airway
Is the airway clear?

No
Chin lift, jaw thrust
(with cervical spine control)
suction

Yes
Give high flow O$_2$

Breathing
Is breathing present?

No
Bag and mask ventilation
intubation

Yes
Is rate and depth
adequate?
Check for pneumothorax

Circulation
Satisfactory?
Check pulse, blood pressure
and capillary refill time
Check for signs of haemorrhage

No
Control external haemorrhage
Insert 2 large-bore IV cannulae
(or insert intraosseous line)
Treat shock with IV colloid
at 20 ml/kg

Yes
Establish IV access

Disability
(Neurological status) rapid
assessment
A—Alert
V—Verbal stimulus response
P—Painful stimulus response
U—Unresponsive pupils

Exposure
Undress the child and then cover with blanket

Management

Recommended first aid is:

- Run cold water over the affected part for 5 minutes.

Admit to burns centre if:

- The extent is over 5% full thickness or over 10% partial thickness.
- A difficult area is involved, e.g. face, hands and feet, perineum or genitalia.
- There is any inhalational injury, e.g. smoke inhalation.
- Chemical or circumferential burns.

The important aspects of management are shown in Fig. 29.9.

Non-accidental injury consideration in burns and scalds

Non-accidental injury (NAI) should be suspected when dealing with cases of burns and scalds if any of the following are present:

- A 'glove and sock' distribution of burns (suggestive of an immersion injury).
- Delay in presentation.

Fig. 29.4 Secondary survey and treatment – multiple trauma

Head	Examine for bruising, lacerations, CSF leak from ears or nose. Mini neurological exam
Face	Look for bruising, fractures and loose teeth
Neck	Cervical spine stabilization. Examine for bony tenderness, bruising or wounds
Chest	Look for wounds, bruising. Feel trachea and auscultate breath and heart sounds
Abdomen	Observe movement, bruising and palpate for tenderness. PR not routinely indicated in children
Pelvis	Inspect perineum and for bony deformity. Look for blood at urethral meatus
Spine	Done by log-rolling: look for swelling, palpate vertebrae and assess motor and sensory function
Extremities	Assess movement, deformity, bruising and tenderness. Test sensation and peripheral circulation
Radiological investigations as necessary and a full history	

Fig. 29.5 Brain damage in head injury

Primary damage	Cerebral laceration and contusion Diffuse axonal injury Dural sac tears
Secondary damage	Ischaemia from shock, hypoxia or raised intracranial pressure Hypoglycaemia CNS infection Seizures Hyperthermia

- Burns or scalds to the buttocks or perineum.
- Other social concerns in the family.

Near drowning

Drowning is more common in boys than girls. It is the third most common cause of childhood accidental death in the UK. In the UK, drowning incidents are more common in freshwater canals and lakes, swimming pools and domestic baths than in the sea.

Fig. 29.6 Indication for immediate head CT in head injuries

Witnessed loss of consciousness >5 min
Three or more vomits
GCS less than 15 (GCS <14 if an infant)
Focal neurological signs or post-traumatic seizures
Clinical features of basal skull fracture or open/depressed skull fracture
Anterograde or retrograde amnesia
Suspicion of non-accidental injury
Dangerous mechanism of injury (e.g. RTA at high speed)

Fig. 29.7 Assessment of the depth of burn

Superficial	Partial thickness	Full thickness
• Red • No blisters • Affects only epithelial layer	• Pink or mottled • Blisters • Some dermal damage	• Painless • White or charred • Full dermal and nerve damage

The two principal problems in near drowning are:

- Hypoxia: laryngospasm results in asphyxia. Only a small amount of water initially enters the lungs.
- Hypothermia: this leads to bradycardia and asystole (extreme hypothermia can be protective).

Haemolysis or electrolyte problems caused by the ingestion or inhalation of large amounts of water can occur.

Management

Skilled resuscitation and warming is vital. Cervical injury should be assumed. All children should be hospitalized for at least 24 hours. Patients admitted in asystole or respiratory arrest should undergo cardiopulmonary resuscitation in the normal way. Resuscitation must be continued until the core temperature has been raised to above 32°C because many arrhythmias are refractory at temperatures below 30°C.

Prognostic indicators of near drowning

The prognostic indicators are shown in Fig. 29.10.

Late respiratory sequelae can occur in the 72-hour period after near drowning. These include pneumonia and pulmonary oedema.

Poisoning

Most cases of poisoning in young children follow accidental ingestion by an inquisitive toddler; in adolescents most poisoning is deliberate self-harm. Children

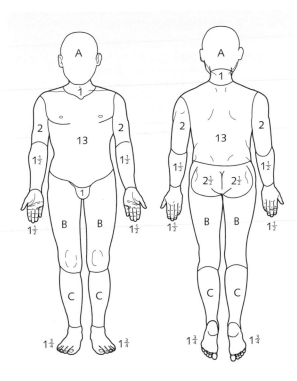

Fig. 29.10	Prognostic indicators for near drowning	
Prognostic indicators	**Poor if:**
Immersion time	Submerged for >10 min
Time to first respiratory effort	No respiratory effort within 3 min
Rectal temperature	<33°C on arrival
Conscious level	Persisting coma
Arterial blood pH	7.0 despite treatment
Arterial blood O_2	<8.0 kPa despite treatment
Type of water	No difference on prognosis

can also be poisoned deliberately by their parents (or inadvertently by their doctors). Although many thousands of children attend hospital each year, very few die as a result of accidental ingestion.

The history should establish:

- What was ingested: identify from carton or bottle.
- Amount ingested: usually an approximation.
- Time ingested: important in relation to management.

The toxicity of the ingested substance can then be assessed (Fig. 29.11) or the Regional Poisons Information Centre contacted if there is any doubt concerning the agent's identity or toxicity.

Clinical features

Examination should include the following:

- Inspect oropharynx and any vomitus.
- Assess level of consciousness.

Area indicated	Surface area at			
	1 year	5 years	10 years	15 years
A	8.5	6.5	5.5	4.5
B	3.25	4.0	4.5	4.5
C	2.5	2.75	3.0	3.25

Fig. 29.8 Assessment of the extent of a burn. The percentage body surface area affected is calculated from this standard body diagram. Note that the area corresponding to head and lower limbs (A, B, C) changes with age. The small child has a relatively big head and short legs

Fig. 29.9	Management of burns
Analgesia	Simple analgesia with escalation of the 'pain ladder' as required
IV fluids	Treat shock with 20 mL/kg If >10% burn will need IV fluids: Normal fluid requirements with additional fluids at: % burn × weight (kg) × 4 per day (half of this given within 8 h) Keep urine output >1 mL/kg/h
Wound care	Sterile towels and avoid excessive re-examination

Fig. 29.11	Poison-specific adverse effects and treatments	
Poison	**Adverse effects**	**Specific treatment**
Iron	Shock, gut haemorrhage	IV desferrioxamine
Paracetamol	Liver failure	IV *N*-acetylcysteine
Salicylates	Metabolic acidosis	Alkalinization of urine with bicarbonate
Ethylene glycol Tricyclic antidepressants	Widespread cellular damage Cardiac dysrhythmias	Ethanol, dialysis if severe Alkalinization of urine with bicarbonate Anti-arrythmics as guided by poisons centre
Ecstasy	Hyperpyrexia and rhabdomyolysis Dysrhythmias	Active cooling Benzodiazepines, e.g. diazepam, to control anxiety

- Look for features specific to various poisons, e.g. small pupils (opiates or barbiturates), tachypnoea (salicylate poisoning) or cardiac arrhythmias (tricyclic antidepressants or digoxin).

Diagnosis

Relevant investigations include:

- Blood levels (at optimum time after ingestion) can be measured for salicylates, paracetamol, digoxin, iron, lithium and tricyclic antidepressants.
- Take a urine specimen for analysis.

Management

If the agent ingested was relatively innocuous the patient can be allowed home after a period of observation. Efforts should be made to remove the poison if there has been a large ingestion of a highly toxic substance. These include:

- Activated charcoal: give 1 g/kg, if necessary by nasogastric tube. It binds a wide range of toxic drugs, with the exception of iron and lithium. It is most efficacious if used within 1 hour of ingestion.

Specific treatment is indicated for certain drugs and toxins (see Fig. 29.11).

Deliberate self-poisoning in older children

This is a serious occurrence that may reflect a significant underlying psychiatric disorder such as depression. In most cases, there is no serious suicidal intent. All children who deliberately poison themselves should be admitted to hospital and assessed by a psychologist or psychiatrist with appropriate follow-up planned prior to discharge.

EMERGENCIES

Children differ from adults in important ways that are relevant to emergency care (Fig. 29.12).

The seriously ill child

A seriously ill child is on one of the pathways leading to cardiopulmonary arrest (Fig. 29.13). Such arrests in children are rarely unheralded but preceded by a period of progressive circulatory, respiratory or central neurological failure. It is vital to recognize such a critically ill child and intervene to prevent the progression to cardiac arrest.

Fig. 29.12 Anatomical and physiological characteristics of young children

Anatomy	Airway Large surface area to volume ratio Small airways and elastic ribs Obligate nasal breathers until 5 months old
Physiology	Increased oxygen consumption and metabolic rate Compliant chest wall: leading to airways collapse Inefficient respiratory muscles Low stroke volume: cardiac output dependent on heart rate

Rapid assessment

An initial ABCD assessment should be carried out to identify features of:

- Airway and breathing: airway obstruction and hypoxia.
- Circulation: shock.
- Disability.

Airway and breathing

A critical state is indicated either by:

- An increase in the work of breathing (respiratory distress).
- Absent or decreased respiratory effort (exhaustion or respiratory depression).

Key signs include (Fig. 29.14):

- Efficacy of breathing.
- Effort of breathing.

Circulation

Signs of potential circulatory failure (shock) include:

- Tachycardia.
- Pulse volume reduction: absent peripheral pulses and weak central pulses are serious signs of advanced shock.
- Capillary refill time of over 2 seconds.
- Blood pressure: hypotension is a late and preterminal sign of circulatory failure.

The effects of circulatory failure encompass:

- Metabolic acidosis with increased respiratory rate.
- Skin: mottled, cold, pale skin peripherally.
- Mental state: agitation followed by drowsiness due to reduced cerebral perfusion.
- Urine output: oliguria due to renal hypoperfusion.

HINTS AND TIPS

Always reassess airway, breathing and circulation (ABC) if the child's condition changes.

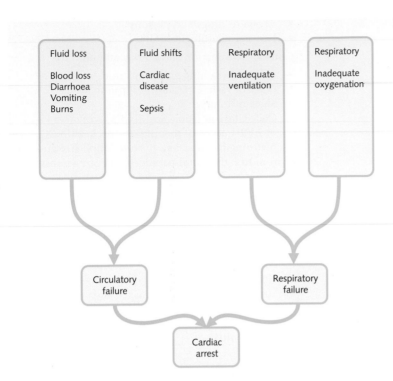

Fig. 29.13 The critically ill child: pathways to cardiopulmonary arrest

Fig. 29.14	Respiratory assessment
Effort of breathing	Respiratory rate Inspiratory or expiratory noises Grunting Use of accessory muscles Nasal flaring Recession (intercostal and subcostal)
Efficacy of air entry	Presence of breath sounds Pulse oximetry
Adequacy of oxygenation	Heart rate Skin colour Mental status

Disability

Concerning signs include:

- Level of consciousness: reduced or falling (see Hints and tips box).
- Posture: most are hypotonic; seizures reflect brain dysfunction.
- Pupils: most sinister signs are dilatation, unreactivity and inequality.

Neurological failure has important effects on both respiration and circulation:

- Respiratory depression.
- Abnormal respiratory patterns.

- Systemic hypertension with sinus bradycardia (Cushing's response) indicates herniation of the cerebellar tonsils through the foramen magnum.

Cardiorespiratory arrest

A standard procedure exists for applying basic life support in the event of a cardiorespiratory arrest (Figs 29.15–29.20). In addition, there are also protocols for the various peri-arrest cardiac arrhythmias.

> **HINTS AND TIPS**
>
> Hypoxia is the cause of the majority of arrests and a primary cardiac cause is rare.

After basic life support procedures, it might be necessary to proceed to:

- Intubation and ventilation.
- Circulatory access: venous or intraosseous.
- ECG monitoring: to identify the rhythm, asystole is most common. The protocol for drug use in asystole is shown in Fig. 29.17.

> **HINTS AND TIPS**
>
> Asystole is the most common arrest rhythm in children.

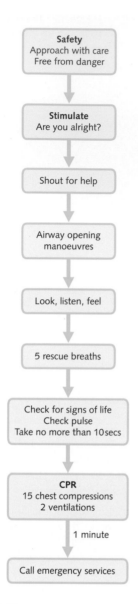

Fig. 29.15 Basic life support

Neurological emergencies

Coma

There are many causes of a reduced conscious level. Evaluation is done by the Glasgow Coma Scale or AVPU (see Chapter 8). Some are self-evident but others might be identified only after careful clinical evaluation and special investigations.

Assessment

A focused history should include information about:

- Chronic medical conditions such as epilepsy and diabetes mellitus.

- Access to drugs and poisons.
- Normal neurological state.

Clinical examination should pay attention to:

- Airway, breathing and circulation.
- Fever or rash: especially a purpuric rash.
- Signs of injury.
- CNS: Glasgow Coma Scale (GCS) score (see Fig. 5.5) or AVPU, signs of meningism (neck stiffness), focal neurological signs and posture, pupil size and reaction to light, fundi-papilloedema or haemorrhages.

Diagnosis

Investigations are determined by the clinical evaluation and may include:

- Blood analysis for glucose, urea, electrolytes, full blood count and acid–base balance.
- Group and save sample for transfusion.
- Urine for toxins.
- Lumbar puncture for suspected meningitis (exclude raised intracranial pressure prior to lumbar puncture).
- Brain imaging: cranial CT or magnetic resonance imaging (MRI).

> **HINTS AND TIPS**
>
> Check blood sugar in a comatose or convulsing child to identify treatable hypoglycaemia as hypoglycaemia is an important cause of both. Recognition and treatment is simple. If missed, brain damage can result.

Management

Initial management should be directed towards identifying and correcting problems with the airway, breathing and circulation. Further specific treatment depends on aetiology. All children with a GCS <8 or P on the AVPU scale need airway protection with endotracheal intubation.

Secondary brain damage is minimized by maintaining oxygenation and perfusion.

Convulsions

The causes of a seizure vary with age (Fig. 29.20). The most common cause in young children is a 'febrile convulsion' (see Chapter 20).

A continuous seizure lasting more than 30 minutes, or repeated seizures without recovery of consciousness between attacks, is called 'convulsive status epilepticus' (CSE).

Prolonged seizures can result in brain damage or death from hypoxia. Cerebral blood flow and oxygen consumption increase five-fold to meet the extra metabolic demand. Oxygen delivery to the brain will be impaired if there is inadequate ventilation or hypotension.

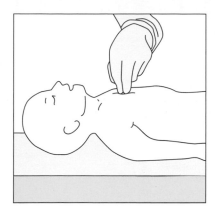

A Infant chest compression: Two finger technique

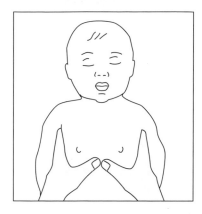

B Infant chest compression: Hand-encircling technique

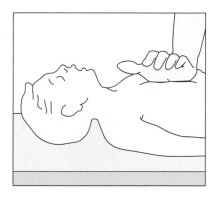

C Chest compression in small children

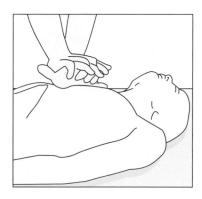

D Chest compression in older children

Fig. 29.16   Cardiac compression techniques

History

- Duration of seizure and any medications administered.
- History of recent trauma.
- Known epileptic? If so, medication regimen.
- Preceding illness or relevant past medical history.

Examination

- Cardiorespiratory status.
- Signs of head trauma.
- Fever, petechial rash, meningism.
- Nature of convulsion: generalized or focal.

Management

An algorithm for management of the convulsing child is shown in Fig. 29.21. While initiating emergency management, establish the history and examine the child. If the seizure persists for longer than 5 minutes then give anticonvulsants. No more than two doses of benzodiazepine should be given due to the risk of respiratory depression.

If benzodiazepines fail to stop the seizure, further options include, in order:

1. Paraldehyde: rectal administration as 10% solution 1 mL/year of age. Safe and usually effective within 5 minutes.
2. Summon senior anaesthetic help.
3. IV phenytoin: give as an infusion under ECG and blood pressure monitoring.

Status epilepticus (convulsive)

Protracted convulsions (of over 30 minutes) can occur in:

- Epilepsy.
- Febrile convulsion.

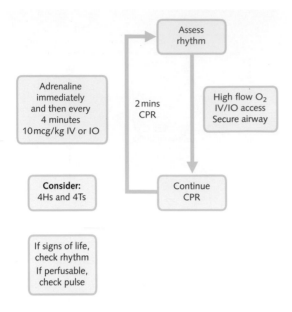

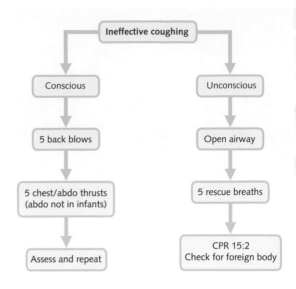

Fig. 29.19 Protocol for the choking child

Fig. 29.17 Protocol for drug use in asystole and pulseless electrical activity

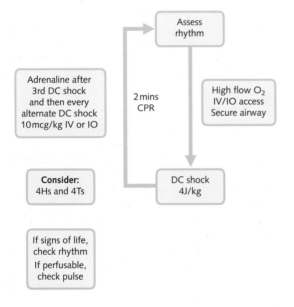

Fig. 29.20	Causes of convulsions
Age	**Causes**
All ages	Hypoglycaemia Head injury Poisoning Meningitis Epilepsy
Birth to 6 months	Hypoglycaemia Hypocalcaemia Inborn errors of metabolism Meningitis
6 months to 5 years	Febrile convulsion Meningitis
>5 years	Epilepsy (most common cause)

Fig. 29.18 Protocol for ventricular fibrillation and ventricular tachycardia

- Head injury.
- Intracranial infection: meningitis or encephalitis.
- Metabolic seizures: hypoglycaemia or poisoning.

Cardiac emergencies

Cardiac emergencies in children occur more commonly than previously thought, although hypoxia still predominates as a cause of cardiorespiratory arrest. The causes and management of heart failure are considered elsewhere (see Chapter 5), as is the management of circulatory failure (shock) and cardiac arrest. Cardiac arrhythmias, uncommon but treatable conditions in childhood, are considered in Chapter 16.

Respiratory emergencies

The pattern of severe respiratory illness in children is determined by features of the anatomy and physiology of their respiratory system, including:

- Small airways: easily obstructed with rapid increase in airways resistance.

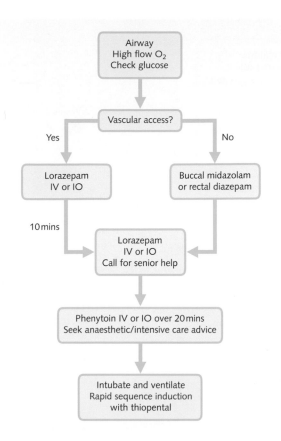

Airway
High flow O_2
Check glucose

Vascular access?

Yes

No

Lorazepam
IV or IO

Buccal midazolam
or rectal diazepam

10 mins

Lorazepam
IV or IO
Call for senior help

Phenytoin IV or IO over 20 mins
Seek anaesthetic/intensive care advice

Intubate and ventilate
Rapid sequence induction
with thiopental

Fig. 29.21 The convulsing child

- Compliant thoracic cage: reduced breathing efficiency.
- Respiratory muscles fatigue more quickly.
- Susceptibility to infection.

HINTS AND TIPS

Not all respiratory distress has a respiratory cause:
- Metabolic acidosis causes deep, rapid breathing.
- Heart failure is associated with tachypnoea.

The illnesses most commonly presenting as emergencies are:

- Upper airway obstruction: croup, acute epiglottitis.
- Lower airway obstruction: asthma, bronchiolitis.
- Pneumonia.

Upper airways obstruction

The cardinal sign of upper airway obstruction is stridor. This is a noise associated with breathing and due to obstruction of the extrathoracic airway. It tends to be worse on inspiration but may also be biphasic.

Fig. 29.22 Features of severe upper airway obstruction
Clinical features
Exhaustion
Decreased conscious level
Poor air entry on auscultation
Tachycardia
Cyanosis
Chest wall recession

The important common causes of acute stridor are:

- Croup: acute laryngotracheobronchitis.
- Inhaled foreign body.
- Epiglottitis and bacterial tracheitis.

Features suggesting severe upper airway obstruction are shown in Fig. 29.22. Epiglottitis has become uncommon since the introduction of Hib vaccination. It is very important NOT to examine the child's throat when suspecting upper airways obstruction.

Croup

This is dealt with in detail in Chapter 17. The key principles of its acute management include:

- Gentle, confident handling.
- Monitoring of O_2 saturation and heart rate.
- O_2 therapy.
- Nebulized budesonide or oral dexamethasone.
- Nebulized adrenaline (epinephrine): gives transient relief of severe obstruction and helps to buy time for the steroids to work or for intubation if needed.

Acute epiglottitis

This is dealt with in Chapter 17. The principles of management of acute epiglottitis include:

- Call for help – paediatric team, senior anaesthetist, ear, nose and throat (ENT) surgeon.
- Any distress to the child – examination, venepuncture, etc. can further compromise the airway and should be deferred until full support is available.
- Arrange examination under anaesthesia.
- Once the diagnosis is confirmed, secure the airway by endotracheal intubation; take blood cultures and start intravenous antibiotics (e.g. ceftriaxone).

Lower airways obstruction

Acute asthma

An algorithm for the management of acute asthma is given in Fig. 29.23. Features of life-threatening asthma are shown in Fig. 29.24.

β_2 Bronchodilators, steroids and oxygen are the mainstays of treatment of acute asthma:

- Inhaled bronchodilator therapy given by spacer is as effective as nebulized bronchodilators, although in severe cases it is given by nebulizer due to ease of giving O_2.

Fig. 29.23 Management of acute severe asthma

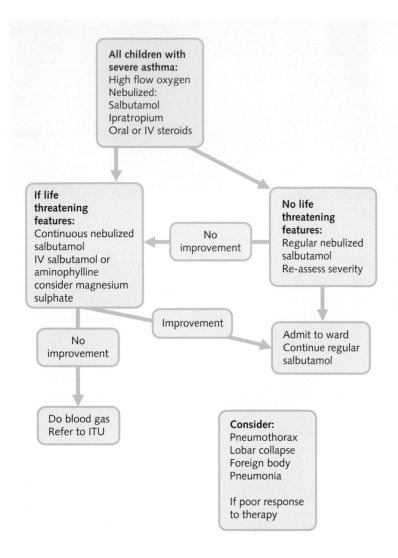

Fig. 29.24 Clinical features of life-threatening asthma

Decreased conscious level
Exhaustion or agitation
Poor respiratory effort
Silent chest
Oxygen saturation <85% in air
Peak-expiratory flow rate (PEFR) <33% of predicted

- Short course (3–4 days) oral steroids can reduce the severity of the attack and should be given early as they take up to 6 hours to act. If the child cannot take oral steroids or is vomiting, intravenous hydrocortisone can be given.
- If the child does not respond adequately to appropriate doses of inhaled bronchodilators, then

intravenous salbutamol, magnesium sulphate or aminophylline can be used.
- Nebulized bronchodilators can cause hypokalaemia, sinus tachycardia and feelings of anxiety.
- If intravenous fluids are required it should be restricted to two-thirds of normal requirement as there is often excess ADH secretion.

Occasionally intubation and ventilation is required and should be managed by a senior anaesthetist.

Bronchiolitis

This is the commonest serious respiratory infection in infancy, characterized by tachypnoea (rate >60), crackles, wheeze and/or recurrent apnoea. Hypoxia may occur requiring oxygen therapy. The management is mainly supportive and involves:

- Monitoring O_2 saturation, respiratory rate and heart rate.
- Humidified O_2 by headbox or nasal cannulae to maintain O_2 saturation above 92%. Continuous positive airway pressure (CPAP) may be indicated for worsening respiratory distress with carbon dioxide retention followed by ventilation if there is no improvement or deterioration on CPAP.
- Maintaining adequate fluid and nutrition intake by giving nasogastric or intravenous fluids.

Antibiotics may be warranted if there is clinical evidence of infection.

Shock (circulatory failure)

Shock is a clinical syndrome resulting from acute failure of circulatory function leading to poor tissue perfusion. It tends to progress through three phases (Fig. 29.25):

- Compensated.
- Uncompensated.
- Irreversible.

The two common causes of shock are hypovolaemia and septicaemia (Fig. 29.26).

Clinical features

A brief history might identify the cause. The early physical signs of shock include:

- Pallor: due to vasoconstriction.
- Tachycardia with reduced pulse volume.
- Poor skin perfusion: capillary refill time >2 seconds, core/toe temperature difference of >2°C.

The late physical signs include:

- Rapid deep breathing: response to metabolic acidosis.

Fig. 29.25 Three phases of shock

Phase	Clinicopathological features
Compensated shock	Vital organ function (brain, heart) is preserved by sympathetic response Pallor, tachycardia, cold periphery, poor capillary return but systolic blood pressure is maintained
Decompensated shock	Inadequate perfusion leads to anaerobic metabolism, metabolic acidosis, and, on occasion, a bleeding diathesis. Blood pressure falls, acidotic breathing, very slow capillary return, altered consciousness, anuria
Irreversible shock	A retrospective diagnosis. Damage to heart and brain irreversible, with no improvement even if circulation is restored

Fig. 29.26 Causes of shock

Mechanism	Causes
Hypovolaemia	Fluid loss • Haemorrhage • Burns • Diarrhoea and vomiting • Diabetic ketoacidosis Fluid shifts • Septicaemia • Anaphylaxis • Peritonitis
Cardiogenic	Arrhythmias Heart failure

- Agitation, confusion: due to brain hypoperfusion.
- Oliguria: urine flow less than 2 mL/kg/h in infants and 1 mL/kg/h in children.
- Hypotension.

Management of shock: general

(See algorithm Fig. 29.27.) If there is no rapid improvement or if there is evidence of organ failure, transfer to an intensive care unit for assisted ventilation, intensive monitoring and inotropic support.

> **HINTS AND TIPS**
>
> Poor capillary refill should not be used in isolation to diagnose shock. The clinician must look at heart rate, blood pressure, base excess and clinical signs of organ perfusion, e.g. conscious level and urine output.

Specific shock syndromes

The three important specific syndromes in which shock occurs are:

- Anaphylactic shock.
- Septicaemic shock.
- Diabetic ketoacidosis.

Anaphylactic shock

See Chapter 14 for the features of anaphylaxis. The major problems are airway obstruction, bronchospasm and shock.

A protocol for management is shown in Fig. 29.28.

Septicaemic shock

Septicaemia is an important cause of shock in children. The main pathogens include:

- *Neisseria meningitidis*.
- *Haemophilus influenzae* (rare if Hib immunized).

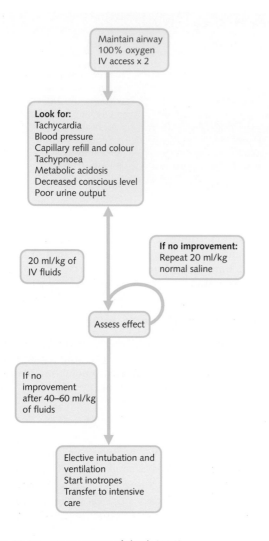

Fig. 29.27 Management of shock (ABC)

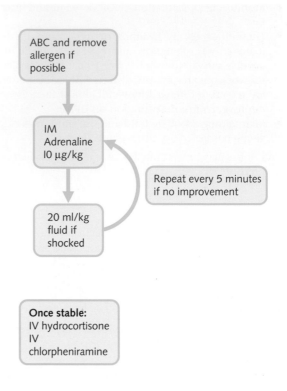

Fig. 29.28 Management of anaphylactic shock

- Staphylococci, pneumococci, streptococci.
- Gram-negative bacteria.

Meningococcal septicaemia is the most fulminant variety. Death can occur within hours of the first symptom; early diagnosis is vital.

Bacterial toxins trigger the release of various mediators and activators, which can:

- Cause vasodilatation or vasoconstriction.
- Depress cardiac function.
- Disturb cellular oxygen consumption.
- Cause 'capillary leak' with hypovolaemia.
- Promote disseminated intravascular coagulation.

Clinical features The clinical features progress from early (compensated) to late (decompensated) shock:

- 'Early' shock: increased cardiac output, decreased systemic resistance, warm extremities, high fever and mental confusion.

- 'Late' shock: reduced cardiac output, hypotension, cool peripheries and metabolic acidosis.

The cardinal sign of meningococcal septicaemia is a petechial or purpuric rash. This might be subtle in the early stages and a careful search for petechiae is required (in 10% of cases a blanching erythematous rash might occur first). Systemic antibiotics should be given immediately if a diagnosis of meningococcal septicaemia or meningitis is suspected.

Management Key points in initial management include:

- Oxygen: 100% O_2 by face mask.
- Fluids: 20 mL/kg of colloid or crystalloid given as a bolus. This can be repeated but if more than 40 mL/kg is required then assisted ventilation is likely to be needed.
- Investigations (Fig. 29.29).
- Antibiotics: broad-spectrum intravenous antibiotics (depending upon local policy), e.g. IV ceftriaxone.

> **HINTS AND TIPS**
>
> Outcome in septic shock is improved with aggressive fluid resuscitation and early referral to intensive care.

Fig. 29.29	Investigations in septic shock
Full blood count (FBC) Electrolytes and liver function Glucose Blood gas Lactate Coagulation screen	These define the severity of disease
Blood culture Urine culture Throat swab Rapid antigen testing and PCR Chest X-ray Abdominal ultrasound if indicated	Looking for the focus of infection

Fig. 29.30	Physical signs in diabetic ketoacidosis
Dehydration	Dry mucous membranes Loss of skin turgor Tachycardia, hypotension if severe
Acidosis	Ketones on breath Kussmaul breathing: rapid, deep, sighing respiration
Cerebral oedema	Headache Slowing of pulse rate and hypertension Decreased conscious level Seizures and focal neurological signs

In severe illness, intensive care facilities are required to allow continuous monitoring of circulatory parameters (including central venous pressure), urine output and pulse oximetry. Assisted ventilation, inotropic agents and renal replacement therapy might be required.

Diabetic ketoacidosis

This is an important and life-threatening complication of insulin-dependent diabetes mellitus. The majority of episodes are seen in patients known to have type 1 diabetes mellitus but can be a presenting feature.

Diabetic ketoacidosis represents the end stage of insulin deficiency. Deficiency of insulin blocks use of glucose leading to hyperglycaemia. As glucose levels exceed the renal threshold, an osmotic diuresis ensues with severe dehydration and electrolytes losses (sodium and potassium). Without insulin, fat is used as a source of energy leading to the generation of ketones and metabolic acidosis.

Clinical features The clinical features evolve as the severity of dehydration and acidosis worsens:

- The new diabetic has a history of polyuria, polydipsia and weight loss. This is followed by the rapid development of vomiting, lethargy and abdominal pain.
- The known diabetic might have an intercurrent illness with vomiting, poor control and documented hyperglycaemia and ketonuria.

Characteristic physical signs are listed in Fig. 29.30.

Diagnosis Essential initial investigations include:

- Blood glucose and ketones.
- Urea and electrolytes.
- Blood gas analysis.
- Urine glucose and ketones.

The typical metabolic abnormalities in diabetic ketoacidosis, which will be revealed by these investigations, include:

- Hyperglycaemia: blood glucose over 15 mmol/L and glycosuria.
- Ketoacidosis: ketonuria, positive blood ketones and metabolic acidosis on blood gas analysis (pH is low, $[HCO_3]$ is reduced, $PaCO_2$ is low, there is respiratory compensation with hypocapnia).
- Dehydration: raised urea.
- Sodium and potassium depletion: serum sodium concentration is often slightly reduced; serum potassium concentration might be low, normal or high, depending on renal function and the degree of acidosis.

> **HINTS AND TIPS**
>
> In diabetic ketoacidosis:
> - Total body potassium depletion is always present.
> - Cerebral oedema is rare but associated with a high mortality. Its prevention is by slow metabolic correction and rehydration and vigilance for early signs (e.g. headache or change in GCS).
> - Serum potassium concentration falls with treatment as potassium is driven into cells (with insulin action and correction of acidosis) and renal function improves.
> - IV fluids need to include potassium to avoid hypokalaemia as treatment proceeds.

Management The mainstays of management are the slow and careful restoration of fluid and electrolyte status, and insulin (Fig. 29.31). If there are signs of shock (e.g. poor perfusion, tachycardia, delayed capillary refill time), then give a 10 mL/kg bolus of normal saline and repeat as necessary to a maximum of 30 mL/kg.

The acidosis will usually correct with correction of fluid balance and insulin therapy. Administration of bicarbonate is rarely used. A nasogastric tube should be

Fig. 29.31	Management of diabetic ketoacidosis
Fluids	Treat shock Maintenance fluids: rehydrate over 48 h 0.9% saline with potassium initially Change to 0.45% saline once glucose has fallen <15 mmol/L
Insulin	Start IV at 0.1 units/kg/h Adjust depending on glucose: avoid drops >5 mmol/L/h
Additional	Monitor electrolytes regularly Monitor conscious level

passed if there is vomiting or evidence of gastric dilatation.

Careful monitoring is required of:

- Fluid status: weight, input and output.
- Electrolytes: check urea and electrolytes regularly (i.e. at least 4-hourly initially).
- Acid–base status: (check 2-hourly initially).
- Blood glucose: monitor hourly.
- ECG monitoring allows early identification dysrhythmias secondary to electrolyte imbalances.
- Vital signs and neurological observations.

It is essential that all fluids given during resuscitation are subtracted from the maintenance calculation of fluids to be given over 48 hours.

Complications Major complications include:

- Cerebral oedema: manifested by reduced conscious level, headache, irritability and fits. Attempt to prevent this by avoiding *rapid* falls in blood glucose or serum sodium concentrations.
- Cardiac dysrhythmias: usually secondary to electrolyte (potassium) disturbances. Acute renal failure is uncommon.

Once the biochemical markers have stabilised oral fluids and the normal regimen of insulin can be restarted. It is important to take this opportunity to review the family's understanding of diabetes and ensure concordance with therapy.

Further reading

National Institute for Health and Clinical Excellence (NICE), September 2007. Triage, assessment, investigation and early management of head injury in infants, children and adults (CG56). http://www.nice.org.uk/CG56.

Samuels, M., Wieteska, S., March 2011. Advanced paediatric life support: the practical approach, fifth ed. Advanced Life Support Group.

Nutrition, fluids and prescribing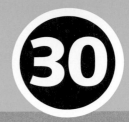

30

Objectives

At the end of this chapter, you should be able to:
- Know the different types of infant feeds and their advantages and disadvantages
- Understand various malnutrition and deficiency states
- Calculate the normal fluid requirements in children
- Understand the metabolism of drugs in children

Infants and children are more vulnerable than adults to inadequate nutrition or the derangement of fluid and electrolyte balance. A higher surface area to volume ratio is associated with a higher metabolic rate, larger calorific requirements and corresponding rapid fluid turnover.

Globally, malnutrition is directly or indirectly responsible for a third of all deaths of children. Conversely in the developed world obesity is increasing in children and likely to shorten life expectancy in the long term.

> **HINTS AND TIPS**
>
> Breast feeding in early infancy saves lives in developing countries due to the risk of waterborne diseases for formula fed infants.

Dehydration associated with diarrhoeal diseases is a major killer worldwide and its treatment with oral rehydration solution represented a major advance. However, attention to fluid and electrolyte status is an important aspect of many childhood illnesses.

Prescribing for infants and children involves many considerations unique to this age group. The route and frequency of administration must be adapted to the age, and dosage must take into account bodyweight, surface area and age-dependent changes in drug metabolism and excretion.

NUTRITION

Normal nutritional requirements

A satisfactory dietary intake should meet the normal requirements for energy and protein, together with providing an adequate supply of vitamins and trace elements. A neonate requires 115 kcal/kg/day which falls during childhood to 50 kcal/kg/day by the age of 18.

Infants and children are vulnerable to undernutrition because of:
- Low stores of fat and protein.
- Nutritional demands of growth (at 4 months of age, 30% of an infant's energy intake is used for growth; by 3 years of age this has fallen to 2%).
- Brain growth: the brain is proportionally larger in infants and is growing rapidly during the last trimester and first 2 years of life. It is vulnerable to energy deprivation during this period.

Infant feeding

An infant's primary source of nutrition is milk, either human breast milk or so-called 'formula' milk, usually based on modified cow's milk.

Breast feeding

This is the preferred method for most infants. Galactosaemia is the only absolute contraindication. HIV-positive mothers should not breast feed in the developed world due to risk of transmission. The many advantages, and few disadvantages, of breast feeding are listed in Fig. 30.1.

> **HINTS AND TIPS**
>
> Establishing breast feeding:
> - The baby should be put to the breast as soon as possible after birth.
> - Thereafter the baby should be fed on demand (indicated by crying).
> - Frequent suckling promotes lactation.
> - Advice with positioning helps to establish feeding.
> - Colostrum (high content of protein and immunoglobulin) rather than milk is produced in first few days.
> - The interval between feeds gradually lengthens from 2–3 hours to approximately a 4-hourly schedule.

Fig. 30.1 Advantages and disadvantages of breastfeeding

Advantages
Health benefits: lower rates of infection, constipation, SIDS, atopic conditions
Convenience: always available at correct temperature, no need for sterilizing equipment. Cost
Emotional: promotes maternal–infant bonding
Reduction in risk of maternal breast cancer
Disadvantages
Volume of intake uncertain
Transmission of drugs: illicit and prescribed
Nutrient deficiencies: (vitamin K and D)
Emotional: failure to establish breastfeeding may be a cause of emotional upset, cannot share the feeding

Fig. 30.3 Introduction of solids

Age	Feeding
6 months (not less than 4 months)	Smooth purees (fruit, vegetables, rice, meat, dairy products – avoid gluten)
6–9 months	Thicker consistencies and finger foods (fruit, vegetables, rice, meat, dairy products, cereals)
9–12 months	Mashed, chopped and minced consistencies (encourage variety of tastes and textures)
12 months	Mashed and chopped foods (encourage finger foods, can introduce whole cow's milk)

The composition of breast milk, cow's milk and infant formula differs significantly (Fig. 30.2). Unmodified, whole, pasteurized cow's milk is unsuitable as a main diet for infants under the age of 1 year because:

- It contains too much protein and sodium.
- It is deficient in iron and vitamins.

Modified cow's milk formulas have a modified casein to whey ratio, reduced mineral content and are fortified with iron and vitamins.

A typical scheme for the introduction of solids is shown in Fig. 30.3.

Special milks

A variety of specialized milks exist that are used in infants who are intolerant of specific constituents. Examples include:

- Low phenylalanine milk: phenylketonuria.
- Lactose free milk: lactose intolerance.
- Hydrolysed milk: cow's milk protein allergy.

Soya was used previously in cow's milk protein allergy but there is cross reactivity in up to 40% of children and so it not is not advised.

Malnutrition

Worldwide, malnutrition due to inadequate intake (starvation) is responsible for millions of childhood deaths. However, malnutrition can also exacerbate many childhood diseases resulting in impaired immunity, slower recovery time and developmental delay. Causes of malnutrition are listed in Fig. 30.4.

Assessment of nutritional status

Evaluation involves:

- Dietary history.
- Anthropometry and clinical examination.
- Laboratory investigations.

Dietary history

The food intake, as recalled by the parents or recorded in a diary, is determined over a period of several days.

Anthropometry

This involves measurement of:

- Height: height for age is reduced (stunted growth) in chronic malnutrition.

> **HINTS AND TIPS**
>
> Breast feeding mothers might be concerned about whether their baby has had an adequate milk intake and this is best measured by the baby's weight gain and wet nappies.

Weaning

The WHO advise the introduction of solid foods (weaning) at 6 months but it can be safely done from 4 months. At this age the infant can coordinate swallowing and has reasonable head control.

Fig. 30.2 Composition of different milks (per 100 mL)

	Breast milk	Cow's milk	Infant formula
Protein (g)	1.3	3.3	1.5
Casein:whey	40:60	60:40	Variable
Carbohydrate (g)	7.0	4.5	7.0–8.0
Fat (g)	4.2	3.6	2.6–3.8
Energy (kcal)	70	65	65
Sodium (mmol)	0.65	2.3	0.65–1.1
Calcium (mmol)	0.87	3.0	1.4
Iron (μmol)	1.36	0.9	10
Vitamin D (pg)	0.6	0.03	1.0

Fig. 30.4 Malnutrition in childhood – causes

Inadequate intake
Starvation due to famine or poverty
Restrictive diets – parental, iatrogenic, self-inflicted
Anorexia nervosa
Loss of appetite due to chronic illness

Malabsorption
Pancreatic disease, e.g. cystic fibrosis
Coeliac disease
Short gut (postoperative)

Increased energy requirements
Cystic fibrosis
Malignant disease
Burns
Trauma

- Weight: reduced weight with normal height (wasting) is an index of acute malnutrition.
- Mid upper arm circumference: an indication of skeletal muscle mass.
- Skinfold thickness: triceps skinfold thickness is a measure of subcutaneous fat stores.

Clinical syndromes of protein-energy malnutrition include:

- Marasmus: wasted (weight less than 60% of mean for age), wizened appearance, withdrawn, and apathetic.
- Kwashiorkor: occurs in children weaned late from the breast and fed on a relatively high-starch diet. It can be precipitated by an acute intercurrent infection. Features include wasting, oedema, sparse hair and depigmented skin, angular stomatitis and hepatomegaly.

Laboratory investigations

Useful laboratory tests include:

- Serum albumin: reduced in severe malnutrition.
- FBC: low haemoglobin and lymphocyte count.
- Blood glucose.
- Calcium, phosphate and vitamin D levels.
- Serum potassium and magnesium levels.

Management

Nutrition can be supplied:

- Enterally, via the gastrointestinal tract: this route is preferred wherever possible.
- Parenterally, directly into the circulation.

In many cases, malnutrition is due to inadequate intake and can be managed by the provision of supplementary enteral feeds given via a nasogastric or gastrostomy tube.

Examples of chronic diseases requiring such supplemental feeding include:

- Cystic fibrosis.
- Congenital heart disease.
- Cerebral palsy.
- Chronic renal failure.
- Malignancy.
- Inflammatory bowel disease.
- Anorexia nervosa.

Vitamin deficiencies

Several important vitamin deficiency diseases still occur in childhood. These include in particular:

- Vitamin D deficiency: rickets.
- Vitamin A deficiency: blindness.
- Vitamin K deficiency: haemorrhagic disease of the newborn.

> **HINTS AND TIPS**
>
> The most common dietary deficiencies in the UK are of iron and vitamin D.

Scurvy due to vitamin C deficiency is now extremely rare in developed countries.

Vitamin D deficiency: rickets

The effects of vitamin D deficiency on growing bone cause rickets. The bone matrix (osteoid) of the growing bone is inadequately mineralized, giving rise to the clinical features described in Fig. 30.5. The undermineralized bone is less rigid resulting in the classic bowed legs.

The normal pathways of vitamin D absorption and metabolism are shown in Fig. 30.6.

The most important source of vitamin D is from sunshine. It is difficult to correct deficiency by dietary

---

Fig. 30.5 Clinical features of rickets

General
Misery
Hypotonia
Developmental delay especially delayed walking
Growth failure and late eruption of teeth

Skeletal
Craniotabes (thin, soft, skull bones, delayed fusion of fontanelle)
Enlarged metaphyses (especially wrists and knees)
Rickety rosary (enlarged costochondral junctions)
Bowing of legs (caused by weight-bearing)

---

manipulation alone. The minimum daily requirement of vitamin D is 400–600 international units (IU) and this might not be attained in infants who are breast fed for a protracted period. Decreased sun exposure is exacerbated by:

- Infants with pigmented skin.
- Urban living conditions.
- Winter.

Much less common causes of rickets include:

- Inherited abnormalities of vitamin D metabolism or of the vitamin D receptor.
- Mineral deficiency, e.g. X-linked hypophosphataemia.
- Chronic renal disease.
- Decreased activity of 1α-hydroxylase in the kidneys leads to rickets as one component of renal osteodystrophy.

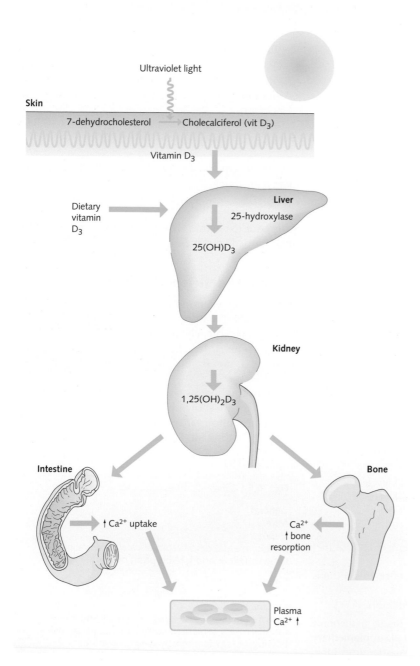

Fig. 30.6 Normal pathways of vitamin D metabolism and action

Rickets of prematurity is a metabolic bone disease in the premature infant that occurs if the milk used contains inadequate calcium and phosphate (1α-dihydroxycholecalciferol levels are elevated because of the hypophosphataemic stimulus, but there is osteopenia and inadequate mineralization of growing bone).

Diagnosis

This is confirmed by X-ray imaging and blood biochemistry. X-ray of the wrist shows cupping and fraying of the metaphysis and a widened metaphyseal plate (Fig. 30.7).

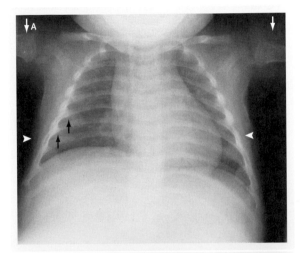

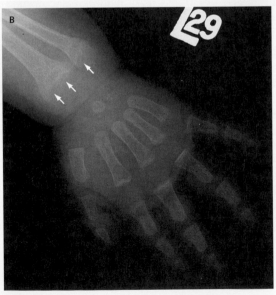

Fig. 30.7 X-ray appearance of rickets. (A) Chest X-ray of a young child with partially treated rickets. Note (i) changes at the metaphyses (white arrows), (ii) periosteal reaction on several ribs (white arrowheads), and (iii) bulging of anterior rib ends, the rickety rosary (black arrows). (B) Left wrist X-ray. Note the irregular 'cupped' metaphyses with loss of bone density (white arrows).

The biochemical changes in classic nutritional rickets include:

- Serum calcium: low or normal (may be normalized by secondary hyperparathyroidism).
- Serum phosphate: low.
- Serum alkaline phosphatase: elevated.
- Serum parathormone (PTH): elevated.
- Serum 1,25-dihydroxycholecalciferol: low.

Treatment

Prevention is obviously preferred and this is achieved by health education, exposure to sunlight and supplementation of the diet with minerals and vitamin D when indicated.

Treatment of nutritional rickets is with vitamin D3 (1,25-dihydroxycholecalciferol) 6000–10 000 IU/day initially for several weeks, followed by provision of 600 IU/day in the diet.

Higher doses might be required in the inherited forms. Biochemistry and radiography monitor the effect of therapy.

Vitamin A (retinol) deficiency

Vitamin A is necessary for membrane stability and it plays a role in vision, keratinization, cornification and placental development. The body's need for vitamin A can be met by milk, butter, eggs, liver and dark green or orange-coloured (e.g. carrots) vegetables.

Worldwide, about 150 million children are at risk of vitamin A deficiency and it has been calculated that up to a third of a million children go blind each year from vitamin A deficiency. In addition, vitamin A deficiency carries increased mortality from infection and poor growth.

The eye disease develops insidiously with impaired dark adaptation followed by drying of the conjunctiva and cornea (xerophthalmia).

Obesity

In 1998 the World Health Organization stated that obesity is a global epidemic. It results from numerous social and environmental factors that are difficult to alter. Obesity in children is increasing in prevalence and treatment is often disappointing. Prevention of obesity remains the optimal solution.

> **HINTS AND TIPS**
>
> - Most obese children are tall and above the 50th centile for height.
> - In Cushing syndrome or hypothyroidism, obesity is associated with low growth velocity and short stature.

The body mass index is a useful measurement of obesity and should be plotted on a BMI chart to assess if a child is obese. Aetiological factors include:

- Excess caloric intake.
- Reduced activity levels.
- Prevalence of obesity in family.

Rarely, an endocrine or chromosomal cause is present such as Cushing syndrome, hypothyroidism or Prader–Willi syndrome.

Obesity has several deleterious consequences including:

- Long-term health risks (diabetes, hypertension, ischaemic heart disease).
- Emotional disturbance: many psychological problems are associated with obesity.
- Obstructive sleep apnoea leading to poor school performance.

Management

A large number of interventions have been tried and involvement of the family as a whole is necessary. An aim to maintain the same weight while linear growth occurs may be more successful than attempting weight loss. Psychological support should be offered. For a small number of morbidly obese adolescents bariatric surgery may be required.

FLUIDS AND ELECTROLYTES

Basic physiology

It is useful to know how fluid is distributed between the different compartments of the body and what the normal requirements for fluid and electrolytes are. Important changes occur with age as the ratio of surface area to volume alters.

Fluid compartments

These are shown in Fig. 30.8. Infants have a greater water content than adults with a higher proportion of fluid in the extracellular space. The percentages can be expressed as volumes: e.g. 70% is equivalent to 700 mL/kg bodyweight (see Hints and tips box).

Blood volume is about 80 mL/kg at birth and falls to about 60 mL/kg by adulthood.

HINTS AND TIPS

- As body density is close to that of water, and 1 litre of water weighs close to 1 kilogram, weights and volumes are freely interchangeable. For example 1000 mL = 1000 g (1 L = 1 kg).
- Changes in bodyweight are the best guide to short-term changes in fluid balance (e.g. a weight loss of 500 g indicates a fluid deficit of 500 mL).

Normal requirements

Fluid requirement is that needed to make up for normal fluid losses, which include essential urine output and 'insensible' losses through sweat, respiration and the gastrointestinal tract. In pathological states there will be additional abnormal losses, such as those associated with diarrhoea or vomiting.

A simple formula for calculating normal fluid requirements according to bodyweight is shown in Fig. 30.9.

There are obligatory electrolyte losses in the stools, urine and sweat, and these require replacement. The maintenance requirement for sodium is about 3 mmol/kg/day and for potassium is 2 mmol/kg/day.

Intravenous fluids

These can be divided into colloids, which include large molecules such as proteins, and crystalloids, which usually contain dextrose (glucose) and electrolytes. Although concerns about colloids have been raised they are still in widespread use for volume expansion in sepsis.

Fig. 30.8 Body fluid compartments (as a percentage of bodyweight)

Age	Total body water	Extracellular fluid	Intracellular fluid
Newborn	70	35	35
12 months	65	25	40
Adult	60	20	40

Fig. 30.9 Normal fluid requirements

Body weight	Fluid requirement per 24 hours
First 10 kg	100 mL/kg
Second 10 kg	50 mL/kg
Further kg	20 mL/kg
Example: 24-hour requirement for child weighing 25 kg	
10 kg at 100 mL/kg	= 1000 mL
10 kg at 50 mL/kg	= 500 mL
5 kg at 20 mL/kg	= 100 mL
Total	= 1600 mL

The compositions of commonly available crystalloid fluids for intravenous use are shown in Fig. 30.10.

Important features of intravenous solutions

- Deaths and neurological damage occur due to erroneous fluid prescriptions in children.
- Regular measurement of urea and electrolytes is required for children on intravenous fluids (not less than 24-hourly).
- 0.9% saline is the resuscitation fluid of choice in all circumstances apart from blood loss.
- Isotonic solutions (0.9% saline or 0.9% saline/5% dextrose) are the safest solutions to use for replacement and maintenance fluids. They can be given in hyponatraemia and hypernatraemia.
- 0.45% dextrose and 5% dextrose can be used as maintenance fluid but only if the electrolytes are normal.
- Neonates require 10% dextrose with electrolytes added.
- 0.18% saline should never be used in paediatric medicine due to its hypotonicity.

Specific fluid and electrolyte problems

These are mostly considered elsewhere:

- Dehydration (see Chapter 18).
- Diabetic ketoacidosis (see Chapter 29).
- Burns (see Chapter 29).

Important features concerning certain electrolyte disturbances are considered here.

Sodium

Serum sodium levels reflect extracellular water shifts:

- Hyponatraemia is seen in the syndrome of inappropriate secretion of ADH (where excess extracellular water is present) and in gastroenteritis treated with water instead of salt solutions.

- Hypernatraemia is less common but is seen in neonates who become dehydrated as a result of poor breast feeding and in diabetic ketoacidosis.
- It is important to avoid rapid changes in sodium concentration because cerebral oedema or myelinosis might result.

Potassium

Hypokalaemia is usually a result of gastrointestinal loss, salbutamol therapy or iatrogenic inadequate intake. It is treated by supplementing IV fluids or oral potassium.

Hyperkalaemia is potentially dangerous, but children and neonates are less vulnerable to hyperkalaemia than adults. The most common cause is renal failure, but it also occurs in:

- Severe acidosis.
- Hypoaldosteronism.
- Iatrogenic potassium overload.

Immediate management involves:

- Calcium gluconate to stabilize myocardium: this does not remove potassium.
- Promotion of cellular potassium uptake by nebulized or IV salbutamol. An alternative is insulin and dextrose.
- Ion-exchange resins, e.g. oral or PR calcium resonium.
- Dialysis or haemofiltration if the above measures fail.

PAEDIATRIC PHARMACOLOGY AND PRESCRIBING

Great variability exists between children and adults in the pharmacology of drugs; differences also exist between the preterm neonate, neonate and older children. It is therefore important that clinicians recognize that much of the information that applies to adults is not always applicable to children, and must be cautious in extrapolating adult data into paediatric practice. Most paediatric doses are calculated based on the child's weight or body surface area, though the latter is used infrequently (Fig. 30.11).

Fig. 30.10 Isotonic crystalloid fluids: composition

Fluid	Sodium (mmol/L)	Potassium (mmol/L)	Chloride (mmol/L)	Energy (kcal/L)
0.9% saline (resuscitation fluid)	150	0	150	0
0.9% saline/5% dextrose (maintenance and suitable in electrolyte abnormalities)	150	0	150	200
0.45% saline/5% dextrose (maintenance if electrolytes in normal range)	75	0	75	200

Fig. 30.11 Bodyweight and body surface area (BSA) by age

Age	Weight (kg)	BSA (m²)
Newborn	3.5	0.25
6 months	7.7	0.40
1 year	10	0.50
5 years	18	0.75
12 years	36	1.25
Adult	70	1.80

HINTS AND TIPS

Water-soluble drugs, e.g. most antibiotics, require a larger initial dose in neonates because they have the greatest amount of total body water. The large volume also means delayed excretion so doses are less frequent.

Many drugs currently used in paediatric practice remain unlicensed. Thus, pharmacokinetic and pharmacodynamic data are rarely available. A paediatric version of the British National Formulary is available.

Absorption and administration

The oral route is most commonly used for administering medication because it is easy, safe and cheap. Its limitations are that many children find certain drugs unpalatable and tablets need to be crushed.

The IV route is reliable and effective but requires venepuncture. The PR route is useful in emergencies, and diazepam and paracetamol can be given this way. Intramuscular injections are rarely used except for immunizations.

In neonates and infants, gastric absorption is altered as normal gastric acid secretion is reduced until 3 years of age; gastric motility is also delayed.

Metabolism and excretion

Hepatic metabolism differs from that in adults in that it is slow at birth but increases rapidly with age; the metabolic processes also differ. For example, paracetamol is metabolized by sulphation whereas adults use the glucuronidation pathway. Thus paracetamol toxicity in children is less than in adults.

The renal handling of drugs also differs because the glomerular filtration rate in children does not approach adult levels until 9–12 months age.

Further reading

British Dietetic Association – 'Food facts' factsheets on breast feeding, weaning and a healthy diet for children. http://www.bda.uk.com/foodfacts/index.html.
National Patient Safety Agency – Patient Safety Alert – Reducing the risk of hyponatraemia when administering intravenous fluids to children. 2007. http://www.nrls.npsa.nhs.uk/resources/?EntryId45=59809.

SELF-ASSESSMENT

Best of fives questions (BOFs)

1. A 14-month-old girl is brought into the emergency department with a 7-day history of fever and general malaise. On examination, she is very miserable, has bilateral conjunctivitis, cracked lips and bilateral cervical lymphadenopathy. A maculopapular rash is noted over her trunk. What is the most likely diagnosis?
   A. Measles
   B. Erythema infectiosum ('fifth disease')
   C. Kawasaki disease
   D. Staphylococcal scalded skin syndrome
   E. Chickenpox

2. A 9-year-old boy is 'blue-lighted' into the emergency department by ambulance with an acute history of reduced consciousness. His mother described him complaining of headache and fever earlier in the day. On examination, he is pyrexial with a GCS of 14/15 and is cardiovascularly stable. A few petechiae are noted on his legs. What is the single most effective immediate management for this child?
   A. Arrange an urgent CT brain scan
   B. Give a 20 mL/kg normal saline fluid bolus
   C. Give a 3 mL/kg 10% dextrose fluid bolus
   D. Gain intravenous access, take blood cultures and administer broad-spectrum antibiotics
   E. Administer vitamin K

3. A paediatrician is called to urgently review a 3-day-old baby on the postnatal ward. On arrival, the baby is profoundly cyanotic and saturations do not improve with high flow oxygen therapy. Examination reveals a single loud second heart sound but no murmur. Intravenous access is secured and the blood gas shows severe metabolic acidosis. A CXR performed shows increased pulmonary vasculature. What is the most likely diagnosis?
   A. Atrial septal defect
   B. Transposition of the great arteries
   C. Patent ductus arteriosus
   D. Tetralogy of Fallot
   E. Ventricular septal defect

4. A 4-year-old girl has been admitted to the ward with an acute febrile illness. A diagnosis of a lower respiratory chest infection has been made and intravenous antibiotics have been commenced. The following morning on the ward round, the medical team note she has an ejection systolic murmur with normal heart sounds and no radiation. She appears clinically well in herself. What would be the single most appropriate management plan?
   A. Proceed to urgently arrange a CXR
   B. Discuss with the local paediatric cardiology centre for advice

C. Once medically fit for discharge, arrange an out-patient ECHO
   D. Explain that this is an innocent murmur and inform the GP to re-evaluate the child once she has recovered from illness
   E. Change the present antibiotic regime

5. A 5-year-old boy is under out-patient review for asthma. His CXR shows hyper-expansion but his symptoms remain unresponsive despite step-wise increase in asthma therapy. Further questioning reveals delayed passage of meconium at birth and finger clubbing is evident on examination. What is the most appropriate next step in the management of this child?
   A. Arrange a CT chest scan
   B. Organize a sweat test
   C. Test lung function using spirometry
   D. Take a per-nasal swab
   E. Send sputum cultures

6. A 2-year-old boy is brought into the emergency department by ambulance at night with an acute history of cough and stridor following a 2-day history of coryzal symptoms. On examination, he is afebrile but has marked intercostal recession with stridor and a 'barking cough' is heard. What is the most likely causative organism?
   A. Adenovirus
   B. Respiratory syncytial virus
   C. Parainfluenza virus
   D. Rhinovirus
   E. Influenza virus

7. A 12-year-old Afro-Caribbean boy has been referred by his GP with a 2-month history of intermittent right-sided painful limp. There is no history of trauma and he is previously fit and well. On examination, his weight is 65 kg (98th–99.6th centile), he is apyrexial and there is painful restricted external rotation of his right hip joint. He has normal inflammatory markers and an X-ray has been requested. What is the likely diagnosis?
   A. Transient synovitis
   B. Osteomyelitis
   C. Perthes disease
   D. Juvenile idiopathic arthritis
   E. Slipped upper femoral epiphysis

8. An 18-month-old female is presented to the emergency department with a 12-hour history of refusal to weight bear on left leg and fever. There is no history of trauma and no other preceding symptoms. On examination, her temperature is 39.5°C, heart rate is 160 beats per minute and she appears

uncomfortable at rest. Her left knee is swollen, erythematous and held in flexion. What is most likely to confirm the diagnosis?
A. X-ray of left knee
B. X-ray of left hip
C. Left knee joint aspiration of fluid
D. Blood tests for inflammatory markers
E. Blood cultures

9. A newborn baby is noted to have coarse facies, a large fontanelle and hypotonia on routine examination. He also has jaundice. His blood sugar levels are normal. Which of the following investigations would be most likely to reveal the underlying diagnosis?
A. Growth hormone
B. Karyotype
C. Thyroid function tests
D. Blood group
E. CK

10. A 7-day-old male baby is brought into the emergency department with a 1-day history of poor feeding and vomiting. He was born at term by spontaneous vaginal delivery weighing 3200 g and his postnatal period was uneventful. On arrival, he appears lethargic and has moderate dehydration. His weight is 2750 g. His blood glucose is 2.0 and his blood gas reveals a sodium of 124 mmol/L and the potassium is 6.8 mmol/L. Following resuscitation and stabilization, what is most likely to confirm the diagnosis?
A. Abdominal ultrasound scan
B. ACTH level
C. Karyotype
D. 17 Hydroxyprogesterone level
E. Chloride level

11. A 12-year-old girl is referred by her GP to the paediatric endocrinology clinic for evaluation of delayed pubertal development. Following clinical assessment, constitutional delay of growth is diagnosed. What investigation is most likely to confirm this diagnosis?
A. MRI brain
B. Thyroid function tests
C. Growth hormone level
D. Bone age
E. Karyotype

12. A 15-year-old girl is referred by her GP to the paediatric endocrinology clinic for assessment of delayed puberty. On examination, her height plots on the 0.4th centile, she has an ejection systolic murmur and widely spaced nipples. Her gonadotrophin levels are also raised. What is the most likely diagnosis?
A. Turner syndrome
B. Kleinfelter syndrome
C. McCune–Albright syndrome
D. Hypothyroidism
E. Silver–Russell syndrome

13. A 3-year-old girl is 'blue-lighted' into the local emergency department with reduced consciousness.

Her mother informs the paramedic that her daughter has been unwell for the last 8 days with vomiting and profuse diarrhoea. On arrival, she is apyrexial, has a heart rate of 170 beats per minute and respiratory rate of 20 per minute. Her systolic blood pressure is 75 mmHg and she has a capillary refill time of 5 seconds. She is barely responsive to pain. Resuscitation begins and a blood gas reveals a pH 6.9, base excess −18 mmol/L and blood sugar of 2.2 mmol/L. What is the most likely clinical syndrome?
A. Anaphylactic shock
B. Septicaemic shock
C. Cardiogenic shock
D. Hypovolaemic shock
E. Neurogenic shock

14. A mother brings her toddler son into the emergency department following a burn. She tells the triage nurse that she had just finished making a cup of tea and left it on the kitchen work top to attend to her crying 4-month-old girl infant. She heard screams from the toddler who had pulled the cup of tea over his right hand. She gave immediate first aid and came to hospital immediately. Mother appears distressed and tearful. Analgesia and suitable dressings are applied. What is the most appropriate next step in the management of this toddler?
A. Discharge home
B. Take blood for routine investigations
C. Give intravenous fluids
D. Call the duty social worker to express your concerns
E. Discuss the case with the regional burns centre

15. A known epileptic is brought into the local emergency department in status epilepticus. The paramedic crew have given rectal diazepam 10 minutes ago but the patient continues to have generalized tonic-clonic seizures. He now has intravenous access and his blood sugar is 5.5 mmol/L. What is the most appropriate next drug treatment to be given?
A. Intravenous lorazepam
B. Intravenous phenytoin
C. Intravenous thiopental
D. Rectal paraldehyde
E. Buccal midazolam

16. A 14-year-old girl self-presents to her local emergency department with a history of deliberate self-poisoning following an argument with her boyfriend. She agrees to blood tests which reveal high paracetamol blood levels necessitating treatment. Which is the appropriate treatment for this teenager?
A. Intravenous desferrioxamine
B. Intravenous N-acetylcysteine
C. Active cooling
D. Alkalinization of urine with bicarbonate
E. Activated charcoal

17. A mother brings her 22-month-old girl to her GP with concerns regarding development. She is able to sit

unsupported and cruises around furniture. She can point to parts of her body, gives her name and puts words together. Mother reports that she takes off her shoes and uses a spoon. During the consultation, the girl is observed to build a tower of five cubes. What is the most appropriate next step in the care of this girl?
A. Reassure mother that her daughter's development is within normal limits
B. Arrange a review appointment in 4 weeks
C. Proceed with investigations
D. Refer her to a general paediatrician for assessment
E. Refer her to a community paediatrician for assessment

18. At a routine health visitor consultation, a 12-month-old boy is noticed to be cruising around furniture, responding to his name and says 'mama' and 'papa'. He is holding a crayon in his left hand and his father informs the health visitor that he only uses his left hand at home. What is the most likely finding here?
A. Gross motor delay
B. Fine motor delay
C. Speech and language delay
D. Play and social delay
E. Global delay

19. A 3-year-old boy is referred to a community paediatrician with concerns regarding development. At assessment, he is able to walk up and down stairs holding the railing and jumps with both feet. The doctor observes poor eye contact and limited speech. The child is also repeatedly opening and closing the drawers in the desk. What is the most likely finding here?
A. Gross motor delay
B. Fine motor delay
C. Speech and language delay
D. Play and social delay
E. Global delay

20. A 15-month-old girl is referred for developmental assessment. She was born at term weighing 3400 g by spontaneous vaginal delivery and required resuscitation at birth with an Apgar score of 3 at 1 minute, 4 at 5 minutes and 7 at 10 minutes. She was admitted to the neonatal unit and required ventilation for 3 days. On assessment, she has global developmental delay. What is the most likely explanation for this finding?
A. Congenital hypothyroidism
B. Meningitis
C. An inborn error of metabolism
D. Intracranial haemorrhage
E. Hypoxic–ischaemic encephalopathy (HIE)

21. A 6-month-old female infant is admitted with a 4-day history of high fever with no focus. A full septic screen is performed which yields negative cultures and normal inflammatory markers. On day 7 of her illness she develops a blanching morbilliform rash all over her body and her fever subsides. What is the most likely diagnosis?
A. Measles
B. Rubella
C. Roseola infantum
D. Scarlet fever
E. Chicken pox

22. A 3-year-old girl of Japanese origin is admitted to hospital with a 7-day history of fever, bilateral conjunctivitis, rash, cervical lymphadenopathy and reddened extremities. Intravenous immunoglobulin and oral aspirin are started. What is the most important investigation in this child's management?
A. Full blood count
B. Throat swab
C. ASOT titre
D. Echocardiogram
E. CXR

23. A 4-month-old male infant has a history of failure to thrive, diarrhoea and has been admitted twice to hospital with pneumonia since birth. On examination, his abdomen is soft with no organomegaly or skin lesions to note. There is evidence of oral thrush. Lymphopaenia is noted on his full blood count. What is the most likely diagnosis?
A. Chronic granulomatous disease (CGD)
B. Selective IgA deficiency
C. Severe combined immunodeficiency (SCID)
D. X-linked agammaglobulinaemia (Bruton's disease)
E. HIV infection

24. A paediatrician is asked to review a heart murmur of a 2-day-old baby born by vaginal delivery following an uneventful period to a primiparous mother, aged 38. The perinatal period was normal and baby has been feeding well. On examination, he is hypotonic, has single palmar creases and epicanthic folds. What is the most likely heart lesion?
A. Atrioventricular septal defect
B. Atrial septal defect
C. Aortic stenosis
D. Coarctation of the aorta
E. Patent ductus arteriosus

25. A mother on the postnatal ward has urgently requested a medical review on her 3-day-old baby who appears blue. On arrival, the baby is deeply cyanosed with cool peripheries and saturations do not improve despite maximum oxygen therapy. Femoral pulses are palpable and a single, loud second heart sound can be heard but no murmur. The baby is brought to the neonatal unit for further care. What is the next most important intervention?
A. Intravenous furosemide
B. Intravenous antibiotics
C. Intravenous fluid bolus of normal saline
D. Intravenous fluid bolus of dextrose
E. Intravenous infusion of prostaglandin E_1

26. A 3-year-old girl with complex congenital heart disease is admitted with fever. On examination, her temperature is 39.5°C and there is a loud ejection systolic murmur. Her CRP is 250 mg/L and a transthoracic echocardiogram confirms vegetations. What is the most likely causative pathogen?
    A. *Streptococcus pneumoniae*
    B. *Streptococcus pyogenes*
    C. *Streptococcus viridans*
    D. Group A haemolytic streptococcus
    E. Group B haemolytic streptococcus

27. A previously well 5-year-old boy is brought in by ambulance to the emergency department with an acute onset of breathing difficulty. On arrival, he appears unwell, pale with audible stridor and is sitting upright unable to speak. His temperature is 40°C. What is the first priority in this child's management?
    A. Lie the child down
    B. Take a throat swab
    C. Obtain intravenous access
    D. Give oral dexamethasone
    E. Summon immediate anaesthetic help

28. A 3-month-old female infant presents with a 2-day history of coryzal symptoms and increased work of breathing. Her mother reports she had two wet nappies over the last 24 hours and is taking half of her bottle feeds. Her heart rate is 150 beats per minute, and she has a respiratory rate of 60 per minute with saturations of 96% in air. On examination she is alert, well perfused and with slight recession. Clinical findings are consistent with bronchiolitis. What is the most appropriate management?
    A. Admit and give supplemental oxygen
    B. Admit and start CPAP
    C. Admit and give naso-gastric feeds
    D. Admit for regular nebulizers
    E. Admit for intravenous antibiotics

29. A 4-year-old girl is under out-patient review for asthma. Her regular treatment consists of a preventative steroid inhaler 200 micrograms BD and a reliever inhaler when required (about fortnightly). However, over the last 3 months she has had to use her reliever inhaler every other day. Her nocturnal coughing has increased resulting in disturbed sleep. What is the appropriate next step in care for this child?
    A. Continue on the same dose of steroid inhaler
    B. Increase the steroid inhaler dose to 400 micrograms BD
    C. Start a course of oral steroids
    D. Start oral theophylline
    E. Add a long-acting beta agonist

30. A 3-year-old girl is admitted with a 3-day history of coryzal symptoms followed by an acute history of breathing difficulty. She is previously fit and well apart from mild eczema and the parents are non-smokers. She is thriving and on examination she has widespread wheeze with no crepitations. What is the most likely diagnosis?
    A. Viral wheeze
    B. Asthma
    C. Heart failure
    D. Bronchiolitis
    E. Recurrent aspiration

31. A 6-week-old baby girl, born by elective caesarean delivery for breech, is brought in to her GP for routine check up with her GP. The history reveals oligohydramnios during pregnancy. On inspection, the baby is noted to have bilateral talipes. For which condition is this baby at greatest risk?
    A. Perthes disease
    B. Scoliosis
    C. Developmental dysplasia of the hip
    D. Torticollis
    E. Arthrogryposis

32. A 7-year-old boy with known sickle cell disease presents to the emergency department with a 3-day history of fever and an immobile left leg. On examination, he is pyrexial at 39.8°C, in pain and refusing to weight bear on his left. What is the most likely diagnosis?
    A. Perthes disease
    B. Transient synovitis
    C. Juvenile idiopathic arthritis
    D. Slipped upper femoral epiphysis
    E. Osteomyelitis

33. A 5-year-old girl is referred to a paediatric specialist by her GP. She has a 7-week history of intermittent left knee and elbow pain which has been becoming more frequent. More recently, she has also been complaining of pain in her right ankle. Her GP performed blood tests that revealed positive antinuclear antibodies. To which sub-specialty should this child be referred as part of her management?
    A. Paediatric cardiology
    B. Paediatric ophthalmology
    C. Paediatric respiratory
    D. Paediatric gastroenterology
    E. Paediatric nephrology

34. A 5-year-old boy is referred to a paediatric specialist by his GP with tall stature and headaches. On examination, he has testicular enlargement and examination of his cranial nerves reveals bilateral papilloedema. What is most likely to confirm the diagnosis?
    A. CT or MRI brain scan
    B. Karyotype
    C. ACTH level
    D. 17-Hydroxyprogesterone
    E. Bone age

35. A 10-year-old boy presents to his GP with short stature. He was admitted to the special care baby unit from birth with hypotonia and required nasogastric

feeding. On examination, his BMI is 26 and he has small genitalia. What is the most likely diagnosis that requires exclusion?

A. Turner syndrome
B. Achondroplasia
C. Silver–Russell syndrome
D. Prader–Willi syndrome
E. Angelman syndrome

36. A 2-day-old baby is admitted to the neonatal unit with respiratory distress and jaundice. A full septic screen is performed which yields *E. coli* positive blood cultures. Opthalmological assessment confirms the presence of cataracts. What is the most likely diagnosis?

A. Galactosaemia
B. Von Gierke's disease
C. Phenylketonuria
D. Medium-chain acyl-coenzyme A dehydrogenase deficiency
E. Maple syrup urine disease

37. A 24-month-old boy is brought into the emergency department by ambulance following a near drowning incident. Resuscitation is in process. Which of the following will indicate a poor prognosis for outcome?

A. Submersion time of 3 minutes
B. Core temperature of 35°C on arrival
C. Arterial pH of < 7.0 post resuscitation
D. Near drowning into seawater
E. No respiratory effort within 90 seconds

38. A 9-year-old boy in asystole is brought in by ambulance to the emergency department. The various members of the cardiac arrest team arrive and resuscitation begins. Which is the most important drug of choice?

A. Adrenaline (epinephrine)
B. Sodium bicarbonate
C. Atropine
D. Amiodarone
E. Lidocaine

39. A 3-year-old girl is brought into the emergency department by ambulance with a 4-hour history of listlessness, high fever and reduced responsiveness. Her temperature is 40.0°C, she has a heart rate of 170 beats per minute, a respiratory rate of 35 per minute and saturations of 100% in 15 litres of high-flow oxygen. On examination, she is responsive to voice and maintaining her airway. Systemic examination is unremarkable; her capillary refill time is 4 seconds. What is the first priority in the management of this child?

A. Intubation and ventilation
B. 10 mL/kg bolus of normal saline
C. 20 mL/kg bolus of normal saline
D. 15 mL/kg packed red cells
E. 3 mL/kg bolus of dextrose

40. A 14-year-old boy is admitted with diabetic ketoacidosis. Intravenous insulin has been running at

0.1 units/kg/h for the last 12 hours alongside a 500 mL bag of 0.9% normal saline. His last blood sugar is 22 mmol/L and he has a good urine output. Which of the following are most likely to be decreased?

A. Serum sodium
B. Serum potassium
C. Serum lactate
D. Serum chloride
E. Serum calcium

41. A 3-year-old boy of Asian origin presents to his GP accompanied by his father. He has a 6-month history of bilateral leg pains and occasionally finds it difficult to walk and has to rest. On examination, he has bowing of his legs but otherwise appears developmentally normal with no other neurological or musculoskeletal findings. His father mentions that his son is also due to see the dentist for 'bad teeth'. What is the most appropriate initial blood test to aid in diagnosis?

A. Bone profile
B. Liver function
C. Full blood count
D. C-reactive protein
E. Renal function

42. A 6-year-old girl is admitted with high fever, headache and neck stiffness. A septic screen is performed and intravenous antibiotics are commenced. Her blood sugar is 6.6 mmol/L. The CSF results are as follows: Cloudy appearance, 8000 polymorphs, CSF protein 2.0 g/L, CSF glucose 2.3. What is the most likely diagnosis?

A. TB meningitis
B. Viral meningitis
C. Bacterial meningitis
D. Encephalitis
E. Not meningitis

43. A 5-week-old baby boy is brought into the emergency department with a 48-hour history of projectile vomiting. The infant is hungry after vomiting and has not opened his bowels in 3 days. Clinical examination reveals a mass in the left upper quadrant region. A blood gas is performed: pH 7.50, pCO_2 5.5 kPa and bicarbonate 30 mmol/L. What does this blood gas represent?

A. Normal findings
B. Metabolic acidosis
C. Metabolic alkalosis
D. Respiratory acidosis
E. Respiratory alkalosis

44. A 4-year-old boy attends the emergency department accompanied by his mother with a 1-week history of abdominal bloating and passing blood-stained urine. His heart rate is 100 beats per minute with a blood pressure of 120/75 mmHg. Clinical examination reveals a non-tender mass in the left loin region and urine dipstick confirms haematuria and proteinuria. What is the appropriate modality of imaging for this child?

A. Plain AXR
B. Plain CT abdomen
C. MRI abdomen
D. Renal ultrasound
E. CT abdomen with contrast

45. A 24-month-old girl is brought into the emergency department by her mother with fever. At triage, her temperature is 38.7°C, other vital signs all within normal limits and she is given antipyretics pending medical review. She is reviewed by the doctor 90 minutes later and her temperature is now 37.7°C. Clinical examination reveals a well hydrated and clinically well child with good social interaction. There are no localizing features and no apparent source for her fever. What is the most appropriate next step in her care?

A. Request a CXR
B. Take bloods for inflammatory markers
C. Take a blood culture
D. Request a urine dipstick
E. Discharge the child home

46. A 2-month-old male infant is brought into the emergency department by her father with fever. At triage, his temperature is 39.5°C and other vital signs are within normal limits. He is quickly assessed by a doctor, which reveals no respiratory distress, a capillary refill time of <2 seconds and good tone and activity. The infant is well perfused and there are no localizing features to indicate a source for his fever. What is the most appropriate next step in this infant's management?

A. A full septic screen followed by IV antibiotics
B. A full blood count and CRP
C. A CXR
D. A clean catch urine sample
E. Admission for observation

47. A 10-year-old boy has a 2-week history of sore throat, fever and lethargy. Upon clinical examination there is pharyngitis, hepatosplenomegaly and bilateral shotty cervical lymph nodes are palpated. Blood tests reveal atypical lymphocytes and an ALT of 190 U/L. What is the most likely causative pathogen?

A. Coxsackievirus
B. Herpes simplex virus
C. Varicella zoster virus
D. Epstein–Barr virus
E. Cytomegalovirus

48. A 9-year-old girl is admitted to the ward with a history of chest pain on exertion. She is otherwise fit and well but was admitted to hospital at 3 years of age for a prolonged febrile illness where she was observed and discharged without diagnosis or treatment. An ECG is performed which is abnormal and an echocardiogram reveals diffuse dilatation of the left

coronary artery. What is most likely to have prevented this condition?

A. Antibiotics
B. Antivirals
C. Antifungals
D. Immunoglobulin
E. Immunization

49. A 4-year-old girl is admitted with fever, difficulty breathing and cough. A diagnosis of left lower lobe pneumonia is made and intravenous antibiotics are commenced. What is the most likely pathogen?

A. *Streptococcus pneumoniae*
B. *Haemophilus influenzae*
C. *Mycoplasma pneumoniae*
D. *Chlamydia trachomatis*
E. *E. coli*

50. A 6-month-old female infant with RSV positive bronchiolitis is requiring 1 litre of nasal prong humidified oxygen and nasogastric feeding. Over the last 8 hours her work of breathing has increased and is showing signs of recession. Her oxygen requirement has also increased to 2 litres and she appears tired. A blood gas is performed which shows a pH of 7.30 and pCO_2 of 7.8 kPa. What is the most appropriate next step in management?

A. Salbutamol nebulizer
B. Intravenous antibiotics
C. CPAP
D. Intubate and ventilate
E. Steroids

51. A previously healthy 7-year-old boy is brought in to see his GP with a fever and coryzal symptoms for the last few days. On assessment, the child is clinically well and he has a rash comprised of several distinctive erythematous lesions, both macular and papular and of differing sizes, distributed all over his body. The lesions have a central faded area. What is the most likely diagnosis?

A. Erythema nodosum
B. Erythema toxicum
C. Erythema marginatum
D. Erythema multiforme
E. Erythema chronicum migrans

52. A 24-month-old girl with trisomy 21 attends for her developmental review. Her mother is concerned about her hearing and explains that she has had two recent right ear infections within the last 5 months. An audiogram is carried out which confirms a conductive hearing loss of the right ear. What is the most likely explanation for this finding?

A. Congenital infection
B. Otitis media with effusion
C. Acquired meningitis
D. Antibiotic toxicity
E. Foreign body

53. A 36-hour-old baby is due to have his newborn check prior to discharge. The paediatrician notes that the antenatal serology is incomplete because the mother declined testing. The baby is symmetrically growth restricted, red reflexes are bilaterally absent and a heart murmur is noted. Femoral pulses can be palpated, the baby is pink and otherwise well. What is an echocardiogram most likely to show?
    A. Ventricular septal defect
    B. Coarctation of aorta
    C. Atrial septal defect
    D. Tetralogy of Fallot
    E. Patent ductus arteriosus

54. A 10-year-old boy is admitted with left lower lobe pneumonia. On day 3 of admission, he develops gradual increased work of breathing and a fever of 40°C. On assessment, he has a respiratory rate of 40 per minute and auscultation reveals a clear right lung field but reduced breath sounds throughout his left lung. The percussion note is 'stony dull' and chest expansion is reduced on his left side. What is the most likely diagnosis?
    A. Empyema
    B. Lobar collapse
    C. Lung abscess
    D. Pneumothorax
    E. Cor pulmonale

55. An 8-year-old boy attends the emergency department following a minor injury while playing football. An X-ray confirms a mid-shaft fracture of his tibia. His records show that he has sustained multiple fractures in the past and is under the paediatric ENT team for conductive hearing loss. The astute emergency doctor also notices that his sclerae have a blue tinge to them. What is the most likely diagnosis that needs to be excluded?
    A. Osteogenesis imperfecta type 1
    B. Osteogenesis imperfecta type 2
    C. Osteogenesis imperfecta type 3
    D. Osteogenesis imperfecta type 4
    E. Osteogenesis imperfecta type 5

56. An 11-year-old girl presents to the emergency department with a 4-day history of cough and fever. A working diagnosis of right middle lobe pneumonia is made and she is commenced on intravenous antibiotics and admitted to the ward. Her blood tests reveal a plasma sodium of 127 mmol/L with normal renal function. Further investigations reveal a low plasma osmolality and a raised urinary sodium level. What is the most likely diagnosis?
    A. Syndrome of inappropriate secretion of ADH
    B. Cushing syndrome
    C. Diabetes insipidus
    D. Secondary adrenal insufficiency
    E. Adrenal hyperplasia

57. A 6-year-old boy with known asthma has been brought in by ambulance to the local emergency department with an acute severe exacerbation. He has already received salbutamol and ipratropium nebulizers together with intravenous steroid. Upon reassessment, he appears exhausted with varying responsiveness. Fifteen litres of oxygen are needed to maintain his saturations and auscultation of his chest reveals minimal breath sounds. What is the next most important step in this child's care?
    A. Reassess 30 minutes later
    B. Give intravenous antibiotics
    C. Request a CXR
    D. Give intravenous salbutamol
    E. Admit to ward

58. A 6-week-old female infant has been admitted with an acute febrile illness. A full septic screen is performed and intravenous antibiotics are commenced. The CSF gram stain is reported as Gram-positive cocci in chains. What is the most likely organism?
    A. *Neisseria meningitidis*
    B. *Haemophilus influenzae*
    C. Group B streptococcus
    D. *Staphylococcus aureus*
    E. *Listeria monocytogenes*

59. All of the following infections can cause a rash. However, which one of the following pathogens is not associated with vesicular skin lesions?
    A. Herpes zoster virus
    B. Varicella zoster virus
    C. *Staphylococcus aureus*
    D. Herpes simplex virus
    E. Human herpesvirus

60. It can be possible to assess whether a murmur is significant by its character and associated features. Which of the following is not a feature of an innocent heart murmur?
    A. No radiation
    B. Varies with posture
    C. Systolic
    D. Third heart sound
    E. No symptoms

61. Bronchiolitis is one of the most common respiratory conditions affecting infants. Which of the following is not a clinical feature of bronchiolitis?
    A. Tachypnoea
    B. Apnoea
    C. Wheeze
    D. Fine crackles
    E. Paroxysmal cough

62. Which one of the following is not associated with systemic juvenile idiopathic arthritis?
    A. Hepatomegaly
    B. Lymphadenopathy
    C. Salmon-pink rash
    D. Anterior uveitis
    E. Fever

63. There are many causes of short stature in children. Which one of the following does not cause short stature?
   A. Turner syndrome
   B. Constitutional delay of growth
   C. Rickets
   D. Thyrotoxicosis
   E. Cystic fibrosis

64. Burns are one of the commonest injuries sustained by children and some require specialist care. Which one of the following is not an indication for referral to a specialist burns centre?
   A. Face involvement
   B. Perineal involvement
   C. 5% partial thickness
   D. Inhalation burn
   E. Circumferential burn

65. Developmental milestones vary between children; however, there are normal ranges for each domain. Which of the following is not a developmental concern?
   A. Not visually fixing at 5 weeks
   B. Not sitting unsupported at 7 months
   C. Not using single words at 16 months
   D. Not walking at 17 months
   E. Not copying a line at 24 months

66. Haemoglobin production differs through fetal life and extra-uterine life and the molecule itself changes with age. Which of the following statements regarding haemoglobin is correct?
   A. At birth HbA is predominant
   B. Hb concentration falls after birth until around 7 weeks
   C. Haematopoesis mainly occurs in the liver and spleen at term
   D. The lifespan of a normal red blood cell is 10 days
   E. Fetal haemoglobin has lower affinity for oxygen

67. An 11-month-old caucasian boy attends his GP as his mother has been struggling to wean him. He will drink cow's milk at regular intervals and eats some baby rice but refuses most other solids. On examination he appears very pale but otherwise well. There is no hepatosplenomegaly. A full blood count (FBC) is arranged in view of the pallor which shows: Hb=7.8 g/dL, mean corpuscular volume (MCV)= 69 fL. What is the most likely cause of his anaemia?
   A. Sickle cell anaemia
   B. Thalassaemia
   C. Iron deficiency anaemia
   D. Vitamin B_{12} deficiency
   E. Folate deficiency

68. A 4-year-old boy presents with pain in his abdomen and joints for the past 24 hours. He is afebrile. On examination he has diffuse abdominal tenderness but there are no masses, no lymphadenopathy and no

hepatosplenomegaly. A widespread purpuric rash is present over the legs and buttocks. A urine dip shows 2+ blood. Routine bloods are normal. What is the most likely diagnosis?
   A. Idiopathic thrombocytopenic purpura
   B. Meningococcal sepsis
   C. Acute lymphoblastic leukaemia (ALL)
   D. Vitamin C deficiency (scurvy)
   E. Henoch–Schönlein purpura

69. A 3-year-old Afro-Caribbean girl presents with severe pain in her hands and abdomen. On examination there is mucosal pallor, yellow sclera, generalized abdominal tenderness with hepatosplenomegaly. Bloods were taken including a FBC: Hb=6.1 g/dL, MCV=78 fL, white cell count (WCC)=6.0 × 109/L, platelets=300 × 109/L. What is the most likely cause of her anaemia?
   A. Thalassaemia
   B. Iron deficiency anaemia
   C. Sickle cell disease
   D. Anaemia of chronic disease
   E. Glucose-6-phosphate dehydrogenase deficiency

70. A 9-year-old girl with known sickle cell disease presents with a 4-day history of fever, coryza and myalgia. Over the past 24 hours she has developed a lacy rash particularly over her hands and feet and has become more lethargic. Her mother reports her looking more pale. A FBC reveals: Hb 5.9 g/dL, WCC 1.0 × 109/L, platelets 50 × 109/L. What is the most likely cause for her blood results?
   A. Splenic sequestration crisis
   B. Painful crisis
   C. Chest crisis
   D. Parvovirus B19 infection
   E. Pneumococcal sepsis

71. An 8-month-old girl with Greek-Cypriot parents is brought to her GP as her parents are worried she is not growing well and is very pale. On examination there is pallor and mildly icteric sclera. She has a distended abdomen with hepatosplenomegaly and there is mild frontal bossing. She was born on the 25th centile and her weight has fallen to below the 2nd centile. Blood tests show a microcytic hypochromic anaemia. What is the likely diagnosis?
   A. Sickle cell disease
   B. Hereditary spherocytosis
   C. Thalassaemia major
   D. Glucose-6-phosphate dehydrogenase deficiency (G6PD)
   E. Iron deficiency anaemia

72. A 14-month-old boy is brought to accident and emergency by his mother with pain and swelling in his right knee. He is unable to weight bear and on examination several large bruises are noted over the lower limbs and arms. He has blood tests, including a FBC and clotting screen, which show: Hb 10.5 g/dL, WCC 11 × 109/L, platelet count 340 × 109/L,

prothrombin time 13.3 sec, APTT >120 sec. Which is the most likely diagnosis?
A. Vitamin K deficiency
B. Haemophilia A
C. Von Willebrand disease
D. Immune (idiopathic) thrombocytopenic purpura
E. Non-accidental injury

73. A 5-year-old boy attends accident and emergency with a nosebleed that his mother has been unable to stop for the past 45 minutes. He saw his GP for a viral upper respiratory tract infection 1 week ago but is otherwise well. His nosebleed is stopped with pressure but on examination he is noted to have multiple petechiae on his chest, legs and abdomen. Blood tests reveal: Hb 10.4 g/dL, WCC 13 × 109/L, platelet count 15 × 109/L, clotting screen normal. The most likely diagnosis is which of the following?
A. Henoch–Schönlein purpura
B. Haemophilia B (Christmas disease)
C. Immune (idiopathic) thrombocytopenic purpura (ITP)
D. Meningococcal septicaemia
E. Haemolytic uraemic syndrome (HUS)

74. A 7-year-old Ghanaian boy presented to accident and emergency, 3 days ago, on his return from holiday in West Africa, with high fever and rigors. A diagnosis of malaria was made and he was started on primaquine. His mother is concerned that he has begun to look increasingly jaundiced. On examination there is deep jaundice, and he is looking pale and breathless. A FBC and film are taken which show: Hb 5.5 g/dL, WCC 15 × 109/L, platelet count 200 × 109/L, blood film: red cell fragments and bite cells with Heinz bodies on staining. The most likely underlying diagnosis is which of the following?
A. Glucose-6-phosphate dehydrogenase deficiency (G6PD)
B. Pyruvate kinase deficiency
C. Sickle cell disease
D. Beta-thalassaemia
E. Hereditary spherocytosis

75. A 4-year-old girl is undergoing chemotherapy for acute lymphoblastic leukaemia. She presents 8 days after her last treatment with a fever of 39°C. She has a portacath in situ. Her FBC shows a WCC 1.0 × 109/L, neutrophils 0.4 × 109/L, platelets 100 × 109/L, Hb 10 g/dL. What is the most important step in her management?
A. Packed red blood cell transfusion
B. Platelet transfusion
C. Administration of G-CSF
D. Antipyretics
E. Intravenous antibiotics

76. ALL is the commonest form of childhood leukaemia and carries a 5-year survival rate of over 80%. However, prognosis depends on a number of factors.

Which of the following is a good prognostic factor in acute lymphoblastic leukaemia?
A. White cell count (WCC) >50 × 109/L at diagnosis
B. Age >10 at diagnosis
C. Age <1 year at diagnosis
D. Non-B cell, non-T cell leukaemia
E. Presence of translocations, e.g. Philadelphia chromosome

77. A 14-year-old boy presents with a history of lethargy, constipation and shortness of breath on lying flat. On examination he has an enlarged, fixed lymph node in his left neck. He is investigated with bloods and a CXR which demonstrate anaemia and a large mediastinal mass. A biopsy is taken from the mass in the neck which shows the presence of Reed–Sternberg cells. What is the likely diagnosis?
A. Tuberculosis of lymph nodes
B. Non-Hodgkin's lymphoma
C. Hodgkin's lymphoma
D. Sarcoidosis
E. Epstein–Barr infection

78. There are a number of syndromes that predispose to specific forms of malignancy and require vigilance and screening to make an early diagnosis. Which of the following conditions is not associated with an increased risk of malignancy?
A. Down syndrome
B. Beckwith–Wiedemann syndrome
C. Ataxia telangectasia
D. Li Fraumeni syndrome
E. Turner syndrome

79. Brain tumours are the most common solid tumour of childhood and presentation may be insidious leading to late diagnosis. Which of the following statements regarding brain tumours in childhood is true?
A. They are usually supratentorial
B. Signs of raised intracranial pressure are rare
C. Astrocytomas carry poor prognosis
D. Medulloblastomas are the most common type
E. Metastasis is common

80. A 3-year-old boy is brought to his GP with abdominal distension. He is otherwise well. There is no family history of note. On examination there is a large, smooth mass palpable in the left flank. There is no lymphadenopathy. Urinalysis shows 2 + blood, urinary catecholamines are not raised. What is the most likely diagnosis?
A. Nephroblastoma (Wilms' tumour)
B. Neuroblastoma
C. Polycystic kidney disease
D. Multicystic kidney disease
E. Horseshoe kidney

81. A 2-year-old boy undergoes a CT scan for abdominal mass. The scan demonstrates a large mass arising from

the renal parenchyma. Following surgical resection a histological diagnosis of nephroblastoma is made. Which of the following statements regarding nephroblastoma is true?
A. It usually causes hypertension
B. It is associated with Beckwith–Wiedemann syndrome
C. A susceptibility gene is found on chromosome 22
D. Metastasis at presentation is common
E. Presentation is usually with abdominal pain and weight loss

82. A 2-month-old baby is brought to the GP as a family photo shows a discrepancy in her eyes. On examination a red reflex is present in one eye only. She is otherwise healthy. Which of the following is the most likely diagnosis?
A. Retinoblastoma
B. Retinopathy of prematurity
C. Congenital cataracts
D. CMV retinitis
E. Glaucoma

83. A 15-year-old boy presents with a 6-week history of pain in his lower leg. On examination there is a painful swelling in the proximal tibia. X-ray of the limb shows a sunburst appearance. What is the most likely diagnosis?
A. Ewing's sarcoma
B. Rickets
C. Osteosarcoma
D. Osteomyelitis
E. Chondrosarcoma

84. An 8-year-old girl is brought to hospital following ingestion of a cereal bar containing peanuts. She is noted to have a widespread urticarial rash and swelling of the face and lips. She is finding it difficult to speak and there is widespread wheeze on auscultation. The single most important step in her management is which of the following?
A. Intramuscular 1 microgram/kg adrenaline (epinephrine) (1:1000)
B. Intravenous adrenaline (epinephrine), 1 microgram/kg (1:10 000)
C. Intravenous hydrocortisone
D. Oxygen
E. Chlorphenamine

85. A 1-year-old child is brought to the GP by his mother. He has a history of severe egg allergy with previous confirmed anaphylactic reaction. Mum is concerned about him receiving his MMR vaccination as she has heard it contains egg. What is the most appropriate advice to give her?
A. He can safely receive all vaccines
B. He must not be given the MMR as it contains egg and he is at risk of severe allergic reaction
C. He should avoid all live vaccines as they may precipitate a reaction

D. He can safely receive the MMR, preferably in hospital, but should not receive the influenza or yellow fever vaccines
E. He can be given the MMR but should receive antihistamine at the same time

86. A 4-year-old girl with a family history of atopy attends her GP. Her older brother suffers from nut allergy and hay fever from grass and pollen. Her mother is very keen to have her tested before introducing her to nuts and requests skin-prick testing. Which of the following statements is true regarding skin-prick testing?
A. The severity of an allergic reaction is accurately predicted by the size of skin-prick reaction
B. It is suitable for identifying both IgE and non-IgE mediated allergy
C. It is more accurate than blinded food challenge
D. Positive (histamine) and negative (saline) controls should be injected, along with other allergens to confirm success of testing
E. Tests for levels of specific IgE to allergens in the serum

87. A 6-month-old boy attends clinic with a history of bloody diarrhoea and failure to thrive. There is no vomiting and examination is normal. A diagnosis of cow's milk allergy is suspected. Which of the following statements regarding food allergy is true?
A. It is commonly non-IgE mediated
B. RAST testing will accurately identify all food allergies
C. A positive skin prick test to soya means that the child is allergic
D. Elimination/reintroduction programme is unhelpful
E. It is rare for children to outgrow their allergies

88. Many allergens have cross-reactivity due to the similarity in the proteins. This results in children being at risk of reacting to other allergens. The following are examples of allergen cross-reactivity, except which one?
A. Grass and peanut
B. Peanuts and soya beans
C. Latex and banana
D. Lentils and peanuts
E. Fish and kiwi

89. A 9-year-old girl presents with haematuria. She is usually fit and well but was treated for tonsillitis last week by her GP. On examination there is peripheral oedema and hypertension but no abdominal mass. Urine dipstick is positive for blood and protein. What is the likely diagnosis?
A. Post-streptococcal glomerulonephritis
B. Haemolytic uraemic syndrome
C. Systemic lupus erythematosus (SLE)
D. Henoch–Schönlein purpura
E. Minimal change nephropathy

90. A 7-year-old girl presents with oedema of the face and legs, and abdominal pain. Urine dipstick shows 4+ protein. A diagnosis of nephrotic syndrome is made and she is started on prednisolone. What would be the likely finding on biopsy and light microscopy?
A. Focal-segmental glomerulosclerosis
B. Mesangiocapillary glomerulonephritis
C. Crescentic glomerulonephritis
D. Minimal change disease
E. Membranous glomerulonephritis

91. On routine newborn examination a baby is noted to have bilaterally undescended testes. Genitalia appears to be male. Which is the most important initial investigation?
A. Karyotype with FISH for sex-determining region of the Y chromosome
B. Abdominal ultrasound scan
C. Abdominal CT scan
D. 17-Hydroxyprogesterone levels
E. Urea and electrolytes (U&Es)

92. An 11-year-old girl presents following 6 days of fever, abdominal pain and bloody diarrhoea. She has become increasingly irritable and lethargic. Blood tests reveal: Hb 7.5 g/dL, WCC 15 × 109/L, platelets 40 × 109/L, urea 9.0 mmol/L, creatinine 200 μmol/L, blood film shows red blood cell fragments. The most likely diagnosis is which of the following?
A. Ulcerative colitis
B. Glucose-6-phosphate dehydrogenase deficiency
C. Haemolytic uraemic syndrome
D. Dehydration
E. Viral gastroenteritis

93. A 12-year-old boy presents to accident and emergency with a history of groin pain for the past 4 hours. He is complaining of nausea and has vomited twice. On examination there is tenderness and swelling of the scrotum and right testicle, with absence of the cremasteric reflex on that side. There is no fever or erythema. Routine blood tests are normal. He describes several previous episodes of pain which were short lived. What is the most likely diagnosis?
A. Testicular torsion
B. Torsion of the hydatid of Morgagni
C. Inguinal hernia
D. Renal stone
E. Epididymo-orchitis

94. A 3-month-old baby girl presents with a fever of 38.6°C, crying and with vomiting. A dipstick demonstrates white cells and protein in her urine. Which of the following organisms is most likely to be responsible for her urinary tract infection?
A. *Enterococcus* spp.
B. *Pseudomonas*
C. *Proteus*
D. *Escherichia coli*
E. *Klebsiella*

95. Many conditions that require surgery can be deferred until the risk of the anaesthetic has lessened with age. However, some require surgery in early infancy. Which of the following would require surgery within the first 6 months of life?
A. Hydrocele
B. Umbilical hernia
C. Posterior urethral valves
D. Inguinal hernia
E. Single undescended testis

96. A 2-month-old girl is brought to clinic following an admission for a urinary tract infection. When discussing the results with her mother which of the following statements regarding urinary tract infection (UTI) is true?
A. Is more common in girls under the age of 3 months
B. Can be diagnosed with >105 white blood cells/mL urine
C. Presents with specific urinary features in young children
D. Is most commonly due to enterococci
E. Risk is increased by constipation

97. A 6-year-old boy is diagnosed with nephrotic syndrome and admitted to hospital to initiate steroid therapy and monitor him for potential complications. Which one of the following complications is he unlikely to be at risk of?
A. Bacterial infection
B. Hypovolaemia
C. Reduced glucose tolerance
D. Pleural effusion
E. Pulmonary embolus

98. A 15-year-old girl attends her GP with lethargy and irregular menstruation. She has also been experiencing intermittent palpitations. She has previously had regular periods and has developed secondary sexual characteristics. On examination she is slim and has firm parotid swelling bilaterally. There is poor dental hygiene. Blood tests are arranged which show: sodium (Na) 134 mmol/L, potassium (K) 3.0 mmol/L, chloride 90 mmol/L. What is the most likely diagnosis?
A. Mumps
B. Polycystic ovarian syndrome
C. Anorexia nervosa
D. Bulimia nervosa
E. Hypothyroidism

99. A 14-year-old girl is brought to her GP by her mother who is concerned that she has been losing weight. Her weight has dropped noticeably over the past year and she has become increasingly withdrawn. She is very active and plays for her school netball team. She makes her own meals at home, rather than eating with the family. She has not reached menarche. On examination her BMI is 15 and fine lanugo hair is noted over her upper body. The most likely cause for her weight loss is which of the following?
A. Hyperthyroidism
B. Anorexia nervosa

C. Malabsorption
D. Diabetes mellitus
E. Depression

100. An 8-year-old boy is referred by the educational psychologist with a suspected diagnosis of ADHD (attention deficit hyperactivity disorder). He has been struggling at school and finds it hard to concentrate on an activity. Teachers have been finding it hard to manage his behaviour as he is restless and constantly running around the classroom. Which of the following would suggest a diagnosis other than ADHD?
A. Easily distracted by other children
B. Difficulty waiting for his turn
C. Symptoms only present at school
D. Constantly talking often interrupting others
E. Fidgeting with his hands or objects while sitting still

101. A 4-year-old boy is referred to his GP by his teacher at nursery. She has noticed that he has delayed speech and has only a handful of words. He struggles with imaginative play and usually plays alone. He becomes upset if there is a change to the daily routine. In the surgery he does not make eye contact. There are no dysmorphic features. What is the most likely diagnosis?
A. Selective mutism
B. Normal development
C. Autism
D. Speech delay
E. Fragile X

102. A 6-year-old boy is brought to the GP with bedwetting. His mother is concerned that he has never been dry at night and wants to know if this is normal. When counselling his mother which of the following statements regarding nocturnal enuresis is correct?
A. It is commonly due to urinary tract infection
B. Children are commonly dry at night by age 4
C. Primary nocturnal enuresis is commonly related to stressful events
D. Cutting down fluid in the evening is ineffective
E. Bell-alarms may be helpful in children who sleep very deeply

103. A 14-month-old is seen in clinic as his mother is concerned that he may be having seizures. The episodes occur when he is angry or upset. He has colour change followed by collapse and occasional jerking movements. The most likely diagnosis is?
A. Breath holding spells
B. 'Tet' spells
C. Myoclonic epilepsy
D. Non-epileptic seizure
E. Vasovagal syncope

104. A 6-year-old boy is falling behind at school. His mother is concerned he is inattentive. She describes him daydreaming frequently, during which time it is difficult to attract his attention. Routine blood tests are normal. An EEG demonstrates spikes at 3 Hz. The likely diagnosis is which of the following?
A. ADHD – inattentive form
B. Absence seizures
C. Juvenile myoclonic epilepsy
D. Daydreaming
E. Non-epileptic seizures

105. A 5-month-old boy is brought in by his mother. She is concerned that he is frequently irritable. She is worried he may be in pain as he tenses and bends his head up, flailing his arms for a few seconds at a time. An EEG is performed which shows large-amplitude slow waves with spikes and sharp waves. The most likely diagnosis is which of the following?
A. Absence seizures
B. Benign rolandic epilepsy
C. Gastro-oesophageal reflux
D. West syndrome (infantile spasms)
E. Breath holding attacks

106. A 12-year-old girl with known epilepsy is brought in by ambulance. She has been fitting for 15 minutes. Her parents administered buccal midazolam after 5 minutes as part of her rescue regimen. On arrival, tonic-clonic movements are ongoing. The ambulance crew have inserted a cannula and are giving high flow oxygen via facemask. What is the next step in management?
A. Intravenous lorazepam
B. Rectal diazepam
C. Rapid sequence induction
D. Loading dose of phenytoin
E. Intravenous phenobarbital

107. An 8-year-old girl presents with a second generalized tonic-clonic seizure. It required lorazepam to terminate the seizure and a decision is made to start anti-epileptic treatment. Which of the following is first line therapy?
A. Phenobarbital
B. Sodium valproate
C. Vigabatrin
D. Ethosuximide
E. Phenytoin

108. A 9-year-old girl is brought to her GP with a 2-month history of headaches. Which of the following features of her headaches is not a red-flag symptom?
A. Associated with vomiting
B. Morning headache
C. Worse on lying down
D. Presence of focal neurology
E. Symmetrical, band-like in nature

109. A 2-year-old boy is referred to out-patients by his GP as there is a family history of neurofibromatosis type 1. Which of the following features would be diagnostic of this condition?
A. Presence of three café-au-lait patches
B. Acoustic neuroma
C. Ash-leaf spots

D. Lisch nodules
E. Adenoma sebaceum

110. Duchenne muscular dystrophy is the most common muscular dystrophy seen in children. Which of the following statements regarding Duchenne muscular dystrophy is true?
    A. It is an autosomal dominant condition
    B. The average age at onset is 14 years
    C. Gower's sign is an uncommon feature
    D. Mutation is in the dystrophin gene
    E. Calf pseudohypertrophy is rare

111. A 4-year-old boy presents to accident and emergency with fever, irritability, headache and neck stiffness. A diagnosis of meningitis is suspected and lumbar puncture is performed. Blood sugar is 4.3 mmol/L. Which of the following CSF results is most suggestive of bacterial meningitis?
    A. WCC 18 × 106/L (20% neutrophils), red cells 6 × 106/L, protein 0.8 g/L, glucose 3.0 mmol/L
    B. WCC 20 × 106/L (80% neutrophils), red cells 5 × 106/L, protein 1.6 g/L, glucose 1.0 mmol/L
    C. WCC 22.0 × 106/L (25% neutrophils), red cells 4 × 106/L, protein 2.4 g/L, glucose 1.2 mmol/L
    D. WCC 5 × 106/L, RBC 4000 × 106/L, protein 0.4 g/L, glucose 3.0 mmol/L
    E. WCC 2.0 × 106/L, red cells 5 × 106/L, protein 0.3 g/L, glucose 3.1 mmol/L

112. An 18-month-old girl is seen on the post take ward round following her first febrile seizure. When counselling her parents about the diagnosis which of the following statements regarding simple febrile convulsions is true?
    A. They are often focal in nature
    B. Children frequently go on to develop epilepsy
    C. Occur between ages of 6 months and 5 years
    D. Should always be investigated with lumbar puncture
    E. May occur without fever

113. An 8-year-old boy is referred for developmental assessment. He has been struggling at school, particularly in maths, and finds it difficult to concentrate. On examination his face is long and narrow, he has a prominent forehead and ears. What is the likely cause of his delay?
    A. Down syndrome
    B. Prader–Willi
    C. ADHD
    D. Fragile X
    E. Rett syndrome

114. Common forms of inheritance include autosomal dominant and autosomal recessive patterns. Which of the following conditions is autosomal dominant?
    A. Neurofibromatosis type 1
    B. Cystic fibrosis

C. Sickle cell disease
D. Haemophilia A
E. Duchenne muscular dystrophy

115. A 6-year-old boy attends the out-patient clinic with a diagnosis of Down syndrome. He has been pale and lethargic for the last 4 weeks and has some bruises on his shins. Which of the following conditions is it important to rule out in view of his underlying diagnosis?
    A. Parvovirus infection
    B. ITP
    C. Haemophilia A
    D. Acute leukaemia
    E. Henoch–Schönlein purpura

116. Down syndrome is the most common form of trisomy encountered in children and occurs on chromosome 21. Which of the following statements is true?
    A. Most babies with Down syndrome are born to older mothers
    B. Males are frequently infertile
    C. The incidence is 1 in 1400
    D. Epicanthic folds are pathognomonic
    E. The majority have severe intellectual impairment

117. A 14-year-old girl attends clinic as she is concerned about her height. She is on the 9th centile for height. On examination she has not yet developed secondary sexual characteristics, she has a square-shaped chest, webbing of the neck and short 4th metacarpals. What is the likely cause for her short stature?
    A. Hypothyroidism
    B. Constitutional short stature
    C. Turner syndrome
    D. Growth hormone deficiency
    E. Russell–Silver syndrome

118. A midwife refers a newborn baby boy with concerns that he has dysmorphic features. He has a number of abnormalities that suggest a diagnosis of Edwards syndrome (trisomy 18). Which of the following is not a feature of Edwards syndrome?
    A. Microcephaly
    B. Rocker-bottom feet
    C. Hypertelorism
    D. Developmental delay
    E. Brushfield spots

119. A pregnant mother is being consented for an amniocentesis and wants to know which conditions it can diagnose. Which of the following can not be accurately diagnosed by amniocentesis?
    A. Sickle cell disease
    B. Down syndrome
    C. Fragile X syndrome
    D. Spina bifida
    E. Cystic fibrosis

120. A 13-year-old boy attends his GP as he is concerned that he is developing breast tissue. On examination

he is tall with clear gynaecomastia. There is sparse pubic hair and small testes. He has been struggling with his school work and is behind his peers. What is the likely diagnosis?
A. Marfan syndrome
B. Klinefelter syndrome
C. Congenital tall stature
D. Hyperthyroidism
E. Growth hormone excess (gigantism)

121. Specific terms are used to describe dysmorphic features to ensure consistency. Which of the following definitions of dysmorphic features is correct?
A. Hypertelorism – increased distance between the eyes
B. Clinodactyly – webbing of the fingers
C. Brachycephaly – flat forehead
D. Micrognathia – small tongue
E. Epicanthic folds – up-slanting of the separation between upper and lower eyelids

122. A mother on the postnatal ward is concerned that her toddler has got chicken pox. The rash developed 2 days ago. She has not previously had chicken pox. What is the most appropriate management of the baby?
A. Check maternal antibodies, if negative give VZIG (varicella zoster immunoglobulin)
B. Observe on postnatal ward for development of chicken pox
C. Discharge home, advise avoid contact with toddler until lesions crusted
D. No precautions necessary
E. Treatment of neonate with aciclovir

123. An 18-month-old baby boy is brought to clinic with features of spastic diplegia. When counselling the parents on the diagnosis of cerebral palsy which of the following statements is correct?
A. The insult usually occurs during delivery
B. Cerebral palsy is a disorder of motor and sensory function due to a static brain injury
C. Reflexes are reduced or absent
D. Botulinum toxin may be useful to treat spasticity
E. MRI scan is diagnostic

124. A newborn baby is delivered by caesarean following an obstructed labour. He requires full resuscitation including adrenaline (epinephrine) and his initial capillary blood gas shows a pH of 6.9 (normal range 7.35–7.45) Which of the following is unlikely to be related to the perinatal asphyxia?
A. Hypotension
B. Renal failure
C. Necrotizing enterocolitis
D. Seizures
E. Heart murmur

125. A male infant born at 29 weeks is now 4 hours old. He has developed an increased oxygen requirement, there is tachypnoea and severe intercostal and subcostal recessions. CXR demonstrates a ground glass appearance. The most likely diagnosis is which of the following?
A. Transient tachypnoea of the newborn
B. Respiratory distress syndrome
C. Congenital pneumonia
D. Pneumothorax
E. Congenital heart disease

126. A female infant born at 28 weeks is now 10 days old. She had been doing very well and breast milk was started 2 days ago via nasogastric tube. She has become increasingly unwell over the past 12 hours with abdominal distension, temperature instability and bile stained aspirates from the NG tube. Some blood is noted in the stools. AXR shows air within the bowel walls. What is the most likely diagnosis?
A. Sepsis
B. Intestinal obstruction
C. Necrotizing enterocolitis
D. Malrotation
E. Duodenal atresia

127. A 3-day-old male infant is noted to have a cardiac murmur. Four limb blood pressures are normal but oxygen saturation is 78% and does not improve with oxygen therapy. Which of the following congenital heart defects is the most likely diagnosis?
A. Patent ductus arteriosus
B. Tetralogy of Fallot
C. Ventricular septal defect
D. Atrial septal defect
E. Coarctation of the aorta

128. A 2-month-old infant is brought to the GP by his mother. She is concerned that he vomits after every feed. She has noticed that his abdomen has become distended. On further questioning he opens his bowels infrequently every 3–4 days and did not pass meconium until 72 hours of age. Abdominal X-ray shows distended loops of bowel with no air in the rectum. The most likely diagnosis is which of the following?
A. Hirschsprung's disease
B. Constipation due to dehydration
C. Pyloric stenosis
D. Cow's milk protein allergy
E. Intussusception

129. A term female baby is seen on the postnatal ward. She is 18 hours old and has not been feeding well. Her mother was told she needed to have antibiotics prior to labour but delivered too quickly to receive them. She is admitted to the neonatal unit with suspected sepsis and CXR confirms congenital pneumonia. What is the most likely causative organism?
A. *Streptococcus pneumoniae*
B. *Escherichia coli*
C. *Listeria monocytogenes*
D. Group B haemolytic streptococcus
E. *Chlamydia pneumoniae*

130. A term infant born by home delivery is brought to accident and emergency on day 4. His mother has noticed a small amount of bleeding from the umbilical stump, which is still oozing some blood at present. His mother mentions that her other children received vitamin K in the hospital but she cannot recall her newborn receiving this. Which of the following blood results is likely to be abnormal?
    A. Platelets
    B. Prothrombin time (PT)
    C. Activated partial thromboplastin time (APTT)
    D. Haemoglobin
    E. Antiplatelet antibodies

131. A 7-month-old infant presents with a 12-hour history of intermittent inconsolable crying; he is mottled, has cool peripheries and has vomited several times. Examination reveals a mass in the right upper quadrant of the abdomen. What is the most likely cause of his symptoms?
    A. Colic
    B. Incarcerated hernia
    C. Gastroenteritis
    D. Intussusception
    E. Gastro-oesophageal reflux

132. A 9-year-old presents with a 6-month history of non-bloody diarrhoea associated with 4 kg of weight loss. His mother says he is less energetic than before and looks paler than normal. There is no history of foreign travel. Blood tests show a microcytic anaemia (Hb 8.9 g/dL, MCV 72) but normal inflammatory markers. What is the most likely diagnosis?
    A. Crohn's disease
    B. Salmonella infection
    C. Coeliac disease
    D. Cow's milk protein allergy
    E. Ulcerative colitis

133. An 8-year-old girl presents with a 6-month history of pain most days around the umbilicus which lasts for an hour and responds to paracetamol syrup. It does not occur at weekends usually. She opens her bowels daily and passes a soft stool. She is thriving with her weight and height on the 75th centile. Which of the following options is the appropriate next step?
    A. Abdominal radiograph
    B. Referral to a paediatric gastroenterologist
    C. Inflammatory markers and liver function tests
    D. Reassurance and no further investigation
    E. Prescription for laxatives

134. A 13-year-old boy with a 3-month history of bloody diarrhoea, abdominal pain and 4 kg weight loss undergoes an endoscopy and colonoscopy. The results show patchy inflammation affecting the ileum and colon. What is the most likely diagnosis?
    A. Crohn's disease
    B. Coeliac disease
    C. Ulcerative colitis
    D. Infective colitis
    E. Intussusception

135. A newborn infant with features of Down syndrome develops vomiting on day 1 of life. The pregnancy was complicated by polyhydramnios. On examination he is well perfused and his abdomen is soft with no masses palpable. His anus is patent but he has not opened his bowels yet. Which of the following is the most useful initial investigation to make a diagnosis?
    A. Plain abdominal radiograph
    B. Abdominal ultrasound scan
    C. CT abdomen
    D. MRI abdomen
    E. Barium follow through

136. A 4-year-old boy attends accident and emergency with a history of 3 days of non-bilious vomiting and diarrhoea; today he has had two vomits with streaks of blood in. He has a mild temperature (38.2°C) but is well hydrated and tolerates a fluid challenge. What is the most likely diagnosis?
    A. Gastro-oesophageal reflux
    B. Oesophagitis
    C. Peptic ulcer disease
    D. Gastroenteritis
    E. Mallory–Weiss tear

137. A 15-year-old boy attends accident and emergency with a 2-day history of bloody diarrhoea associated with abdominal cramps and lassitude. He has a fever of 38.8°C. His parents have similar symptoms and they all ate at the same takeaway chicken shop 3 days before. He has not travelled abroad recently. Which organism is most likely responsible for his symptoms?
    A. Rotavirus
    B. *Shigella*
    C. Amoebiasis
    D. *E. coli*
    E. *Campylobacter*

138. A 3-year-old girl of Irish parents presents with a history of diarrhoea since birth. The stool is pale and offensive smelling. She was born on the 25th centile but is now on the 0.4th centile for weight and height. She has been admitted on four occasions with pneumonia and has a chronic cough. Which investigation is most likely to yield her diagnosis?
    A. Sweat test
    B. Coeliac antibodies
    C. Stool reducing substances
    D. Stool for microscopy and culture
    E. Endoscopy and colonoscopy

139. A 6-month-old baby attends with a history of constipation since birth. Her mother has been using glycerine suppositories every 3 days to help her defecate. When she inserts the suppository a gush of liquid stool is passed. Her mother remembers she did not open her bowels until she was 3 days old. Which of the following investigations would confirm the diagnosis?
    A. Thyroid function tests
    B. Barium enema

C. Bone profile
D. Abdominal film
E. Suction biopsy of the rectum

140. A 4-week-old formula fed girl presents with jaundice. Her mother reports that her urine looks dark and her stools are pale. She has failed to regain her birth weight. Her total bilirubin is 135 (normal <100 μmol/L) the conjugated fraction is 65 (normal <20 μmol/L). Her full blood count and reticulocytes are normal. What is the most likely diagnosis?
A. Physiological jaundice
B. Biliary atresia
C. Spherocytosis
D. G6PD deficiency
E. Urinary tract infection

141. A 6-day-old baby who is breast feeding well and thriving is referred by the midwife because she appears jaundiced. She has pigmented stools and is passing urine normally. Examination is unremarkable. Her bilirubin is 68 (normal <100 μmol/L) with a conjugated level of 8 (normal <20 μmol/L). Which of the following would be your management of this infant?
A. Complete a prolonged jaundice screen
B. Commence phototherapy
C. Top up feeds with formula milk
D. Repeat the bilirubin level in 8 hours
E. No treatment required

142. A 9-year-old boy attends hospital with a 24-hour history of abdominal pain initially around the umbilicus and now in the right iliac fossa. His mother says he has not eaten today and has been listless. He finds it difficult to stand up straight. He is tender on palpation of his abdomen and guarding. What is the next step in management?
A. Referral to surgical team
B. Abdominal radiograph
C. Intravenous antibiotics
D. Full septic screen
E. Admit to the ward for review on the ward round

143. A 6-week-old male infant presents with a week of worsening non-bilious vomiting. His mother reports the vomit is projectile in nature and seems to be getting gradually worse. He is eager to feed after the vomits but is having fewer wet nappies than usual. On examination he is afebrile, appears hungry and looks mildly dehydrated. What is the most likely diagnosis?
A. Cow's milk protein intolerance
B. Gastroenteritis
C. Meningitis
D. Pyloric stenosis
E. Malrotation and volvulus

144. There are very few absolute contraindications to live vaccinations. Which of the following is not a contraindication to vaccination with a live vaccine?
A. Acute fever >38°C
B. On high dose steroid therapy

C. Previous severe local reaction
D. Impaired cell mediated immunity
E. Less than 2.5 kg in weight

145. A 3-month-old baby is found dead in a Moses basket sleeping on her back. She was born in July at 41 weeks to a mother who smoked during the pregnancy and afterwards. Which of the following factors is the most likely to have influenced her sudden infant death?
A. Maternal smoking
B. Sleeping in a 'Moses basket'
C. Supine sleeping position
D. Born in summer months
E. Post-term delivery

146. A 5-month-old baby with no previous attendances at hospital is brought to the hospital by his distraught parents with a swollen left upper arm. Both parents tell you separately that he was playing on the floor and fell to one side. They noticed he was crying so phoned an ambulance to come to hospital. A radiograph of the arm shows a spiral fracture of his left humerus. Which of the following features suggest non-accidental injury?
A. Immediate presentation at hospital
B. History of incident does not fit with injury
C. Parents appearing distraught
D. Both accounts of the incident matching
E. No previous attendances at hospital

147. A 13-year-old girl is made to stay at home to clean the house while her two younger sisters attend ballet lessons on Saturday mornings. Her mother tells her she has to do it as she is too fat and clumsy to go to ballet. What category of abuse does this fit most closely?
A. Physical abuse
B. Neglect
C. Emotional abuse
D. Sexual abuse
E. Fabricated and fictitious illness

148. A 16-year-old girl is admitted to hospital and diagnosed with appendicitis. She is due to undergo an appendicectomy. She is accompanied by her mother and stepfather and her birth father. Which of the following are best placed to provide consent for the operation?
A. The doctor performing the procedure
B. Her mother
C. The girl herself
D. Her stepfather
E. Her birth father

149. A 3-month-old baby is seen in clinic with a severe nappy rash. The rash covers the perineal area including the skin folds and features satellite lesions. There is also a white coating to the baby's tongue. Otherwise the baby is well and thriving. Which of the following is the most appropriate treatment?
A. Topical flucloxacillin preparation
B. 1% hydrocortisone ointment

C. Barrier cream, e.g. zinc and castor oil cream
D. Antifungal preparation, e.g. miconazole
E. Emollient, e.g. white soft paraffin

150. An 8-month-old develops an itchy rash which seems most distressing at night. His mother has started to develop similar symptoms. On examination the rash is affecting the whole body but worst on the soles of the feet, head and neck. The lesions are small fluid filled vesicles and excoriations are visible. What is the most likely diagnosis?
A. Seborrhoeic eczema
B. Scabies
C. Tinea capitis
D. *Molluscum contagiosum*
E. Impetigo

151. A 3-year-old boy has a crop of six small pedunculated lesions with a central punctum on his trunk. They are not itching and he is otherwise well and thriving. His older sister has similar lesions on her trunk. Which of the following is the most appropriate management?
A. Laser removal of the lesions
B. Topical steroid therapy
C. No treatment required
D. Investigation of immune function
E. Silver nitrate cautery of lesions

152. A 5-year-old boy is referred by the school nurse as his weight and height are on the 99th centile at school entry weighing. He appears a healthy child with tall parents. He has no birth marks and his blood pressure is normal. Which of the following actions is appropriate?
A. Thyroid function tests
B. 9 a.m. cortisol level
C. Calculate mid-parental height
D. Dietary assessment
E. Genetic studies for Prader–Willi syndrome

153. Breast feeding is the best for babies and there are very few contraindications. Which of the following is an absolute contraindication to breast feeding in the UK?
A. Galactosaemia
B. Phenylketonuria
C. Neonatal jaundice
D. Cleft palate
E. ABO incompatability

154. A 12-year-old boy returns from a holiday to Kenya with a febrile illness. It is associated with a headache and rigors. On examination he has hepatomegaly, is jaundiced and there are some lesions on his arms and legs that look like insect bites. Which of the following investigations is most likely to confirm the suspected diagnosis?
A. Blood culture
B. Full blood count
C. Blood film for malaria parasites
D. Hepatitis serology
E. Liver function tests

155. A 6 week old baby is referred by the health visitor as she has only just regained her birth weight. She is being fed with formula milk and her stools are normal. On examination she appears thin but otherwise normal. She is admitted to the ward and fed by the nursing staff for a week as her mother is readmitted with an infection. She demonstrates excellent weight gain during this period. What is the most likely cause for her initial poor weight gain?
A. Cow's milk protein intolerance
B. Gastro-oesophageal reflux
C. Cystic fibrosis
D. Inadequate intake/neglect
E. Urinary tract infection

156. A 15-year-old boy presents to hospital with malaise, fever and mild jaundice over the last week. He says two other girls at his school have the same symptoms following a recent ski trip to France. On examination he has tender hepatomegaly and cervical lymphadenopathy. What is the most likely cause of his illness?
A. Acute myeloid leukaemia
B. Leptospirosis
C. Hepatitis A infection
D. Non-Hodgkins lymphoma
E. Epstein–Barr infection (EBV)

157. A 14-month-old baby girl is brought to the outpatient clinic as her parents are concerned about her size. She is on the 2nd centile for weight and height and head circumference. She was born on the 2nd centile. She is taking cow's milk and is fully weaned, her stool is normal and examination unremarkable. Her parents are concerned as they are both short and do not want her to be small when she is older. Which of the following is the most likely cause of her size?
A. Constitutionally small
B. Cow's milk protein enteropathy
C. Hypothyroidism
D. Growth hormone deficiency
E. Skeletal dysplasia

158. A 15-year-old girl attends clinic concerned about her episodic abdominal pain and loose stool over the last year. She dates it back to when she changed schools and says it occurs more often on school days. She describes crampy abdominal pain followed by the need to pass a stool which happens about twice a month. Her bowel habit is normal on the other days. There has never been any blood and she has not lost any weight. Which of the following is most likely to be the underlying cause of her symptoms?
A. Cow's milk protein intolerance
B. Coeliac disease
C. Ulcerative colitis
D. Irritable bowel syndrome
E. Overflow diarrhoea secondary to constipation

159. An 18-month-old exclusively breast fed infant has not started standing or walking yet. On examination she has swelling of her wrists and an open fontanelle. She has yet to erupt any teeth. Which of the following is the most likely cause?

A. Vitamin A deficiency
B. Vitamin B deficiency
C. Vitamin C deficiency
D. Vitamin D deficiency
E. Vitamin E deficiency

160. A newborn baby girl is born following a pregnancy complicated by oligohydramnios with bilateral talipes and requires ventilation for pulmonary hyposplasia. She fails to pass urine in the first 24 hours of life. Which of the following is likely to be the cause?

A. Nephrotic syndrome
B. Posterior urethral valves
C. Bilateral renal agenesis
D. Autosomal dominant polycystic kidney disease
E. Duplex kidney

Extended-matching questions (EMQs)

For each scenario described below, choose the single most likely diagnosis from the list of options given above. Each option may be used once, more than once or not at all.

1. Rashes

A. Chickenpox (varicella zoster)
B. Impetigo
C. Meningococcal septicaemia
D. Measles
E. Henoch–Schönlein purpura
F. Urticaria
G. Eczema
H. Erythema infectiosum ('fifth disease')
I. Erythema nodosum

1. A 10-year-old girl is brought into her local emergency department by ambulance with a 6-hour history of high fever, lethargy and neck stiffness. A non-blanching rash is noted on her lower extremities.
2. A 4-year-old boy is presented to his GP with a 3-day history of fever, reduced oral intake and rash. Several erythematous macules and papules are noted of varied distribution across his face and trunk. He seems to be uncomfortable and itching.
3. A 7-year-old boy has a 3-day history of fever, cough and conjunctivitis. He has now developed a blotchy, confluent rash and appears very miserable.
4. An 18-month-old girl is brought to her GP with tiny blisters around her nose and mouth. She appears clinically well in herself and a few of the lesions are noted to have a golden-crusted appearance to them.
5. A 12-year-old boy who recently returned from Pakistan gives a history of cough and night sweats. On examination, he is noted to have erythematous tender nodular lesions on both shins.

2. Heart disease

A. Aortic stenosis
B. Ventricular septal defect
C. Tetralogy of Fallot
D. Coarctation of the aorta
E. Patent ductus arteriosus
F. Atrial septal defect
G. Transposition of the great arteries
H. Supraventricular tachycardia
I. Infective endocarditis

1. An 8-week-old infant presents to the emergency department with intermittent cyanotic episodes. A loud ejection systolic murmur is noted and CXR reveals a 'boot-shaped' heart appearance.
2. A 2-week-old baby, born at 27 weeks' gestation, has been difficult to extubate from conventional ventilation. On examination, a continuous murmur is heard underneath the left clavicle.
3. A 5-day-old baby boy is brought into the emergency department by ambulance. He is tachypnoeic, pale and poorly perfused. No murmur can be heard but femoral pulses are weak.
4. An 18-month-old boy is admitted to the ward for observation following an accidental head injury. On routine examination, he is noted to have a systolic murmur, loudest at the lower left sternal edge. His father mentions that he is under review by a paediatric cardiologist but no definitive operation has been planned.
5. A 4-month-old infant has been brought to her local emergency department with an acute history of poor feeding and tachypnoea. Mother reports that she also seems sweaty during feeds. She is attached to a pulse oximetry monitor and the heart rate reads 230 beats per minute.

3. Tachypnoea

A. Bronchiolitis
B. Asthma
C. Croup
D. Lobar pneumonia
E. Cystic fibrosis
F. Pertussis (whooping cough)
G. Viral wheeze
H. Inhaled foreign body
I. Tuberculosis infection

1. A 5-month-old ex-premature female infant is presented to her GP with a 48-hour history of difficulty breathing and poor feeding. Her 3-year-old sibling has recently had a coryzal illness. On examination, she has a dry cough, a respiratory rate of 70/minute and intercostal and subcostal recession. Auscultation reveals widespread fine crackles and expiratory wheeze.
2. A 2-year-old boy has a 36-hour history of low-grade fever and cough. He is brought to the emergency department at 2 a.m. with acute onset of breathing difficulty. Parents describe him as having a 'barking cough' and harsh breathing. On examination, he is tachypnoeic with inspiratory stridor at rest.

3. An 11-year-old boy presents with a 7-day history of fever and cough. He was seen by his GP 5 days ago who prescribed amoxicillin but his condition has not improved. He is normally fit and well and there is no history of foreign travel or infectious contacts. On examination, his temperature is 39°C with a respiratory rate of 30/minute. His saturations are 92% in air and auscultation reveals reduced air entry at his right lung base with dull percussion note.

4. A 6-year-old girl is brought to her GP with a 3-month history of nocturnal cough and exertional breathlessness. During the history taking, her father mentions that she had eczema during infancy and mother is a smoker. On examination she appears thin and short for age with Harrison sulci.

5. A 10-week-old infant is admitted to hospital with a 5-day history of paroxysms of cough culminating in occasional vomits and blue episodes. She missed her 8-week primary set of immunizations as the family were abroad at that time. She appears mildly tachypnoeic at rest with normal saturations. Blood tests are unremarkable other than a lymphocytosis is noted.

4. Limp

A. Septic arthritis
B. Perthes disease
C. Trauma
D. Leukaemia
E. Osteomyelitis
F. Slipped upper femoral epiphysis
G. Juvenile idiopathic arthritis
H. Developmental dysplasia of the hip
I. Transient synovitis

1. A 6-year-old boy attends the emergency department accompanied by his mother. He has been unwell with coryzal symptoms for the last 5 days and has now developed a painful left hip. Examination reveals reduced external rotation of his left hip. He is systemically well and inflammatory markers are not raised.

2. A 22-month-old girl is brought to her GP with a 1-day history of high fever and non-weight-bearing on her right leg. On examination, she is febrile at 38.8°C and her right leg is held in a fixed position. There is marked tenderness on passive movements and her hip joint feels warm to palpate.

3. A 2-year-old boy presents with a 3-week history of painless limp on his left side. He was born as a breech delivery and mother had 'bone problems' when she was a child. Examination reveals asymmetric skin creases but no other abnormalities.

4. An 8-year-old boy is referred to the paediatric orthopaedic team by his GP with a 4-month history of intermittent limp on his right side. An X-ray reveals increased density of his right femoral head with some height reduction.

5. A previously healthy 4-year-old girl is brought to the emergency department accompanied by her father with a 4-week history of painful limp. Father informs the doctor that she has had frequent epistaxis and occasional bleeding gums over the last 6–8 weeks. On examination, her weight is 12 kg (0.4th–2nd centile) with marked pallor. No focal findings are noted when examining both legs.

5. Endocrine disorders

A. Hypothyroidism
B. Hyperthyroidism
C. Congenital adrenal hyperplasia
D. Diabetes mellitus
E. Cushing syndrome
F. Turner syndrome
G. Phenylketonuria
H. Mucoploysaccharidoses
I. Galactosaemia

1. An 8-year-old boy is urgently referred by his GP to the emergency department with a 4-week history of polyuria and polydipsia. At the GP's surgery, his urine dipstick revealed 3+ ketones and 3+ glucose and his random blood sugar level was 17 mmol/L.

2. A 20-month-old female infant is seen in clinic with a history of global developmental delay and two previous afebrile seizures. On examination, she plots on the 2nd centile (compared with a weight that plotted on 25th centile 6 months prior) and has fair skin and light hair. On further questioning, mother does not recall a Guthrie test ever being carried out on her daughter.

3. A 12-year-old girl was noted to have a deterioration in recent school performance. Her teacher describes her as agitated and intolerant of heat. There is also a history of weight loss and diarrhoea.

4. A 9-day-old baby is brought into the emergency department by ambulance with vomiting and severe dehydration. There is 15% weight loss since birth and clinical evidence of shock. Initial blood gas reveals hyponatraemia and hyperkalaemia.

5. A 3-year-old boy is referred to a specialist for global developmental delay and hearing impairment. On examination, he is noted to have a kyphosis and ophthalmology assessment reveals corneal opacities in both eyes.

6. Emergencies

A. Diabetic ketoacidosis
B. Status epilepticus
C. Acute epiglottitis
D. Acute severe asthma

E. Anaphylaxis

F. Septicaemic shock

G. Cardiorespiratory arrest

H. Head injury

I. Acute poisoning

1. A previously healthy 15-year-old girl is brought into the emergency department by ambulance following a distressed 999 call from her friend. The history from the ambulance crew is limited but they report the patient was at a friend's house at a party with several other teenagers and no adults. On arrival, her temperature is 38°C and heart rate 140 beats per minute. She appears agitated and paranoid and is complaining of chest pain.

2. A 3-year-old boy is brought into the emergency department with prolonged seizures. There is no relevant past medical history other than he had an overnight admission 8 months ago for an afebrile seizure. On examination, generalized tonic-clonic movements are observed. He is apyrexial and his blood sugar is 5.5 mmol/L.

3. A 6-year-old girl is rushed into her local emergency department by her parents with an acute onset of breathing difficulty. The family were eating out at a seafood restaurant when her symptoms developed. On examination, she is tachypnoeic and has swollen lips. Auscultation reveals widespread wheeze throughout.

4. A 10-year-old boy presents to the emergency department with a 6-week history of abdominal pain and weight loss. His urine dipstick reveals glycosuria and ketonuria. His blood gas results are: pH 7.20, bicarbonate 15 mmol/L, base excess −10 and glucose of 22 mmol/L.

5. A 14-year-old boy is brought into the emergency department by ambulance from a local nightclub. On arrival, his GCS is 9/15, heart rate 60 beats per minute and blood pressure 160/100 mmHg. His blood glucose is 8 mmol/L. No focal findings can be made on primary survey although the nurse reports that one pupil is larger and less responsive than the other.

7. Developmental assessment

A. Normal developmental limits

B. Fine motor delay

C. Gross motor delay

D. Fine motor and gross motor delay

E. Speech and language delay

F. Play and social delay

G. Language and fine motor delay

H. Language and gross motor delay

I. Global delay

1. A 20-month-old boy says 'mama' and 'dada' but no other words. He has a palmar grasp and can transfer toys from hand to hand. He is unable to stack two blocks together. He crawls on his hands and knees and finds it hard to hold a spoon.

2. A 7-month-old infant can sit unsupported and has a palmar grasp. He can make speech sounds and turns to his mother's voice. He has hand and foot regard and has a fear of strangers.

3. A 3-year-old girl can build a tower of three bricks and is able to name parts of the body and a few colours. She plays with other children and helps with her dressing. She falls over while running and cannot kick a ball.

4. A 22-month-old has a circular scribble and can build a tower of six bricks. He can pull himself to stand and is able to cruise around furniture. He says 'more juice' and gives his name.

5. A 5-year-old girl skips and can hop forward. She is able to draw a detailed person, is able to eat using a knife and fork and plays games with friends. She gives her name and gender and can count up to 10.

8. Seizures

A. Absence seizures

B. Benign rolandic epilepsy

C. Jacksonian seizures

D. Juvenile myoclonic epilepsy

E. Pseudo-seizures

F. Reflex anoxic seizure

G. Temporal lobe epilepsy

H. West syndrome

1. A 5-month-old girl has frequent episodes (up to 10 per day) where she suddenly jerks her arms and is then stiff for 2–5 seconds. They can occur in response to a startle.

2. A 14-year-old has twitching of his leg muscles especially when he has just woken up, poor concentration, and frequent 'daydreaming' episodes. He has had one generalized tonic-clonic seizure in the morning.

3. A 3-year-old has episodes of stopping and staring for several seconds when she is playing. She recovers quickly and continues playing afterwards.

4. An 11-year-old girl presents with multiple seizures which occur when she is stressed and involve rapid jerking and flailing of her limbs lasting for no more than 30 seconds. There is no post-ictal phase.

5. An 8-year-old has complaints of a 'rising' feeling in her stomach accompanied by staring vacantly and chewing motions. She also reports frequent episodes of déjà-vu.

9. Jaundice

A. ABO incompatibility
B. Glucose-6-phosphate dehydrogenase deficiency
C. Haemolytic uraemic syndrome
D. Hepatitis A
E. Hereditary spherocytosis
F. Rhesus incompatibility
G. Sickle cell disease
H. Thalassaemia

1. A 6-year-old girl, child of Somalian parents, presents with pain in her left leg and right arm not responding to simple analgesia. She is pale, increasingly jaundiced and has hepatosplenomegaly.
2. A term female infant is jaundiced at 5 hours of age and requires an exchange transfusion She is the second child of unrelated parents. Her mother is AB negative.
3. An 8-year-old boy returned from Bangladesh is unwell with diarrhoea and vomiting for the last 10 days. On examination he has jaundice, fever, hepatomegaly and abdominal tenderness.
4. A 3-year-old caucasian girl with anaemia has splenomegaly. She has a positive osmotic fragility test and her blood film shows red cell fragments and spherical blood cells.
5. A 4-year-old boy presents with jaundice. He has fragmented red cells on blood film following ingestion of broad beans. He required phototherapy as a neonate.

10. Genetics

A. Angelman syndrome
B. DiGeorge syndrome
C. Duchenne muscular dystrophy
D. Pierre Robin syndrome
E. Prader–Willi syndrome
F. Spinal muscular atrophy
G. Trisomy 21
H. Trisomy 13 (Patau syndrome)

1. A male newborn infant is admitted with poor feeding. He is noted to have marked micrognathia, cleft palate and a protruding tongue. Cardiovascular and ophthalmology examinations are normal.
2. A newborn female infant is noted to have dysmorphic features. She has a protruding tongue, epicanthic folds and a widened sandal gap. She has been having some difficulty in feeding and is hypotonic on examination. There is a loud systolic murmur.
3. A 6-year-old boy is seen with short stature. He is obese and eats obsessively, throwing tantrums when his parents try to restrict his intake. He has delayed motor milestones, walking at 2½ years.
4. A 2½-year-old boy who was developing well is brought to clinic by his mother who is concerned he cannot climb stairs and seems less confident when walking than before. On examination there is a waddling gait, weakness of the thigh muscles and large calf muscles.
5. A newborn baby is noted to have microcephaly. The eyes are small and forehead is sloping. There is an area of unformed skin on the scalp (cutis aplasia), a large umbilical hernia, cleft lip and palate and rocker-bottom feet.

11. Oncology

A. Acute lymphoblastic leukaemia
B. Ewing's sarcoma
C. Craniopharyngioma
D. Neuroblastoma
E. Non-Hodgkin's lymphoma
F. Osteosarcoma
G. Retinoblastoma
H. Wilms' tumour

1. A 5-year-old girl presents with an abdominal mass. On examination there was a large right-sided, smooth, non-tender mass. A CT scan is arranged which shows a smooth, well defined mass arising from the renal parenchyma.
2. A 6-month-old boy is brought to the GP as his mother has noticed a squint. On examination there is an absent red reflex on the right side.
3. A 10-year-old boy presents with severe left leg pain for the past few weeks. He is normally fit and well. On examination there is swelling and tenderness over the left femur. An X-ray of the femur is arranged which shows an onion-skin appearance in the mid-shaft.
4. A 2-year-old girl presents with a history of bruising with only minor bumps and knocks. Her mother is concerned that she is not gaining weight, despite a good appetite. On examination she is pale and thin. There is bruising over the lower limbs and inguinal lymphadenopathy. A FBC demonstrates: Hb 9.8 g/dL, WCC 52×10^9/L, platelets 100×10^9/L.
5. A 13-year-old boy attended the optician as he has been experiencing daily headaches and is concerned about his vision. He has not previously worn glasses. He is otherwise fit and well, there is no family history of migraine. Visual assessment demonstrates bitemporal hemianopia.

12. Congenital malformations

A. Cystic adenoid malformation
B. Diaphragmatic hernia
C. Duodenal atresia
D. Exomphalos
E. Gastroschisis
F. Myelomeningocele
G. Pulmonary hypoplasia
H. Spina bifida occulta
I. Tracheo-oesophageal fistula

1. A term infant born 8 hours ago is noted to have respiratory distress. There is a history of polyhydramnios. On examination copious frothy secretions are present. Her mother reports that she began coughing during her first breast feed.
2. A 37-week male infant born by caesarean section is seen on the postnatal ward at 24 hours of age. His mother is concerned that he has been vomiting after each feed. On examination his abdomen is distended and the sheets are stained with green vomit.
3. The neonatal SHO is called to see a 38-week female infant born by spontaneous vaginal delivery 2 hours ago. Her mother declined anomaly scan at 20 weeks. She is grunting with recession and head bobbing. On examination her chest is barrel shaped and her abdomen is scaphoid. The apex beat is displaced to the right.
4. A 40-week male infant is born by caesarean section. The midwife reports an abnormality was found at 20-week scan. On examination there is a lesion over the lumbar spine extending towards the sacrum. The area is red with absence of the overlying skin, fluid is leaking from the area and the spinal cord is readily visible.
5. A term neonate is born by planned caesarean section after an abnormality was discovered on routine antenatal scanning. At delivery a sac containing bowel is noted to be protruding from the abdominal wall.

13. Disorders of emotion and behaviour

A. Anorexia nervosa
B. Anxiety
C. Attention deficit hyperactivity disorder (ADHD)
D. Autism
E. Bulimia nervosa
F. Chronic fatigue syndrome
G. Depression
H. Selective mutism

1. A 10-year-old boy is falling behind at school. His teachers are concerned that he is constantly fidgeting and disrupts class. His mother is struggling at home, reporting he is constantly on the go and will not settle to one activity.
2. A 3-year-old boy is referred for assessment by his nursery school teacher as she is concerned about his behaviour. He frequently plays alone and does not like to interact with other children. He will spend hours playing with the toy cars, arranging them by colour and size. His speech is delayed and he uses only a few words.
3. A 4-year-old girl is referred by her nursery school as she has delayed speech. She is able to make her needs understood with gestures but does not speak and is reluctant to play with other children. Her mother describes that at home she plays readily with her older brother and speaks in sentences of more than five words.
4. A 14-year-old girl has become increasingly isolated at school. She was previously a popular member of her class. She has stopped attending netball practice as she no longer enjoys it. She finds it difficult to get to sleep at night and wakes in the early morning. She has lost her appetite and finds it hard to motivate herself as she 'does not see the point of continuing'.
5. A 15-year-old girl presents with weight loss and social withdrawal. She has become obsessed with cooking and spends hours making elaborate meals for her family. She runs several miles each day and dresses in baggy clothes because she 'looks fat'.

14. Gastrointestinal disease

A. Coeliac disease
B. Ulcerative colitis
C. Post-infective lactose intolerance
D. Cystic fibrosis
E. Bilary atresia
F. Peptic ulcer disease
G. Cow's milk protein intolerance
H. Gastro-oesophageal reflux disease
I. Pyloric stenosis
J. Intussusception

1. An 8-month-old girl cries and vomits after most feeds especially if laid flat. However, the symptoms have improved since weaning and growth is adequate.
2. An 11-month-old boy appears in pain with his legs drawn up, and he is crying inconsolably. He is pale mottled and clammy and passes a 'redcurrant jelly' stool.
3. A 3-year-old boy with faltering growth since weaning. He complains of intermittent abdominal pain, bloating after meals and loose stools. He has a microcytic anaemia.

4. A 2-year-old girl has vomiting, diarrhoea and a fever for 5 days then seems to recover but she continues to pass loose stools three to four times a day for a further 2 months.

5. A 13-year-old girl has a 6-month history of abdominal pain accompanied by frequent loose stools which sometimes contain blood. She complains of nausea and has lost 4 kg of weight during this time.

15. Nutrition

A. Vitamin D deficiency

B. Kwashiorkor

C. Marasmus

D. Hyperkalaemia

E. Hyponatraemia

F. Vitamin A deficiency

G. Vitamin C deficiency

H. Obesity

I. Hypernatraemia

J. Vitamin K deficiency

1. A 2-year-old girl has not started to walk yet and has poor dentition. On examination she has bowed legs and swollen wrists. She is still taking mostly breast milk with little solid food.

2. A 6-day-old girl is jaundiced, passing little urine, and has lost 12% of her birthweight. Her mother is struggling to establish breast feeding.

3. A 3-year-old boy living in Malawi complains of deterioration in his vision at night and feels that his eyes have become dryer. Gradually he loses his sight completely.

4. A 12-year-old boy with polycystic kidney disease develops acute on chronic renal failure and is waiting for a transplant.

5. A 3-year-old child in Kenya presents with swelling of his extremities, thinning of his hair and loss of his skin pigmentation. On examination he has ascites and peripheral oedema.

16. Gastroenterology investigations

A. pH/impedance study

B. Colonoscopy

C. Barium enema

D. Abdominal ultrasound

E. Rectal biopsy

F. Plain abdominal radiograph

G. Small bowel biopsy

H. Video fluoroscopy

I. CT abdomen

J. Gastroscopy

1. A 5-week-old boy with vomiting after every feed for the last week, who has a palpable mass in the epigastric region.

2. A 10-month-old girl with a long history of constipation who did not open her bowels until she was 48 hours old.

3. A 13-year-old boy with a 6-month history of weight loss, abdominal pain, malaise and bloody stools.

4. An 8-month-old boy with faltering growth vomits after each feed. He is irritable and cries after feeding.

5. A 2-day-old baby boy has bilious vomiting, a distended abdomen and has not opened his bowels since birth.

17. Renal abnormalities

A. Autosomal recessive polycystic kidney disease

B. Duplex kidney

C. Horseshoe kidney

D. Posterior urethral valves

E. Pyelonephritis

F. Renal agenesis

G. Renal stones

H. Vesico-ureteric reflux

1. A 6-year-old girl presents with a 2-day history of abdominal pain and vomiting. She had an episode of shaking, affecting the whole body, lasting for several minutes. On examination there is tenderness in the right flank and she is febrile at 39 °C.

2. A newborn infant is noted to be lethargic. He has been breast feeding well although his mother has noticed he is passing large amounts of urine. His abdomen is distended and there is a large left-sided abdominal mass. An ultrasound scan is arranged and shows bilaterally enlarged kidneys with multiple cysts.

3. A 2-year-old girl presents with fever, dysuria, vomiting and has frequency of micturition. Urine dipstick is positive for nitrates and leucocytes. Her parents report this is her fourth episode of UTI. Ultrasound scan is arranged which demonstrates dilated ureters and blunting of the calyces bilaterally.

4. A 3-day-old boy is reviewed on the post-natal ward. His mother is concerned that his abdomen is distended. There is no vomiting and he has been feeding well. Examination reveals a grossly distended abdomen with a dull mass in the suprapubic area. His mother does not think he has passed urine yet.

5. A newborn infant is admitted to the neonatal unit with severe respiratory distress. He was delivered by caesarean section and the liquor volume was much reduced. There is a history of oligohydramnios throughout the pregnancy. He is ventilated, requiring very high pressures.

1. C – Kawasaki disease. This child's clinical features satisfy the diagnostic criteria for KD. It is an autoimmune disease in which the medium-sized blood vessels throughout the body become inflamed and is largely seen in children under 5 years of age.

2. D – Gain intravenous access, take blood cultures and administer broad-spectrum antibiotics. Meningococcal sepsis is a catastrophic diagnosis if missed with serious potential long-term complications. The management, as with any emergency, is paying attention to airway, breathing and circulation followed by definitive treatment with broad-spectrum intravenous antibiotics, e.g. ceftriaxone.

3. B – Transposition of the great arteries. TGA often presents in the first days after birth following spontaneous closure of the ductus arteriosus. Babies are often unwell with severe cyanosis and metabolic acidosis. TGA is the most common cyanotic congenital heart lesion that presents in neonates.

4. D – Explain that this is most likely to be an innocent murmur and inform the GP to re-evaluate the child once she has recovered from her hospital admission. This patient has an innocent murmur, which can be more pronounced in the presence of an intercurrent febrile illness. Typical features of innocent murmurs are: soft, systolic, normal heart sounds, an asymptomatic child, no accompanying signs or symptoms suggestive of cardiac disease, no radiation and variation with posture.

5. B – Organize a sweat test. The history of delayed passage of meconium and findings of finger clubbing raise suspicion for cystic fibrosis, which must be excluded. The gold standard for diagnosis is the sweat test and a CF genotype will also detect common mutations.

6. C – Parainfluenza virus. Parainfluenza viruses account for up to 80% of cases of croup. Other viruses that cause croup are adenovirus and RSV. The characteristic symptoms of cough and stridor of croup typically follow symptoms of an upper respiratory tract infection and it has its peak incidence in the second year of life in the winter.

7. E – Slipped upper femoral epiphysis. This is a child with 'risk-factors' for SUFE. He is black, overweight and in the correct age group for children with SUFE to present. The lack of fever does not suggest an infective cause. An X-ray will confirm the diagnosis.

8. C – Left knee joint aspiration of fluid. This is septic arthritis until proven otherwise. Inflammatory markers may be normal at this stage and X-rays may also be non-conclusive. It is vital that joint aspiration be performed as soon as possible followed by broad-spectrum antibiotics to prevent joint destruction.

9. C – Thyroid function tests. The combination of features suggests congenital hypothyroidism. In the developed world this is most commonly due to agenesis or failure of migration. Thyroxine treatment should be started as soon as the diagnosis is confirmed to preserve neurological function.

10. D – 17 hydroxyprogesterone level. This baby has presented with a 'salt-losing' adrenal crisis as reflected by the hyponatraemia and hypoglycaemia. Clinical presentation of CAH can either be classic or non-classic and symptoms are due to androgen excess and cortisol deficiency.

11. D – Bone age. In constitutional delay of growth, bone age will reveal delayed skeletal maturity. In contrast, normal skeletal maturation is seen in familial short stature.

12. A – Turner syndrome. Causes of delayed puberty can be classified into central causes (low gonadotrophins) and gonadal failure (high gonadotrophins). The ejection systolic murmur suggests coarctation of the aorta which is the commonest heart lesion in Turner syndrome.

13. D – Hypovolaemic shock. This girl has hypovolaemic shock likely secondary to gastroenteritis. Her observations, clinical status and blood gas analysis imply decompensated shock and urgent intervention is required in order to prevent irreversible shock and death. An intraosseous needle is likely to be needed due to poor perfusion with aggressive fluid resuscitation (after stabilization of airway and breathing).

14. E – Discuss the case with the regional burns centre. There are no concerns in this case to arouse suspicion for child abuse. Burns involving the face, hands or perineum are an

indication for discussion with the regional burns centre and it is very likely they would want to review the child as soon as possible.

15. A – Intravenous lorazepam. This is the next step in the status epilepticus protocol once intravenous access has been gained. No more than two doses of benzodiazepam should be given to avoid the risk of respiratory depression.

16. B – Intravenous *N*-acetylcysteine. Liver function tests and clotting studies must also be checked as liver failure may occur. Psychiatric evaluation is needed for all children presenting with deliberate poisoning.

17. E – Refer her to a community paediatrician for assessment. This toddler has specific gross motor delay and warrants developmental assessment by a community paediatrician. Always regard concerns raised by parents over their child's development as serious. Investigations are likely to be needed in this case.

18. B – Fine motor delay. This infant is demonstrating left hand preference, which is a worrying sign at 12 months of age. This may signify hemiplegia and warrants further assessment.

19. D – Play and social delay. This child is showing strong signs of a social communication disorder, e.g. autistic spectrum disorder. Autism has a prevalence rate of approximately 1 in 100 people and boys are four times more likely to develop it than girls. The average age at diagnosis is 3 years although speech concerns occur from about 2 years onwards.

20. E – Hypoxic–ischaemic encephalopathy. The poor Apgar score and need for ventilation are consistent with birth asphyxia and HIE. Perinatal events account for approximately 10% of cases of cerebral palsy.

21. C – Roseola infantum. Also known as 'sixth disease'. This is commonly caused by HHV6 or HHV7 and is a well recognized cause of febrile convulsions in 10–15% of cases.

22. D – Echocardiogram. This child is being treated for Kawasaki disease and therefore the most important complication is coronary artery aneurysms which can occur in 20–25% of untreated cases. Aneurysms have a peak frequency at around 4 weeks of onset of illness.

23. C – Severe combined immunodeficiency (SCID). This infant gives a classic presentation for SCID which must be excluded. SCID is an X-linked disorder and treatment is with bone marrow transplantation.

24. A – Atrioventricular septal defect. This baby has clinical features of trisomy 21 and hence, an AVSD is the most likely lesion, accounting for 40% of heart lesions in trisomy 21. The next most common is a VSD which accounts for approximately 30%.

25. E – Intravenous infusion of prostaglandin E1. This baby has congenital cyanotic heart disease until proven otherwise and an infusion of prostaglandin is mandatory for patency of the ductus arteriosus to allow mixing of blood.

26. C – *Streptococcus viridans*. *Streptococcus viridans* accounts for approximately 90% of cases of infective endocarditis (IE). Management consists of a 4–6-week course of intravenous antibiotics. Peripheral stigmata of disease are less commonly encountered in children with IE.

27. E – Summon immediate anaesthetic help. Acute epiglottis is now rare in children following the introduction of the *Haemophilus influenzae* vaccine (Hib) as part of the routine immunizations schedule. It is a life-threatening emergency and securing the airway is of paramount importance prior to intravenous antibiotics.

28. C – Admit and give nasogastric feeds. Her saturations are acceptable and hence, supplemental oxygen is not needed. However, as a general rule, less than 50% of oral intake warrants admission for feeding support and given the minimal recession, nasogastric feeds would be more physiological than intravenous fluids.

29. E – Add a long-acting beta agonist. This child needs escalation of her asthma treatment. She should be reviewed to see if the long-acting beta agonist has been beneficial. The step-wise approach to asthma is available on the British Thoracic Society website within the asthma guidelines.

30. A – Viral wheeze. Asthma cannot be diagnosed in this age group although given the atopic history of this child there may be a predisposition to develop asthma at a later stage. Her age and lack of crackles on examination make bronchiolitis unlikely but still possible.

31. C – Developmental dysplasia of the hip. Risk factors for DDH include first born, female, oligohydramnios, breech delivery, family history of DDH, congenital muscular pathology and congenital foot abnormalities, e.g. talipes and clubfoot.

32. E – Osteomyelitis. Children with sickle cell disease have increased susceptibility to osteomyelitis. Other examination findings may include

erythema of the affected limb with warmth. Acute phase reactants are likely to be elevated.

33. B – Paediatric ophthalmology. This girl has oligoarticular JIA as suggested by the duration of symptoms and asymmetrical joint involvement. These patients are at high risk for developing anterior uveitis and hence ophthalmological screening is very important.

34. A – CT or MRI brain scan. Precocious puberty in boys is always pathological and requires investigation. The headaches and findings of papilloedema suggest an intracranial cause and therefore a brain tumour must be excluded.

35. D – Prader–Willi syndrome. PWS is a genetic syndrome of chromosome 15 in which seven genes (or a subset of these) are deleted or not expressed on the paternal chromosome. Clinical features are present throughout stages of childhood and include reduced fetal movements, hypotonia at birth, hyperphagia (overeating) during childhood and hypogonadism.

36. A – Galactosaemia. This autosomal recessive condition is associated with cataracts, liver failure and *E. coli* sepsis. It is diagnosed by decreased or absent galactose-1-phosphate uridyltransferase in red blood cells. Treatment is by a lactose free diet and no breast feeding.

37. C – Arterial pH of <7.0 post resuscitation. See Fig. 29.10, listing prognostic indicators for near drowning, in Chapter 29.

38. A – Adrenaline (epinephrine). Asystole is the commonest cardiac arrest rhythm in children and adrenaline (epinephrine) is the only drug of choice here, in addition to ongoing CPR and securing the airway and intravenous/ intraosseous access.

39. C – A 20 mL/kg bolus of normal saline. This girl has clinical features of shock (likely septic shock in view of the high fever). As with any emergency, attention must be paid towards ABCD. Her airway is patent and is receiving oxygen. She does, however, have circulatory compromise with tachycardia and delayed CRT and therefore requires a fluid bolus.

40. B – Serum potassium. Insulin drives potassium into cells and therefore serum potassium falls. Intravenous fluids should be given with potassium (i.e. 0.9% sodium chloride and 10 mmol KCL) when treating DKA. Patients with DKA require 6–8-hourly monitoring of urea and electrolytes and blood gases.

41. A – Bone profile. This boy has rickets (vitamin D deficiency) as suggested by the bowing of legs and dental problems. Bone profile will reveal a raised alkaline phosphatase and the serum calcium may or may not be low. The vitamin D level should also be checked.

42. C – Bacterial meningitis. The CSF results reveal typical bacterial meningitis. In viral meningitis, the CSF protein is low and the CSF glucose is normal. With TB meningitis, however, the CSF protein is markedly raised (usually >10 g/L) with a low CSF glucose.

43. C – Metabolic alkalosis. This infant is likely to have pyloric stenosis, which is supported by the history, clinical findings and blood gas results. Serum chloride should be checked (if not available on a blood gas) which would be reduced. An ultrasound scan will confirm or refute this diagnosis.

44. D – Renal ultrasound. This is a concerning presentation and all findings point to a Wilms' tumour, which must be excluded. A renal ultrasound scan is a quick, non-invasive investigation which should be arranged immediately. If a Wilms' tumour is confirmed, then further imaging is likely to be required for staging, etc.

45. D – Request a urine dipstick. This is a well child presenting with fever without apparent focus. The examination findings do not suggest any 'red' or 'amber' features and hence, in accordance with the NICE 'traffic light' guidance of fever management, the next step is to request a urine dipstick and CXR only if there are signs of pneumonia (not in this case). If the urine is clear of infection then the child could be discharged home with advice.

46. A – A full septic screen followed by IV antibiotics. This infant warrants a full septic screen as indicated by the age group of <3 months and high fever. The infant is not unwell and not displaying any signs of shock or compromise. In this type of scenario, inflammatory marker results should be looked at retrospectively so as to not delay investigations and treatment.

47. D – Epstein–Barr virus. Both clinical and biochemical findings point to EBV causing glandular fever. Hepatomegaly occurs in approximately 10% of cases and splenomegaly in about 50% of cases. Treatment is symptomatic and supportive.

48. D – Immunoglobulin. This is a missed case of Kawasaki disease with serious complications. The clue here is the previous admission for prolonged fever without treatment. Kawasaki disease is the commonest cause of acquired cardiac disease in children.

49. A – *Streptococcus pneumoniae*. In pneumonia, age is a good predictor of the likely pathogens. Viruses alone are found as a cause in younger children in up to 50%. In older children, when a bacterial cause is found, it is most commonly *S. pneumoniae* followed by mycoplasma and chlamydial pneumonia.

50. C – CPAP. This infant may be entering the peak stage of her bronchiolitis where typically things can get worse before they get better. In view of her respiratory status and metabolic acidosis, CPAP is the next most effective step.

51. D – Erythema multiforme. The description is highly suggestive of EM. It is usually idiopathic and self-limiting but in this scenario, may be secondary to streptococcal or mycoplasma infection.

52. B – Otitis media with effusion. OME (also known as 'glue ear') is the commonest cause of conductive deafness in children. Other clues in this question are trisomy 21 (which carries a higher incidence of OME) and the repeated ear infections. Surgical treatment of OME is with insertion of grommets.

53. E – Patent ductus arteriosus. This baby has been born to a non-rubella immune mother. Supportive findings include the absent red reflexes (cataracts) and growth restriction. The commonest cardiac lesions in this case are a PDA and pulmonary stenosis.

54. A – Empyema. The clinical findings of worsening respiratory distress and 'stony dull' percussion note suggest an empyema. This is not an uncommon complication of pneumonia and a CXR is needed followed by an ultrasound scan to assess the extent of the empyema. In some hospitals, an ultrasound may be advised as first-line imaging.

55. A – Osteogenesis imperfecta type 1. There are eight types of OI but type I is the commonest and accounts for 50% of all people with OI. Blue sclerae are often present but not always. Diagnosis is by culturing skin fibroblasts that show a reduced amount of type 1 collagen.

56. A – Syndrome of inappropriate secretion of ADH. The laboratory findings here all point to SIADH. This is a common stress response and in this case is secondary to pneumonia. Other causes of SIADH include CNS disease and treatment is by treating the underlying cause and fluid restriction.

57. D – Give intravenous salbutamol. This child has deteriorated and is demonstrating features of life-threatening asthma. Urgent action is required and the next step is to proceed with IV salbutamol bolus followed by an infusion. IV magnesium sulphate is a suitable and sometime preferable alternative.

58. C – Group B streptococcus. *Neisseria* and *Haemophilus* are Gram-negative organisms. *Staphylococcus aureus* is also Gram-positive but occurs in clusters. Listeria is a Gram-positive rod.

59. E – Human herpes virus. HHV is associated with roseola infantum – a common cause of febrile illnesses in infants. The rash is typically a widespread maculopapular rash which appears on the face, neck and trunk. *Staphylococcus aureus* causes impetigo, another common cause of vesicular rash in children.

60. D – Third heart sound. There should be no added sounds with innocent murmurs. Innocent murmurs follow the rule of 'S': soft, short, systolic, symptom-free, signs – none. A split second heart sound is normal.

61. E – Paroxysmal cough. This is a typical feature of pertussis infection.

62. D – Anterior uveitis. Anterior uveitis is a common complication of oligo-articular arthritis, which is why ophthalmological screening is an essential part of management. Systemic JIA can also involve the pleurae and serosal membranes and the fever is typically one of daily spikes.

63. D – Thyrotoxicosis. This would be associated with tall stature rather than short stature. Rickets is another important cause of short stature due to poor skeletal growth and maturation.

64. C – 5% partial thickness. Commonly, >10% partial thickness burn would indicate referral to a burns centre. Other indications include electrical or chemical injuries, hand and feet involvement.

65. C – Not using single words at 15 months. Single words, e.g. mama and dada, should be heard by about 12 months of age. Please refer to the developmental assessment chapter for a figure listing signs of abnormal development: limit ages.

66. B – Hb concentration falls after birth until around 7 weeks. Early fetal haematopoesis begins in the liver, spleen and lymph nodes; however, bone marrow begins production around the fourth month of gestation and is the main source by term. Most haemoglobin is HbF at term – this has a higher affinity for oxygen to facilitate gas exchange at the placenta. A gradual changeover occurs after delivery. Hb concentration is high at birth and falls until around 7 weeks to a nadir of about 9 g/dL.

67. C – Iron deficiency anaemia. Iron deficiency is extremely common in childhood with iron

deficiency anaemia affecting around 3% of toddlers. It is usually dietary, there is often a history of fussy eating. Under 1 s consuming unmodified cow's milk are particularly at risk. It is a microcytic, hypochromic anaemia and is usually asymptomatic. If severe it can lead to lethargy, breathlessness and even cardiomyopathy. There is increasing evidence that iron deficiency impacts cognitive development.

68. E – Henoch–Schönlein purpura. HSP is characterized by palpable purpura in the absence of thrombocytopenia or coagulopathy, abdominal pain, arthralgia and renal involvement. Immune thrombocytopenic purpura (ITP) would have low platelets. A raised white cell count $\pm$ lymphadenopathy would be expected with ALL. Scurvy can cause purpura but there is no indication of this here.

69. D – Sickle cell disease. Sickle cell disease (HbSS) causes an anaemia, often normocytic, which may be quite profound. It is characterized by intermittent 'crises' where the abnormal haemoglobin precipitates leading to 'sickling' of red blood cells which clump together. This produces a variety of clinical manifestations in addition to acute haemolysis. The most common presentation is with painful vaso-occlusive crisis (bone pain). Splenomegaly is present in young children but autosplenectomy occurs in older children.

70. D – Parvovirus B19 infection. Parvovirus B19, aka 'fifth disease', is an erythrovirus. In children it frequently manifests with fever, mild flu-like symptoms and the classic 'slapped cheek' rash. It can produce a transient aplastic anaemia, especially in children with underlying haematological conditions (e.g. hereditary spherocytosis, G6PD, etc.). In children with sickle cell disease the pancytopenia may be particularly severe.

71. C – Beta-thalassaemia major. Beta-thalassaemia is a quantitative defect in haemoglobin production. Homozygous mutation produces thalassaemia major which presents as HbF levels decline in infancy. There is a microcytic hypochromic anaemia and children are transfusion dependent. Frontal bossing is produced by extramedullary haematopoiesis.

72. B – Haemophilia A. Haemophilia A (factor VIII deficiency) is an X-linked recessive condition resulting in abnormal clotting. Infants usually get through birth and the initial neonatal period without significant problems, although intracranial bleeding is a risk.

Presentation is usual during early childhood, often with excessive bleeding (e.g. following circumcision), or, as in this case, with haemarthrosis and easy bruising as the child begins to mobilize.

73. C – Immune (idiopathic) thrombocytopenic purpura (ITP). ITP most commonly presents with bruising or petechiae in an otherwise well child. The platelet count is low (production of platelets is normal but they are rapidly consumed). Around 60% of cases are preceded by a viral infection.

74. A – Glucose-6-phosphate dehydrogenase deficiency (G6PD). This is an X-linked disorder of red cell enzyme. It reduces the ability of the red blood cell to respond to oxidative stress. It is characterized by haemolysis in response to infection, drugs (including primaquine), acidosis (e.g. diabetic ketoacidosis) and fava beans. It is common in Afro-Caribbean groups.

75. D – Intravenous antibiotics. Febrile neutropenia is a common side-effect of chemotherapy. It occurs most frequently 8–10 days post-chemotherapy. Prompt management is vital and would include peripheral and central blood cultures, and rapid initiation of intravenous antibiotics according to local protocol. G-CSF injections can be used to stimulate a rise in the neutrophil count. Supportive treatment with platelet/red blood cell transfusions may be needed but these are not indicated here.

76. D – Non-B cell, non-T cell leukaemia. The non-T cell, non-B cell lineage leukaemia has an improved prognosis over those with either clear T cell or B cell lineage. The other factors listed are associated with higher risk stratification and a poorer prognosis.

77. C – Hodgkin's lymphoma. The differential diagnosis of lymphadenopathy is vast. In this case the histology is diagnostic with Reed–Sternberg cells being pathognomonic for Hodgkin's lymphoma. The shortness of breath is due to superior vena caval obstruction from the mediastinal mass on lying flat.

78. E – Turner syndrome. Beckwith–Wiedemann syndrome has an increased risk of Wilms' tumour, Li Fraumeni syndrome is a mutation in the p53 tumour suppressor gene. Down syndrome has a particularly increased risk of haematological malignancies. Ataxia telangiectasia is a disorder of DNA repair mechanisms.

79. C – Astrocytomas carry poor prognosis. Brain tumours are mainly infratentorial. Diagnosis

is often late, with signs of raised intracranial pressure. Metastasis of CNS tumours is rare. Astrocytomas are the most common form and continue to have poor prognosis despite treatment.

80. A – Nephroblastoma (Wilms' tumour). The most common renal tumour, presents mainly in the under 5 s with painless, smooth abdominal mass. It is associated with syndromes including Beckwith–Weidemann, hemihypertrophy, WAGR and Denys–Drash. Metastasis at diagnosis is uncommon. Mutations have been found on chromosome 11.

81. B – It is associated with Beckwith–Weidemann syndrome. Beckwith–Weidemann is a genetic overgrowth condition caused by deregulation of genes on chromosome 11. There is gigantism and macroglossia. It is associated with exomphalos and predisposes to tumours, particularly nephroblastoma (Wilms' tumour).

82. A – Retinoblastoma. Retinoblastoma can occur unilaterally but in 40% of cases is bilateral. Checking for a red reflex is one of the most important parts of the newborn and 6–8-week checks.

83. C – Osteosarcoma. Primary malignancies of the bone are rare. They occur most frequently in adolescent boys. The sunburst appearance on X-ray is suggestive of osteosarcoma. Ewing's sarcoma is associated with onion-skin appearance on X-ray. There are no features suggestive of rickets or osteomyelitis. Chondrosarcomas are rare and found mainly in the axial skeleton.

84. A – 1 microgram/kg intramuscular adrenaline (epinephrine) (1:1000). Anaphylaxis is a medical emergency and rapid treatment can be life-saving. Treatment is with the ABC approach. If possible the allergen should be removed (e.g. drug infusion). Intramuscular adrenaline (epinephrine) is the most important pharmacological treatment and may be given by adrenaline (epinephrine) autoinjector if available. Oxygen will be needed but will not stop the reaction. Intravenous steroids (e.g. hydrocortisone) and antihistamine (e.g. chlorphenamine) should also be given but do not take immediate effect and are not the most important step in treatment here.

85. D – He can safely receive the MMR, preferably in hospital, but should not receive the influenza or yellow fever vaccines. The MMR does not contain egg, although it is produced on chick fibroblasts. If there is a history of severe anaphylaxis to egg advice should be sought about location of vaccination. Yellow fever and influenza vaccines contain egg and must not be given to egg allergic children.

86. D – Positive (histamine) and negative (saline) controls should be injected, along with other allergens to confirm success of testing. Size of reaction does not correlate with clinical symptoms. Skin-prick testing is only suitable for diagnosis of IgE mediated allergy. RAST testing measures serum specific IgE levels.

87. A – It is commonly non-IgE mediated. For this reason RAST test (which identifies specific IgE) may not identify food allergies. A positive skin test does not necessarily correlate with clinical allergy (there may be cross-reactivity) and should be taken in context. Children frequently outgrow their allergies (especially cow's milk allergy). An elimination–reintroduction test may be extremely helpful in diagnosing allergy.

88. E – Fish and kiwi. It is important to counsel families about the risk of reacting to other allergens that are known to cross-react to reduce the chance of anaphylaxis.

89. A – Post-streptococcal glomerulonephritis. The description here is of acute nephritis (haematuria, proteinuria, hypertension). The most common cause in childhood is post-streptococcal glomerulonephritis which is indicated by the preceding tonsillitis (this may also be present in IgA nephropathy). Minimal change nephropathy is the most common cause of nephrotic syndrome. There are no features of SLE or Henoch–Schönlein purpura in this case. Haemolytic uraemic syndrome mainly occurs following diarrhoeal illness.

90. D – Minimal change disease. Unlike in adults the most common cause of nephrotic syndrome in childhood is minimal change disease. There is no abnormality seen on light microscopy although podocyte changes are visible on electron microscopy. Minimal change disease is usually steroid sensitive and renal biopsy is not indicated unless there is steroid resistant or frequently relapsing nephrotic syndrome or other abnormal features.

91. E – Urea and electrolytes (U&Es). In an infant with bilaterally undescended testes it is important to consider complex genital anomaly. The most common cause for this is congenital adrenal hyperplasia (CAH). A number of investigations are warranted including rapid FISH for sex determination,

ultrasound of the abdomen to determine placement of the testes (or identify female internal genitalia) and 17-hydroxyprogesterone (raised in the most common form of CAH). However, the immediate risk to the infant is a CAH salt-wasting crisis, therefore U&Es should be done as soon as possible.

92. C – Haemolytic uraemic syndrome. This is usually associated with diarrhoea, particularly *E. coli* 0157 (shiga-toxin producing). Onset is around 5–10 days after development of diarrhoea. There is a triad of microangiopathic haemolytic anaemia, thrombocytopenia and renal failure. Clinical features can mimic ulcerative colitis and dehydration may produce renal failure in gastroenteritis; however, these would not cause haemolysis.

93. A – Testicular torsion. Testicular torsion occurs when the testis turns on the remnant of the processus vaginalis and blood supply is restricted. It presents most commonly with testicular pain of less than 12 hours duration, although lower abdominal or inguinal pain can also occur. There may be swelling of the testis and overlying erythema. Epididymo-orchitis is often associated with urinary symptoms. Doppler of the testis may help differentiate these (blood flow reduced in torsion and increased in epididymitis). Torsion of the hydatid of Morgagni presents similarly to testicular torsion but is much less common.

94. D – *Escherichia coli*. *E. coli* is the most common cause of urinary tract infection in the structurally normal kidney.

95. C – Posterior urethral valves. Failure to treat posterior urethral valves (by temporary urinary drainage followed by definitive surgical management) leads to irreversible renal damage. Hydroceles and umbilical hernias usually resolve spontaneously. A unilaterally undescended testicle warrants surgical referral if undescended at the age of 1 year. Inguinal hernias frequently require repair but there is no urgency to do this within the first 6 months of life.

96. E – Risk is increased by constipation. UTI is more common in boys under the age of 3 months (due to increased frequency of urinary tract abnormalities). The most common cause is *E. coli* and presentation is frequently non-specific. A raised urinary WCC alone is insufficient to diagnose UTI. Risk factors for UTI include: vesicoureteric reflux (VUR),

obstructive uropathy, e.g. ureterocoele, urethral valves, neuropathic bladder, e.g. spina bifida, habitual infrequent voiding and constipation.

97. B – Reduced glucose tolerance. Nephrotic syndrome (NS) predisposes to bacterial infection, predominantly through loss of immunoglobulins. Hypoalbuminaemia can lead to ascites or pleural effusions along with massive third space losses and hypotension. NS is a hypercoagulable state and both arterial and venous thromboembolism are reported in up to 3% of children. Reduced glucose tolerance is a side-effect of steroid therapy but not directly of nephrotic syndrome.

98. D – Bulimia nervosa. Bulimia nervosa is characterized by binge-eating and purging (often through vomiting and excessive exercise). There is abnormal body image and obsession with food and bodyweight, although BMI may be normal. Vomiting can lead to electrolyte imbalances as seen in this case, particularly hypokalaemia, hypochloraemia and metabolic alkalosis. The parotid swelling and enamel erosion are also sequelae of recurrent vomiting.

99. B – Anorexia nervosa. Anorexia nervosa is characterized by low bodyweight and a fear of weight gain. There is distorted body image and pubertal delay or amenorrhea may be a feature. The differential diagnosis for weight loss would include all of the other answers; however, the fixation with food, social withdrawal and excessive exercise make anorexia the most likely cause.

100. C – Symptoms present only at school. The core features of ADHD are inattention, hyperactivity and impulsiveness. Features of these must be present in more than one setting (e.g. at school and at home) for a period of more than 6 months. The term has become increasingly popular with parents and the diagnosis should only be made following careful evaluation, including exclusion of other conditions, e.g. autism or developmental delay, and consideration of psychosocial factors.

101. C – Autism. Autism is a pervasive developmental disorder characterized by speech delay and poor social communication skills. It is part of a spectrum of disorders including Asperger's syndrome. Autistic children struggle to interpret non-verbal communications and to form relationships with peers. Autistic behaviours are

associated with a number of syndromes including fragile X, untreated phenylketonuria and Williams syndrome.

102. E – Bell-alarms may be helpful in children who sleep very deeply. Primary nocturnal enuresis (where a child has never been dry) is usually secondary to deep sleep and failure to wake to a full bladder or inadequate ADH secretion. Secondary enuresis is more commonly associated with emotional stress. Conditions such as UTI, neuropathic bladder and constipation may lead to enuresis but are uncommon.

103. A – Breath holding spells. These occur in children between 6 months and 2 years and are triggered by high emotion (tantrums, etc.). The child holds their breath, becomes pale or cyanotic, loses consciousness and falls to the floor. There may be tonic-clonic movements. History is vital in distinguishing this from other forms of syncope. 'Tet' spells are episodes of increased cyanosis occurring in tetralogy of Fallot.

104. C – Absence seizures. Absences can occur very frequently during the day and may be mistaken for poor concentration or daydreaming. The EEG is characteristic. First-line treatment is with sodium valproate or ethosuximide.

105. D – West syndrome (infantile spasms). This seizure disorder presents in infancy, often with the salaam seizures described here, and has a characteristic EEG (hypsarrhythmia). It is treated with vigabatrin or ACTH.

106. A – Intravenous lorazepam. The protocol for status epilepticus is described in Chapter 29. First-line treatment is with benzodiazepines. The first dose has been given in the community as buccal midazolam. A second dose is indicated if the seizures are continuing 10 minutes after administration of first dose. This could be given as rectal diazepam but intravenous access has already been obtained and thus lorazepam is the drug of choice.

107. B – Sodium valproate. First-line therapy for generalized tonic-clonic seizures include carbamazepine, valproate, lamotrigine and topiramate. Phenytoin is generally avoided in view of its side-effect profile. Ethosuximide is useful in absence seizures.

108. E – Symmetrical, band-like in nature. Most headaches are benign; however, there are some sinister causes. 70% of brain tumours present as headache. Red flag symptoms are those of raised intracranial pressure, focal neurology, weight loss, sudden onset or progressive in nature.

109. E – Lisch nodules. Diagnostic criteria for neurofibromatosis type 1 include at least two of the following: six or more café-au-lait patches, two or more neurofibromas (or one plexiform neurofibroma), axillary freckling, Lisch nodules, optic glioma, first-degree relative with NF-1. Acoustic neuromas are a feature of NF-2, ash-leaf macules and adenoma sebaceum are features of tuberous sclerosis.

110. D – Mutation is in the dystrophin gene. Duchenne muscular dystrophy is X-linked. It is associated with calf pseudohypertrophy, proximal muscle weakness (with positive Gower sign) and cardiomyopathy. Onset is generally early with most patients wheelchair bound by 12 years of age.

111. B – WCC 20×10^6/L (80% neutrophils), red cells 5×10^6/L, protein 1.6 g/L, glucose 1.0 mmol/L. This shows a neutrophilia with raised protein and low glucose characteristic of bacterial meningitis. A suggests viral meningitis, C tuberculous meningitis, D subarachnoid haemorrhage with E representing normal CSF values.

112. C – Occur between ages of 6 months and 5 years. Simple febrile convulsions are short-lived tonic-clonic seizures occurring in children between 6 months and 5 years in response to rapid rise in temperature. They should not be focal or occur without fever. Most children will not go on to develop epilepsy. Where there is a clear focus for the fever a lumbar puncture may not be indicated.

113. D – Fragile X. Fragile X is the most common form of inherited intellectual disability. It is caused by a trinucleotide repeat sequence on the X chromosome. Once the expansion is large enough symptoms become apparent. There is a wide phenotypic variation. Some female carriers have mild intellectual impairment. Physical features include narrow face, prominent chin and forehead, large ears and testes, and hyperlaxity.

114. A – Neurofibromatosis type 1. Cystic fibrosis and sickle cell disease are examples of autosomal recessive conditions. Fragile X and Duchenne muscular dystrophy are X-linked.

115. D – Acute leukaemia. Down syndrome is associated with an increased risk of leukaemia and the presence of pallor and

purpura should prompt a full blood count and film to be performed to look for leukaemia cells.

116. B – Males are frequently infertile. Overall incidence of Down syndrome (DS) is 1 in 700. Despite increased incidence in older mothers, the majority of DS occurs in infants of younger mothers. Intellectual disability is typically in the mild to moderate range. Epicanthic folds are a feature of DS but are not pathognomonic. Males are frequently infertile (although cases of offspring have been reported).

117. C – Turner syndrome. All of the above are causes of short stature; however, failure to develop secondary sexual characteristics in combination with the dysmorphic features mentioned suggests Turner syndrome.

118. E – Brushfield spots. Phenotypic features of Edwards syndrome include microcephaly, low set ears, micrognathia, cleft palate/lip, palpebral fissures, hypertelorism, ptosis, clenched hands, rocker bottom feet, abnormal nails and absent radii. Brushfield spots are associated with Down syndrome.

119. D – Spina bifida. Analysis of fetal DNA from amniocentesis can be performed for all of the above except spina bifida which is diagnosed on ultrasound. For cystic fibrosis screening it is important to know the mutations in parents. Fragile X can be diagnosed with amniocentesis but chorionic villous sampling may be unreliable.

120. B – Klinefelter syndrome. Boys with Klinefelter syndrome (47, XXY) are tall (particularly long legs). They often have small testes and gynaecomastia, learning and attention difficulties are common. Hyperthyroidism would explain the height and gynaecomastia but not the small testes or learning difficulties.

121. A – Hypertelorism – increased distance between the eyes. Clinodactyly is an inwards curving of the little finger towards the 4th finger, brachycephaly describes a short, broad head, micrognathia describes a small jaw, epicanthic folds are folds in the upper eyelid which cover the inner corner of the eye.

122. A – Check maternal antibodies, if negative give VZIG (varicella zoster immunoglobulin). Exposure to varicella in utero can produce congenital varicella syndrome. However, the neonate is at risk if a mother is exposed 5 days pre to 2 days post birth (transmission of virus without time for mother to develop protective antibodies). If mother has been previously exposed the baby will be protected by passive immunity. If mother is not immune VZIG should be given. Aciclovir is given if lesions develop in the newborn.

123. D – Botulinum toxin may be useful to treat spasticity. Cerebral palsy (CP) is a disorder of posture and motor function secondary to static brain injury. The timing of insult in CP is usually unknown but birth asphyxia is an uncommon cause. The diagnosis is clinical (with hypertonia and hyperreflexia), MRI may be helpful but is not diagnostic.

124. E – Heart murmur. Perinatal asphyxia affects all the organs of the body and can produce liver and renal dysfunction. In the brain it is manifested as seizures or change in conscious level. In the heart it can cause muscle damage which causes hypotension but does not usually cause a murmur.

125. B – Respiratory distress syndrome. Many conditions can produce respiratory distress in the newborn infant. Transient tachypnoea of the newborn occurs in the first 4 hours post-delivery due to inadequate fluid clearance from the lungs. Premature infants may develop spontaneous pneumothoraces or one may develop secondary to resuscitation or mechanical ventilation. The X-ray changes here are suggestive of respiratory distress syndrome (surfactant insufficiency). Management is with artificial surfactant, oxygenation and ventilatory support.

126. C – Necrotizing enterocolitis. Necrotizing enterocolitis (NEC) occurs in up to 6% of babies born at <1.5 kg. Risk factors include prematurity, low birthweight, and early feeding (especially with formula milk). It presents with general features of sepsis (lethargy, temperature instability, hypotension, glucose intolerance) and abdominal symptoms including distension, blood in the stool and bile stained aspirates. Pneumatosis (air within the bowel wall) is highly suggestive of NEC.

127. B – Tetralogy of Fallot. Tetralogy of Fallot comprises pulmonary stenosis, overriding aorta, ventricular septal defect and right ventricular hypertrophy. Congenital cyanotic heart disease is less common than acyanotic heart disease. Other forms include: transposition of the great arteries, tricuspid atresia, total anomalous pulmonary drainage and hypoplastic left

heart. Infants with cyanotic heart disease are often dependant on the ductus arteriosus and it is vital to keep this open with prostaglandin infusion until surgery can be performed.

128. A – Hirschsprung's disease. The delayed passage of meconium, infrequent passage of stool and lack of air in the rectum are all suggestive of Hirschsprung's disease. The segment of bowel which is aganglionic may be small or involve most or all of the colon. The timing of presentation and severity of disease will depend on the length of bowel involved. Treatment involves surgical resection of the aganglionic segment.

129. D – Group B haemolytic streptococcus. The organisms listed are all causes of neonatal sepsis; however, in view of the previous history group B haemolytic streptococcus is the most likely causative organism. Approximately 30% of women are colonized with this and require intrapartum antibiotics to reduce the chances of infection in the neonate.

130. D – Prothrombin time. The bleeding is caused by vitamin K deficiency also called haemorrhagic disease of the newborn. Low vitamin K levels result in a prolonged prothrombin time and so a raised INR. Neonates usually receive vitamin K at birth either via the intramuscular or oral route. If the latter it needs to be a total of three doses.

131. B – Intussusception. Intussusception occurs when a part of the bowel telescopes inside itself. It is thought that an initial infection may lead to an increase in size of the lymphoid tissue in the bowel which can act as the lead point. Peak age of onset is 6–9 months. Symptoms include episodic severe abdominal pain, pallor and eventually shock and redcurrant jelly stool. Treatment is by air reduction enema or surgery if this is not effective.

132. C – Coeliac disease. Coeliac disease is a gluten-mediated immunological disorder affecting the gut predominantly but also other organs. Damage occurs to the villi of the proximal small intestine leading to atrophy and loss of the absorptive surface. Symptoms include loose stools, faltering growth and abdominal bloating. Blood tests may show a microcytic anaemia and tissue transglutaminase IgA antibodies are raised. Treatment is to exclude gluten completely from the diet.

133. D – Reassurance and no further investigation. Functional abdominal pain is the most likely diagnosis and no further investigation is required. Reassuring features in the history include the fact that the pain is short lived and responds to simple analgesia and that she is thriving. It is of note that it does not occur at weekends. The nearer the pain is to the umbilicus the less likely it is to be significant. Often after a thorough assessment simple reassurance is all that is required.

134. A – Crohn's disease. The symptoms described may be common to Crohn's disease and ulcerative colitis; however, the findings at endoscopy and colonoscopy point to Crohn's disease as it can affect any part of the intestinal tract and tends to occur in skip lesions. Ulcerative colitis affects the colon only usually.

135. A – Abdominal radiograph. The most likely diagnosis is duodenal atresia as the vomiting started so early and it is a cause of polyhydramnios in pregnancy. It is more common in infants with Down syndrome. A plain abdominal radiograph can be obtained easily and is likely to show the classical 'double bubble' sign which is pathognomonic of duodenal atresia. Treatment is by surgical correction.

136. E – Mallory–Weiss tear. A Mallory–Weiss tear is a small tear in the oesophageal mucosa after prolonged forceful vomiting. It can lead to blood in the vomit and is a complication of gastroenteritis. It is a self-limiting condition that requires no treatment. Other causes of haematemesis are rare in children but can occur due to liver disease.

137. E – *Campylobacter*. The symptoms described are of an infective colitis. *Campylobacter* typically causes a bloody diarrhoea and is transmitted by infected chicken among other foods. The fact that other members of the family are affected and the timing of onset in symptoms after the takeaway are classical. No treatment is usually required but the Health Protection Agency should be informed.

138. A – Sweat test. The most likely diagnosis is cystic fibrosis due to the combination of respiratory symptoms and faltering growth and diarrhoea. Many cases are now diagnosed via the newborn screening programme. However, a sweat test is the test of choice at this age. Cystic fibrosis is more common in Celtic populations.

139. E – Suction biopsy of the rectum. The most likely diagnosis is Hirschsprung's disease. This is an aganglionic segment of the intestine. Constipation from a young age is classical. Often if the initial obstruction to the passage of stool is overcome (i.e. by the suppository) the stool that is passed is soft or liquid and may gush out. Histology of a biopsy of the rectum will show an absence of ganglionic cells.

140. B – Biliary atresia. This infant has prolonged jaundice which is conjugated and associated with pale stools and faltering growth which is caused by biliary atresia until proved otherwise. This is a serious condition which requires surgical correction via the Kasai procedure as soon as possible for the best outcome. If it is not diagnosed early the Kasai procedure may not be successful and then liver transplantation is required.

141. E – No treatment is required. This baby has physiological jaundice of a low level that does not require any treatment. It may be exacerbated by breast feeding but this does not mean breast feeding should not be encouraged. Breast milk may delay the maturation of the liver enzymes involved in the metabolism of bilirubin but should be continued. The conjugated fraction of the jaundice level is low suggesting it is a predominantly unconjugated jaundice.

142. A – Referral to surgical team. The history of the pain is classical of appendicitis. Often the pain starts more centrally and then moves towards the right iliac fossa. Guarding suggests peritonitis and warrants prompt intervention. A surgical review is required to evaluate if an appendicectomy is required. The surgical team may ask for further investigations to be done but these should not delay their review.

143. D – Pyloric stenosis. Pyloric stenosis is a thickening of the pylorus muscle around the outflow of the stomach. This leads to difficulty in emptying of the stomach and non-bilious vomiting. The peak incidence is between 2 and 6 weeks of age and occurs more commonly in boys. Classically the vomiting occurs after a feed and the infant is immediately eager to feed again. Surgical correction is required but any dehydration or electrolytes need to be corrected first.

144. E – Less than 2.5 kg in weight. There is no specific weight an infant needs to be prior to vaccination and preterm infants are vaccinated with respect to their chronological age rather than corrected age. Vaccinations can occur if the child is mildly unwell but should be deferred if a fever of >38 °C is present. High dose steroid therapy means that the appropriate immune response to the vaccination will not occur. Severe local reactions are a contraindication but not small lumps at the injection site. Live vaccinations should not be given if a cell-mediated immunodeficiency is suspected.

145. A – Maternal smoking. Maternal smoking during pregnancy and after pregnancy has been shown to increase the rates of sudden infant deaths. Parents should be counselled about this prior to conception. The infant should be placed supine in a cot or Moses basket to sleep and not in the parental bed. Neonates born very early or late have higher rates of sudden infant death but this is less of a factor than smoking.

146. B – History of incident does not fit with injury. A spiral fracture suggests a twisting force has been applied to the arm. This is unlikely from falling from a sitting position. A spiral fracture at this age is unusual and raises the suspicion of non-accidental injury. Immediate presentation at hospital and the attitude of the parents are not concerning.

147. C – Emotional abuse. Emotional abuse can be manifested as persistent and malicious criticism. In this case the girl is made to feel that she is not worthy of ballet lessons like her siblings as she is clumsy and fat. This can lead to behaviour problems and self-esteem and confidence issues in later life.

148. C – The girl herself. At the age of 16 a young person has the same rights to consent as an adult. Therefore she can consent to the treatment irrespective of her parents' wishes; however, it is good practice for them to be aware of her decision if she agrees. The only difference is that she cannot choose to refuse life-saving treatment until she is 18 years old.

149. D – Antifungal preparation, e.g. miconazole. The most likely diagnosis is candidiasis. The hallmarks of this rash are satellite lesions and the fact it is affecting the tongue and nappy area. Treatment using an antifungal preparation is indicated and can be given orally and to the nappy area to ensure eradication.

150. B – Scabies. *Sarcoptes scabiei* is a mite that can be transmitted from person to person by skin to skin contact. It causes intense itching and

can affect the whole body in infants. The classical hallmarks are burrows visible on the wrists or between the fingers. It may affect other members of the family.

151. C – No treatment required. The lesions are suggestive of *Molluscum contagiosum* which is caused by a pox virus. If they are all over the body then an immune work up may be indicated but small crops are common in childhood. They resolve spontaneously and no treatment is required.

152. C – Calculate mid-parental height. It is reassuring that his height and weight are both on the 99th centile. Most endocrine causes of obesity are associated with short stature. As his parents are tall it is likely that he is the appropriate weight and height for his age but calculation of the mid-parental height would confirm this.

153. A – Galactosaemia. Galactosaemia is a disorder of the metabolism of galactose which can result in liver dysfunction, coagulopathy and cataracts. Treatment is by removing any source of galactose from the diet including breast milk. Breast feeding can be continued safely in the other conditions.

154. C – Blood film for malaria parasites. The history of travel to a malarial area in conjunction with a febrile illness means that malaria must be excluded. Hepatomegaly and jaundice add weight to the likelihood. A blood film or smear for malarial parasites should be performed and ideally repeated to confirm or refute the diagnosis.

155. D – Inadequate intake/neglect. There is no suggestion of an organic illness in the history. The fact that the infant gained weight quickly when adequate intake was offered makes previous inadequate intake likely. This may have been due to lack of understanding of the needs of the baby or neglect but it needs thorough assessment before discharge.

156. E – Epstein–Barr infection (EBV). The combination of lymphadenopathy, fever and malaise suggests EBV, also called glandular fever. It is known as the kissing disease as it can be passed from person to person and occurs in teenagers. Hepatomegaly is common and contact sports should be avoided until recovery.

157. A – Constitutionally small. This baby is following the centile she was born on and has small parents. There is no suggestion of any organic illness and she is healthy. Some parents request treatment to increase height but the use of growth hormone is restricted to a few very specific indications.

158. D – Irritable bowel syndrome. Irritable bowel syndrome can causes symptoms in response to stressful situations. The fact that she gets pain and diarrhoea infrequently, and most often on school days, makes a more serious diagnosis unlikely. In addition she is growing well which is reassuring.

159. D – Vitamin D deficiency. Vitamin D is an increasingly recognized problem and can lead to rickets, as in this case. The signs of rickets are altered mineralization of the bones resulting in swelling of the wrists, delayed dentition and closure of the fontanelle. Vitamin D replacement is the treatment of choice and supplementation should be offered to breast feeding mothers.

160. C – Bilateral renal agenesis. This causes Potter syndrome which is incompatible with life. The oligohydramnios is due to a lack of fetal urine and causes the pulmonary hypoplasia.

EMQ answers

1. Rashes

1. C – This is a diagnosis not to be missed. Children can present acutely and the haemorrhagic rash may be a late sign.
2. A – The rash in VZV it typically itchy, vesicular and follows a brief coryzal period. It starts on the scalp or trunk and goes through stages of papules, vesicles, pustules and crusts.
3. D – Measles is highly infectious. Koplik's spots are pathognomonic and appear 3–4 days before the onset of the rash. Measles can be particularly severe in immunocompromised children.
4. B – Impetigo is usually caused by *Staphylococcus aureus* and can be worse in children with pre-existing skin disease.
5. I – Important causes of erythema nodosum are TB and streptococcal infection.

2. Heart disease

1. C – Tetralogy of Fallot is one of the most common congenital heart disorders. Tetralogy of Fallot results in an inadequate flow of blood to the lungs for oxygenation (right-to-left shunt). The four typical features are right ventricular outflow tract obstruction (infundibular stenosis), ventricular septal defect (VSD), over-riding aorta and right ventricular hypertrophy.
2. E – The ductus arteriosus usually closes at around day 3 or 4 after birth. Failure to close will lead to shunting of blood from the aorta to the pulmonary artery. Bounding pulses may be present due to wide pulse pressure. Premature babies who are symptomatic from a PDA can be treated medically or surgically.
3. D – Coarctation of the aorta can be preductal, ductal or postductal and can present in later childhood with hypertension. It is twice as common in boys as in girls and more common in girls with Turner syndrome.
4. B – VSDs account for approximately 30% of all congenital heart disease and are often isolated but other heart defects may coexist. Smaller lesions will have louder murmurs.
5. H – Most infants are asymptomatic. Treatment consists of vagal stimulation and/or intravenous adenosine.

3. Tachypnoea

1. A – Bronchiolitis is the commonest respiratory infection affecting infants and occurs as winter epidemics. The causative organism is respiratory syncytial virus (RSV) in the majority of cases and diagnosis can be confirmed on a nasopharyngeal aspirate.
2. C – Croup is a viral laryngotracheal infection usually caused by parainfluenza infection. Typically, there is a preceding cough and coryzal illness followed by the characteristic 'barking cough' and stridor which is worse at night.
3. D – This child is likely to have an atypical lobar pneumonia, e.g. secondary to mycoplasma pneumonia, given his age and lack of improvement to first-line antibiotics. He would benefit from an intravenous macrolide, e.g. clarithromycin and a CXR if complications were clinically suspected.
4. B – This child has probable asthma, as suggested by her prior atopic history and presenting symptoms, and wheezing may not always be heard.
5. F – In infants, the characteristic 'whoop' is often absent although apnoea can be a common complication. Diagnosis can be made on a per-nasal swab and erythromycin can be given but this does not shorten the duration of the illness.

4. Limp

1. I – Transient synovitis or 'irritable hip' is often caused by a viral infection and is self-limiting with analgesics and antipyretics. The child is clinically well with no evidence of raised inflammatory markers.
2. A – Septic arthritis presents with an unwell infant or child and clinical findings may not always be present. The most common causative organism is staphylococcus and this condition should be treated promptly to avoid joint destruction.
3. H – DDH is the likely diagnosis in this case. Suggestive pointers include the breech delivery and family history, also suggestive of DDH in mother.
4. B – Perthes disease has an insidious onset of limp and hip X-rays are diagnostic.
5. D – This child's history is suspicious of bone marrow disease, e.g. leukaemia, given the concerning

history suggestive of thrombocytopenia and findings of pallor and likely weight loss. A full blood count and blood film is essential here to confirm or refute pancytopenia and blast cells.

5. Endocrine disorders

1. D – This is a classic history for DM. It is important to check that this child is not in diabetic ketoacidosis (DKA) by performing a blood gas. DKA is a medical emergency and approximately 10–15% of newly diagnosed type 1 diabetics will present in DKA.

2. G – PKU is a rare autosomal recessive condition in which those affected are missing an enzyme called phenylalanine hydroxylase, which is needed to break down an essential amino acid called phenylalanine. Phenylalanine plays a role in the production of melanin and therefore infants with PKU often have fair skin and light hair. Screening for PKU is performed nationally on the Guthrie test.

3. A – Juvenile hypothroidism is commonly due to Graves' disease and clinical features are similar to those of adults.

4. C – This presentation is a classic 'salt-losing' crisis seen in male newborns with CAH. Treatment involves fluid resuscitation with glucocorticoid replacement. Long-term management is aimed at cortisol and mineralocorticoid replacement.

5. H – The mucopolysaccharidoses (MPS) are a group of multisystem disorders primarily affecting the neurological, skeletal, cardiovascular and ophthalmological systems. Examples include Hurler and Hunter syndromes.

6. Emergencies

1. I – This girl has acute poisoning and her symptoms of agitation, chest pain and evidence of pyrexia point towards ecstasy ingestion. Management is aimed at cooling and consideration of benzodiazepine use to control anxiety. Discussion with the local poisons centre is mandatory.

2. B – Status epilepticus is defined as continuous seizure activity lasting longer than 30 minutes without the regaining of consciousness. The past history of an afebrile seizure may now suggest a diagnosis of epilepsy.

3. E – The clue in the history here is eating at a seafood restaurant. Ingestion of an allergen (e.g. probable shellfish in this scenario) has provoked symptoms of anaphylaxis and this child may benefit from an EpiPen at discharge.

4. A – This is the child's first presentation of diabetes as DKA. Abdominal pain and weight loss should always prompt checking of blood sugar level. The blood gas values satisfy the diagnostic criteria for DKA.

5. H – This boy is very likely to have been involved in a fight and sustained a severe head injury. Immediate action needs to be taken since his observations of hypertension, bradycardia and one dilated pupil suggest raised intracranial pressure. Anaesthetic help is required and a CT brain scan performed once A, B and C are stabilized.

7. Developmental assessment

1. I – This child has global delay. His gross motor skills are that of a 12-month-old and his fine motor skills equate to an 8-month-old.

2. A – All within normal developmental stages for a 7-month-old.

3. D – A 3-year-old should be able to build a tower of 6–8 bricks and also be able to kick a ball, jump with feet together and use stairs holding onto a banister.

4. C – This child has isolated gross motor delay and should be able to run and sit on a tricycle.

5. E – Speech and language delay. Her speech is appropriate for a 3-year-old.

8. Epilepsy

1. H – Also known as infantile spasms. EEG characteristically shows hypsarrhythmia. West syndrome is often associated with developmental delay or regression.

2. D – This typically onsets during the teenage years and is characterized by myoclonic jerks occurring particularly on waking. There is often a mixture of absence, myoclonic and tonic-clonic seizures.

3. A – These are extremely common in childhood. The child will stare, stop whatever they are doing and be unresponsive. They can happen very frequently and can interfere with school performance. EEG shows a classic 3 Hz pattern.

4. E – Pseudoseizures, also known as psychogenic non-epileptic seizures. Clinically they mimic epileptic seizures but are not associated with any EEG changes.

5. G – Temporal lobe epilepsy. This is the most common form of partial epilepsy. It is frequently preceded by an aura (déjà vu, fear or gastric sensations are most common). There may be secondary generalization.

9. Jaundice

1. G – This is a vaso-occlusive crisis in sickle cell (aka painful or bony) crisis. There is acute haemolysis and jaundice.
2. F – This occurs where a rhesus negative mother has been sensitized by a previous rhesus positive pregnancy (this may include a miscarriage). Antibodies cross the placenta and cause severe haemolysis and jaundice or antenatal hydrops.
3. D – Hepatitis A is transmitted by the faeco-oral route. It has an incubation period of 2–4 weeks and presents with a prodromal illness followed by diarrhoea and vomiting.
4. E – This is usually an autosomal dominant disorder. It has a range of phenotypes with the most severe presenting with anaemia and jaundice in the neonatal period.
5. B – This deficiency in red cell enzymes is X-linked. It is characterized by episodes of acute haemolysis triggered by oxidate stressors in the form of drugs or some foods.

10. Genetics

1. D – Also known as the Robin sequence. Occurs when there is failure of the development of the maxilla in early development. Maxillary hypoplasia in combination with normal size tongue leads to development of a cleft palate.
2. G – This is the most common chromosomal disorder in infants. Dysmorphic features include brachycephaly, epicanthic folds, up-sloping palpebral fissures, single palmar crease, widened sandal gap and protruding tongue.
3. E – This is a rare condition caused by absence of paternal long arm of chromosome 15. It is characterized by hypotonia and feeding difficulty in the neonatal period. In early childhood there is hyperphagia and behavioural difficulties.
4. C – This an X-linked defect in the dystrophin gene which leads to a gradual decline in motor function. It generally onsets between 2 and 3 years of age and progresses at varying rates. By the age of 12 most children are wheelchair bound. Cardiomyopathy is present from the mid-teens and is present in all cases by the age of 18.
5. H – This is a condition is characterized by failure of development of the mesoderm that will become the midface, eye and forebrain. There are usually ocular abnormalities such as microphthalmia, coloboma or cyclops. There is congenital deafness and microcephaly or holoprosencephaly.

11. Oncology

1. H – This is the most common renal tumour of childhood. It is associated with syndromes such as Beckwith–Weidemann and Denys–Drash. It most commonly presents with painless abdominal mass, although pain or haematuria may be presenting features.
2. G – This is an ocular tumour mainly occurring in infancy. It is often picked up as leucocoria or squint. It is caused by mutation of the RB gene on chromosome 13 and may be bilateral at presentation. Early detection usually results in good prognosis.
3. B – This is an undifferentiated sarcoma of the same family as the primitive neuroectodermal tumours. It occurs in younger patients than osteosarcoma and tends to occur in the femur. It has a characteristic onion skin appearance on X-ray.
4. A – This is the most common form of leukaemia in childhood, occurring mainly between 2 and 5 years of age. Common presenting features include bruising or bleeding, bone pain, lymphadenopathy and fever. Blast cells are seen on blood film and bone marrow biopsy is diagnostic.
5. C – This arises from remnants of Rathke's pouch and puts pressure on the optic chiasm above. Presentation is frequently with headache or visual disturbance (mainly bitemporal hemianopia). They interfere with pituitary function and may produce growth failure or diabetes insipidus.

12. Congenital malformations

1. I – These mainly occur in conjunction with oesophageal atresia. There is an abnormal connection between the trachea and oesophagus. Feeding leads to aspiration and respiratory distress. Frothy secretions may be present. Insertion of NG tube and X-ray may demonstrate the abnormal connection.
2. C – The presentation of intestinal atresias depends on the level of obstruction. In distal atresias abdominal distension is the predominant feature whereas in proximal obstruction vomiting occurs earlier. Vomiting will be bilious if the obstruction is distal to the ampulla of Vater (most cases).
3. B – This results from a defect in the diaphragm allowing the abdominal organs to herniate into the chest. It is more frequently left-sided. Presentation depends on the size of the hernia but may be with collapse. In this case the apex beat is displaced to the right by the abdominal contents.

4. F – This is the most common neural tube defect. There is complete failure in closure of the vertebral arch, meninges and overlying skin. A neurological deficit is inevitable. There is CSF leakage from the site and infection is a major risk.

5. D – Exomphalos is a defect in the anterior abdominal wall. There is an intact membrane covering the herniated abdominal contents (unlike gastroschisis). It is frequently associated with other congenital abnormalities such as neural tube defects and congenital heart disease.

13. Disorders of emotion and behaviour

1. C – Attention deficit hyperactivity disorder (ADHD) comprises a triad of symptoms: inattention, hyperactivity and impulsivity. The symptoms must be present in more than one setting, be persistent for more than 6 months and cause significant functional impairment.

2. D – This is a developmental condition affecting social interaction, communication and behaviour. There is difficulty interpreting non-verbal communication and there may be a lack of desire for interaction with peers. Speech is delayed and stereotyped behaviours (e.g. hand flapping and spinning) are common.

3. H – Selective mutism is a form of anxiety disorder characterized by the inability to speak in specific social situations. It usually affects younger children and the majority resolve with time.

4. G – Depression is less common in children than in adults but probably occurs more frequently than has previously been thought. There is persistently low mood, social withdrawal, anhedonia and hopelessness. There may be changes in sleep pattern and appetite with lethargy.

5. A – Anorexia nervosa is characterized by a fear of weight gain despite being underweight and abnormal body image. There is a restrictive diet and often a preoccupation with food. Excessive exercise may be used to control weight and sufferers will often go to extreme lengths to hide their condition.

14. Gastroenterology

1. H – Symptoms often improve when solid food is started and growth can be maintained despite the vomiting. Reassurance can be sufficient if growth is good.

2. J – Redcurrant jelly stool is a late sign and indicates that intervention is required. Air enema reduction can be used at long as the infant is cardiovascularly stable.

3. A – The symptoms of coeliac disease may begin shortly after gluten is introduced at weaning. Treatment is complete exclusion of gluten from the diet.

4. C – Persistent diarrhoea after recovery from gastroenteritis may be due to a temporary lactose intolerance which usually resolves spontaneously. Treatment is to exclude lactose until symptoms resolve.

5. B – Ulcerative colitis is a lifelong disease with a relapsing and remitting course. Treatment is medical but surgery is sometimes required.

15. Nutrition, fluids and electrolytes

1. A – Replacement with vitamin D is required and dietary advice.

2. I – Support to help establish breast feeding is often required.

3. F – This is one of the commonest causes of blindness worldwide and can affect immunity and growth.

4. D – Hyperkalaemia is better tolerated in children than adults but can lead to cardiac arrhythmias.

5. B – The is due to protein malnutrition and can occur in children weaned late or on a predominantly starch based diet.

16. Gastroenterology investigations

1. D – The most likely diagnosis is pyloric stenosis and an ultrasound scan can identify the thickened pylorus muscle.

2. E – A delay in the passage of meconium suggests Hirschprung's disease which is due to absence of ganglionic cells in the bowel wall.

3. B – The symptoms could be due to Crohn's disease or ulcerative colitis but a colonoscopy will differentiate between them.

4. A – Gastro-oesophageal reflux disease can be diagnosed using either a pH or impedance study. The latter is more reliable in infants.

5. F – Bowel obstruction is the most likely diagnosis and a plain abdominal film will help to show where the obstruction is.

17. Renal abnormalities

1. E – Pyelonephritis or upper urinary tract infection. This is suggested by the systemic illness with flank pain and rigors, rather than classical urinary symptoms of dysuria and frequency. It requires treatment with intravenous antibiotics.

2. A – Autosomal recessive polycystic kidney disease previously known as infantile polycystic kidney disease. It is characterized by multiple cysts affecting the renal collecting ducts and the liver (leading to both renal and hepatic failure).

3. H – Vesicoureteric reflux (VUR) occurs where there is backflow of urine into the ureters and renal pelvis. Primary VUR results from abnormal insertion of the ureters into the bladder, reducing the length of ureter in the muscular wall and leading to inadequate closure of the ureters upon bladder contraction.

4. D – Posterior urethral valves are mucosal flaps in the urethra interrupting passage of urine. It may be antenatally diagnosed or present in the neonatal period with distended bladder and poor voiding.

5. F – Renal agenesis is the congenital absence or hypoplasia of the renal parenchyma. It may be unilateral or bilateral and is a frequent cause of miscarriage or still birth. In bilateral cases there is severe oligohydramnios producing pulmonary hypoplasia.

Glossary

Acute epiglottitis life threatening emergency, caused by infection with *H. influenzae* leading to inflammation of the epiglottis and upper air way obstruction.

Acute glomerulonephritis acute inflammation of the glomeruli leading to fluid retention, hypertension, haematuria and proteinuria.

Acute otitis media an acute inflammation of the middle ear due to a viral or bacterial infection.

Apnoea of prematurity episodes of apnoea seen in preterm infants due to immaturity of the respiratory centre.

Attention deficit hyperactivity disorder a condition characterized by lack of attention beyond normal for the child's age, hyperactivity and impulsiveness.

Autistic spectrum disorder a range of conditions usually with onset earlier than 3 years, characterized by impaired social interaction, impaired communication and a restricted pattern of behaviour.

Breath-holding attacks episodes characterized by a screaming infant or toddler holding his/her breath in expiration, goes blue and limp for a few seconds followed by rapid recovery.

Bronchiolitis acute inflammation leading to narrowing of the bronchioles and lower airways, most commonly caused by respiratory syncytial virus.

Caput succedaneum diffuse swelling of the scalp in a neonate that crosses the suture lines, caused by oedema.

Cephalohaematoma subperiosteal haemorrhage into the scalp bones in a neonate, usually associated with birth trauma.

Cerebral palsy a disorder of motor function due to a non-progressive lesion of the developing brain; the manifestations may evolve as the child grows, although the lesion itself remains the same.

Chronic lung disease of prematurity Preterm infant needing oxygen beyond 36 weeks corrected gestation or beyond 28 days of age.

Congenital adrenal hyperplasia a group of disorders caused by a defect in the pathway that synthesizes cortisol from cholesterol, often presenting with female virilization, salt wasting and cortisol deficiency.

Craniosynostosis premature fusion of the cranial sutures.

Croup acute inflammation of the upper airways (larynx, trachea and bronchi) most commonly caused by parainfluenza virus.

Cushing's syndrome syndrome caused by glucocorticoid excess either due to exogenous replacement or endogenous overproduction, characterized by short stature, truncal obesity, skin striae and hypertension.

Developmental dysplasia of the hip progressive malformation of the hip joint leading to varying degrees of actebular dysplasia and dislocation of the femoral head; previously known as congenital dislocation of the hip.

Exomphalos abdominal contents herniate through the umbilical ring, covered in a sac formed by the peritoneum and amniotic membrane.

Febrile convulsions seizure episode associated with fever in a child between 6 months and 6 years of age in the absence of intracranial infection or any other neurological disorder.

Gastroschisis a developmental defect of the abdomen where whole or part of the bowel and viscera, without a covering sac, protrude through a defect in the abdomen adjacent to the umbilicus.

Gillick principle a child under 16 years of age can give consent for a treatment if he or she is of sufficient understanding to make an informed decision and does not wish the parent to be asked.

Global developmental delay a significant delay in two or more developmental domains.

Guillain–Barré syndrome acute demyelinating polyneuropathy, often following a viral or bacterial infection, typically characterized by hyporeflexia and an ascending paralysis.

Haemolytic uraemic syndrome clinical syndrome caused by verocytotoxin producing *E. coli* O157: H7, resulting in microangiopathic haemolytic anaemia, thrombocytopenia and renal failure.

Haemophilia A X-linked recessive coagulation disorder due to reduced or absent factor VIII.

Haemophilia B X-linked recessive disorder of coagulation caused by deficiency of factor IX.

Henoch–Schönlein purpura a multisystem vasculitis of small blood vessels, affecting skin, kidneys, joints and the gastrointestinal tract.

Idiopathic thrombocytopenic purpura immune mediated destruction of platelets leading to thrombocytopenia, for which no other cause is evident.

Inborn errors of metabolism any inherited disorder that results from a defect in the normal biochemical pathways.

Infantile colic recurrent episodes of inconsolable crying of unknown aetiology, often accompanied by drawing up of the legs, seen in the first few months of life.

Infantile spasms (West syndrome) a rare kind of epilepsy which has its onset in late infancy and is characterized by myoclonic spasms and a typical EEG (hypsarrhythmia).

Irritable hip transient inflammation of the lining of the hip joint (transient synovitis), usually following a viral infection.

Juvenile idiopathic arthritis arthritis involving one or more joints in a child, persisting for more than 6 weeks after excluding other causes; previously known as juvenile chronic arthritis/juvenile rheumatoid arthritis.

Kawasaki disease a systemic vasculitis causing fever, redness of eyes, lymphadenopathy, mucosal involvement and rash with a potential for late coronary aneurysms.

Legg–Calve–Perthes disease idiopathic avascular osteonecrosis of the femoral head seen in children between 3 and 12 years of age.

Low birthweight weight less than 2500 g.

Muscular dystrophies group of disorders characterized by progressive degeneration of muscle in the absence of any storage material.

Necrotizing enterocolitis inflammation and necrosis of the intestine, commonly seen in preterm infants and often predisposed by early and rapid introduction of formula feeds.

Neonatal encephalopathy a combination of abnormal consciousness, tone and reflexes, respirations, feeding and seizures in the early neonatal period due to various reasons, not necessarily from intrapartum asphyxia.

Neonatal screening this is done by the neonatal spot blood test, screening for phenylketonuria, hypothyroidism, cystic fibrosis, MCADD deficiency and certain haemolytic anaemias.

Nephrotic syndrome clinical condition characterized by proteinuria, hypoalbuminaemia and oedema.

Neural tube defect range of conditions caused by a failure of fusion of the neural plate, resulting in defects of the vertebra and/or the spinal cord.

Neurodegenerative disease disorders of the central nervous system characterized by delayed development and a loss of acquired skills (developmental regression).

Nocturnal enuresis involuntary voiding of urine during sleep beyond 5 years of age.

Otitis media with effusion persistent fluid in the middle ear due to recurrent middle ear infections or poor Eustachian tube ventilation.

Patent ductus arteriosus a vessel connecting the aorta to the left pulmonary vein that usually closes a few hours after birth.

Persistent fetal circulation high pulmonary vascular resistance leading to right to left shunt across the duct and at the atrial level, in the absence of any other congenital heart defect.

Physiological jaundice of the newborn jaundice occurring between 2 and 14 days of life, in a term infant characterized by predominantly unconjugated hyperbilirubinaemia and a total bilirubin less that 350 μmol/L, in the absence of other causes.

Preterm less than 37 completed weeks' gestation.

Pyelonephritis infection of the upper urinary tract involving the renal pelvis.

Pyrexia of unknown origin documented protracted fever for more than 7 days without a diagnosis despite initial investigations.

Reflex anoxic seizures episodes, usually provoked by pain, where an infant or toddler turns pale and loses consciousness, sometimes associated with a few jerky movements followed by rapid recovery.

Respiratory distress syndrome respiratory distress, usually in a preterm infant, due to surfactant deficiency.

Retinopathy of prematurity abnormal vascular proliferation of the retina occurring in preterm infants in response to various injuries, especially hyperoxia.

School refusal an unwillingness to attend school, usually due to separation anxiety, stressors like bullying or adverse life events; these children usually tend to be good academically, but oppositional at home.

Short stature a height below 0.4th centile for age.

Slipped upper femoral epiphysis uncommon condition characterized by progressive slippage of the femoral head from the neck at the epiphysis, most commonly seen in obese teenagers.

Small for gestational age Birth weight less than 10th centile for gestational age.

Still's disease a systemic variant of juvenile rheumatoid arthritis characterized by high fever, typical rash, lymphadenopathy, hepatosplenomegaly and serositis.

Stridor predominantly inspiratory noise due to narrowing of the extrathoracic airways.

Tetralogy of Fallot cyanotic congenital heart disease characterized by a large VSD, pulmonary stenosis, overriding of the aorta and right ventricular hypertrophy.

Thalassaemia a group of haemolytic anaemias characterized by defective globin chain synthesis.

Transient tachypnoea of the newborn a transient condition characterized by tachypnoea and respiratory distress due to delayed reabsorption of lung fluid.

Transposition of great arteries cyanotic congenital heart disease where the aorta arises from the right ventricle and the pulmonary artery arises from the left ventricle, usually associated with an ASD, VSD or a PDA.

Wheeze predominantly expiratory noise due to obstruction of the intrathoracic airways.

Index